T0093346

NEONATAL INTENSIVE CARE NURSING EXAM PREP STUDY GUIDE

NEONATAL INTENSIVE CARE NURSING EXAM PREP STUDY GUIDE

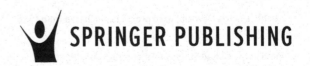

SPRINGER PUBLISHING

Copyright © 2024 Springer Publishing Company, LLC
All rights reserved.

No part of this publication may be reproduced, stored in a retrieval system, or transmitted in any form or by any means, electronic, mechanical, photo-copying, recording, or otherwise, without the prior permission of Springer Publishing Company, LLC, or authorization through payment of the appropriate fees to the Copyright Clearance Center, Inc., 222 Rosewood Drive, Danvers, MA 01923, 978-750-8400, fax 978-646-8600, info@copyright.com or at www.copyright.com.

Springer Publishing Company, LLC
11 West 42nd Street, New York, NY 10036
www.springerpub.com

Acquisitions Editor: Jaclyn Koshofer
Content Development Editor: Julia Curcio
Compositor: Exeter Premedia Services Private Ltd.

ISBN: 978-0-8261-6578-7
ebook ISBN: 978-0-8261-6628-9
DOI: 10.1891/9780826166289

23 24 25 26 / 5 4 3 2 1

The author and the publisher of this Work have made every effort to use sources believed to be reliable to provide information that is accurate and com-patible with the standards generally accepted at the time of publication. The author and publisher shall not be liable for any special, consequential, or exemplary damages resulting, in whole or in part, from the readers' use of, or reliance on, the information contained in this book. The publisher has no responsibility for the persistence or accuracy of URLs for external or third-party Internet websites referred to in this publication and does not guarantee that any content on such websites is, or will remain, accurate or appropriate.

RNC-NIC® is a registered trademark of National Certification Corporation (NCC). NCC does not endorse this exam preparation resource, nor do they have a proprietary relationship with Springer Publishing Company.

Library of Congress Cataloging-in-Publication Data

Title: Neonatal intensive care nursing exam prep study guide.
Description: New York, NY : Springer Publishing, [2024] | Includes
  bibliographical references and index.
Identifiers: LCCN 2023000725 (print) | LCCN 2023000726 (ebook) | ISBN
  9780826165787 (paperback) | ISBN 9780826166289 (ebook)
Subjects: MESH: Neonatal Nursing | Study Guide
Classification: LCC RJ253 (print) | LCC RJ253 (ebook) | NLM WY 18.2 |
  DDC 618.9201--dc23/eng/20230328
LC record available at https://lccn.loc.gov/2023000725
LC ebook record available at https://lccn.loc.gov/2023000726

Contact sales@springerpub.com to receive discount rates on bulk purchases.

Publisher's Note: New and used products purchased from third-party sellers are not guaranteed for quality, authenticity, or access to any included digital components.

Printed in the United States of America by Gasch Printing.

CONTENTS

PREFACE

This *Exam Prep Study Guide* was designed to be a high-speed review—a last-minute gut check before your exam day. We created this review to supplement your certification preparation studies. We encourage you to use it in conjunction with other study aids to ensure you are as prepared as possible for the exam.

This book follows the National Certification Corporation's most recent exam content outline and uses a succinct, bulleted format to highlight what you need to know. The aim of this book is to help you solidify your retention of information in the month or so leading up to your exam. It is written by certified inpatient obstetric nurses who are familiar with the exam and the content you need to know. Special features appear throughout the book to call out important information, including:

- **Complications:** problems that can arise with certain disease states or procedures
- **Nursing Pearls:** additional patient care insights and strategies for knowledge retention
- **Alerts:** need-to-know details on how to handle emergency situations or when to transfer care
- **Pop Quizzes:** critical-thinking questions to test your ability to synthesize what you learned (answers in the back of the book)
- **Two Full-Length Practice Tests:** one printed in the book, one online
- **Free One-Month Access to ExamPrepConnect:** the digital study platform that guides you confidently through your exam prep journey

We know life is busy. Being able to prepare for your exam efficiently and effectively is paramount, which is why we created this *Exam Prep Study Guide*. You have come to the right place as you continue on your path of professional growth and development. The stakes are high, and we want to help you succeed. Best of luck to you on your certification journey. You've got this!

PASS GUARANTEE

If you use this resource to prepare for your exam and do not pass, you may return it for a refund of your full purchase price, excluding tax, shipping, and handling. To receive a refund, return your product along with a copy of your exam score report and original receipt showing purchase of new product (not used). Product must be returned and received within 180 days of the original purchase date. Refunds will be issued within 8 weeks from acceptance and approval. One offer per person and address. This offer is valid for U.S. residents only. Void where prohibited. To initiate a refund, please contact Customer Service at csexamprep@springerpub.com.

1 GENERAL EXAMINATION INFORMATION

OVERVIEW

The RNC-NIC® is administered by the National Certification Corporation (NCC). The NCC was founded in 1975 as a not-for-profit organization and offers multiple specialty certifications, including the subspecialty certification in NICU. The RNC-NIC is a competency-based exam that tests specialty knowledge in caring for acutely and critically ill neonatal patients and their families within an intensive care environment.

CERTIFICATION REQUIREMENTS

To be eligible to sit for the RNC-NIC exam, test takers must have the following requirements:
- A current, active, unencumbered license as an RN in the United States or Canada
- 24 months of specialty experience as a U.S. or Canadian RN comprising a minimum of 2,000 hours, with specialty experience comprising direct patient care, education, administration, or research
- Employment in the specialty sometime within the last 24 months

ABOUT THE EXAMINATION

- This certification is offered via a computer at a computer test center or from home with live remote proctoring.
- The NCC provides a content outline for the RNC-NIC exam on their website, with the percentage distribution of questions per each major content category. This is included as part of the NCC Candidate Guide: Neonatal Intensive Care Nursing RNC-NIC®, which is updated annually.
- The 3-hour, computer-based certification examination contains up to 175 test questions, with 150 of the questions scored and the other 25 questions included as pretest items. The pretest items do not impact the final score of the assessment. All questions are multiple choice with a premise and three possible answers.

CATEGORIES OF QUESTION TOPICS

- **General Assessment (9%):** maternal risk factors and birth history; physical and gestational age assessment
- **General Management (44%):** resuscitation and stabilization; fluids and electrolytes and glucose homeostasis; nutrition and feeding; oxygenation, ventilation, and acid–base homeostasis; thermoregulation and integumentary; pharmacology, pharmacokinetics, and pharmacodynamics; neuroprotective and neurodevelopmental care; infection and immunology
- **Assessment and Management of Pathophysiologic States (39%):** cardiovascular; respiratory; gastrointestinal and gastrourinate; hematopoietic; neurologic/neuromuscular; genetic, metabolic, and endocrine; head, eye, ear, nose, and throat ►

CATEGORIES OF QUESTION TOPICS (*continued*)

- **Psychosocial Support (5%):** discharge management; family-centered care; grieving and palliative care; mental health
- **Professional Issues (3%):** evidence-based practice, legal/ethical, patient safety, quality improvement

HOW TO APPLY

- Applications for the exam are accepted online only on the NCC website. The NCC sends confirmation via email and can take 1 to 14 days to process, review, and approve applications.
- Once approved, applicants have 90 days from the date of the application to take the exam and must schedule within the first 30 days of the eligibility window.
- The exam cost is $325, which is composed of a $50 nonrefundable application submission and a $275 testing fee.

HOW TO RECERTIFY

- NCC certification must be maintained every 3 years.
- Certification that is not maintained will expire.
- The NCC certification maintenance program allows certification holders to continue certification status by obtaining specific hours of continuing education credit as defined in the certification holder's Education Plan, which is generated by their Continuing Competency Assessment (CCA).
- For continuing education credit to be used for certification maintenance, it must be earned after the certification holder has taken their assessment and as defined by their Education Plan before certification maintenance is due.

HOW TO CONTACT THE NATIONAL CERTIFICATION CORPORATION

Website: nccwebsite.org
Email: info@nccnet.org
Mailing address:
National Certification Corporation
676 N. Michigan Avenue, Suite 3600
Chicago, IL 60611

2 ANTEPARTUM AND INTRAPARTUM

PERINATAL HISTORY AND MATERNAL RISK FACTORS

Overview

- Many maternal risk factors may affect fetal development and well-being.
- Risks depend on maternal disease processes and how they affect the developing fetus.
- In general, risk factors for the fetus may include preterm delivery, congenital anomalies, need for Cesarean delivery, and intrauterine growth restriction (IUGR)/low birth weight.

DIABETES

Maternal diabetes may include:

- Type 1
- Type 2
- Gestational diabetes

Complications

Complications for the fetus include higher rates of:

- Preterm birth
- Congenital anomalies
- Macrosomia
- Delayed surfactant synthesis and lung maturation

Complications for the infant include:

- Neonatal hypoglycemia
- Polycythemia
- Respiratory distress
- Low iron stores
- Cardiomyopathy
- Hyperbilirubinemia
- Development of diabetes later in life

THYROID DISEASE

- Untreated thyroid disease during pregnancy is linked to both poor maternal and fetal outcomes. ▶

[🧠] **COMPLICATIONS**

Low birth weight (with or without prematurity) is the main determinant of infant mortality. It affects the development of the newborn and may determine the risk of developing chronic diseases. Maternal conditions such as diabetes, thyroid disease, renal disease, neurologic disorders, heart disease, respiratory disease, malnutrition, and substance use are risk factors for low birth weight. Conditions should be managed expectantly to reduce risk to the developing fetus.

[📝] **POP QUIZ 2.1**

A full-term infant of a patient with uncontrolled diabetes is born with tachypnea, retractions, and nasal flaring. Considering these symptoms, what could be a possible diagnosis and why?

THYROID DISEASE (*continued*)

- The fetus relies on the mother for thyroid hormones during the first few months of pregnancy. Deprivation of the maternal thyroid hormone can have irreversible effects on the fetus and their developing brain.
- Hypothyroidism has been associated with the following risk factors: neuropsychological and cognitive impairment of the fetus, preeclampsia/gestational hypertension, placental abruption, postpartum hemorrhage, and perinatal morbidity and mortality of the pregnant patient and the fetus.
- Hyperthyroidism (most often due to Graves disease) is associated with increased rates of the following: heart failure, preeclampsia, spontaneous abortion, and stillbirth.

PHENYLKETONURIA

- Phenylketonuria (PKU) is caused by a phenylalanine hydroxylase deficiency.
- All infants born in U.S. hospitals are routinely screened for PKU.
- PKU is an inherited disorder that can cause intellectual developmental disabilities if not treated.
- During pregnancy, high levels of a protein called phenylalanine in maternal blood can affect the infant's developing brain.
- An infant with PKU cannot process a portion of phenylalanine, which is in any food containing protein.

[🧠]   **COMPLICATIONS**

The pregnant patient's antibodies can cross through the placenta and cause Graves disease in the newborn. Infants with Graves disease may require hospitalization and intensive care support. Severe cases in the neonate can be fatal. In mild cases, the consequences of Graves disease in the infant are temporary. However, despite intervention, maternal Graves disease may have permanent consequences for the baby. Infants born to mothers with a history of Graves disease should be assessed and monitored following birth.

[⚡]   **ALERT!**

Elevated levels of phenylalanine may cause brain damage. Phenylketonuria can be managed with a specialized formula and a restrictive diet.

SYSTEMIC LUPUS ERYTHEMATOSUS

- Pregnancy in patients with systemic lupus erythematosus (SLE) should be planned during periods of disease dormancy for at least 6 months prior to conception. Active SLE at the time of conception is a strong predictor of adverse outcomes.
- Risks include the following: miscarriage, stillbirth, preeclampsia, and neonatal lupus.
- *Neonatal lupus* is a passively transferred autoimmune disease that can occur in infants born to patients with anti-Ro/ Sjögren syndrome–related antigen A autoantibodies (SSA) or anti-La/ Sjögren syndrome B (SSB) antibodies, who may or may not carry the diagnosis of SLE or Sjögren.
- Congenital heart block is the most serious complication in the neonate. It occurs in approximately 2% of children born to first-time mothers with anti-Ro/SSA antibodies, and the risk of complete heart block increases to 16% to 18% for subsequent pregnancies.

[🌐]   **NURSING PEARLS**

Breastfeeding is encouraged for most patients with systemic lupus erythematosus. The safety of medications should be discussed on an individual level and specific risks considered. Premature or ill infants may be at increased risk of some medication exposures. Medications such as hydroxychloroquine, prednisone, cyclosporine, azathioprine, and tacrolimus are considered compatible with breastfeeding. Methotrexate, mycophenolate mofetil, cyclophosphamide, leflunomide, and small molecules such as tofacitinib are not compatible with breastfeeding.

HEART DISEASE

- In heart disease, there is generally a greater risk to the pregnant patient than to the fetus.
- Risks to the fetus may include respiratory distress, decreased oxygenation, fetal acidosis, hypoxia, and death.
- Continuous electronic fetal monitoring is recommended during labor to assess fetal well-being.

RESPIRATORY DISEASE

- Risk factors for maternal respiratory disease include the following: asthma (maternal bronchial asthma leads to significant increase in risk of childhood asthma), hypoxemia, and stillbirth.
- Maintaining maternal oxygen saturation above 95% is recommended to sustain optimal fetal oxygenation.

RENAL DISEASE

- Depending on the pregnant patient's stage of chronic kidney disease (CKD), there is an increased risk of preeclampsia and a need for Cesarean section.
- Risk factors for the infant include fetal growth restriction, low birth weight, and preterm birth.

MATERNAL NUTRITION

Malnutrition

Malnutrition in pregnancy can impair placental development in the following ways:
- Reduction in placental size
- Reduction in blood flow
- Diminished nutrient delivery to the fetus

Obesity

Obesity in pregnancy leads to many risks for the pregnant patient and the infant. Risks to the infant include:
- Macrosomia
- Congenital anomalies: neural tube defects, cardiac malformations, orofacial defects, limb reduction abnormalities, and anorectal atresia
- Neurodevelopmental disorders
- Asthma
- Increased risk of developing childhood obesity and metabolic disorders

 COMPLICATIONS

Infants of patients with obesity are at an increased risk of macrosomia, which can lead to shoulder dystocia. Shoulder dystocia is considered an obstetric emergency because it can lead to life-threatening infant injuries. Practitioners should consider the risk factors for shoulder dystocia when managing labor and delivery in patients with obesity.

NEUROLOGIC DISORDERS

MATERNAL SEIZURE DISORDERS

- Pregnant patients with seizure disorders, especially epilepsy, are at an increased risk of perinatal complications such as hemorrhage, stillbirth, and development of epilepsy.
- Maternal use of antiepileptic drugs increases the risk of fetal congenital malformations.
- Congenital malformations include neural tube defects, congenital heart abnormalities, urinary tract defects, oral clefts, skeletal abnormalities, and adverse neurodevelopmental outcomes. ▶

MATERNAL SEIZURE DISORDERS (*continued*)

- There is also risk to the fetus from maternal seizures, especially generalized tonic-clonic seizures, including hypoxia, lactic acidosis, and fetal injury.

MULTIPLE SCLEROSIS

- Multiple sclerosis (MS) does not appear to have an impact on a patient's ability to carry a fetus to full term.
- MS diagnosis does not increase rates of premature birth or stillbirth, birth defects, Cesarean delivery, or spontaneous abortion.
- Treatments for MS must be evaluated for risks versus benefits, as many medications for MS are considered unsafe in pregnancy or are associated with adverse effects.

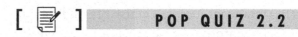

POP QUIZ 2.2

A patient with myasthenia gravis presents with preeclampsia and possible HELLP (hemolysis, elevated liver enzymes, and low platelets) syndrome. The patient needs immediate treatment. What considerations should be made about the treatment?

MYASTHENIA GRAVIS

- Certain medications used to treat myasthenia gravis (MG) can have adverse effects on the fetus. Immunosuppressive medications (azathioprine, cyclosporine, methotrexate, mycophenolate mofetil) should be discontinued or decreased. Intravenous (IV) cholinesterase inhibitors should be avoided as they can cause preterm labor. Magnesium sulfate is not recommended in patients with MG as it can precipitate a myasthenic crisis.
- *Transient neonatal MG* is a vertical transmission of MG from the pregnant patient to the fetus.
- Infants born to patients with autoimmune MG need to be examined immediately after birth and observed for the first 3 to 4 days of life for any signs of transient myasthenic weakness. Some infants may require short-term breathing and feeding support.
- Infants with transient neonatal MG do not continue to have MG once autoantibodies passed from the pregnant patient to the fetus through the placenta have been removed or spontaneously broken down.

MATERNAL SUBSTANCE USE

Overview

- The clinical presentation of infants exposed to substance use in utero is variable and dependent on the substance of exposure, timing, gestational age, sex, and amount of the last maternal consumption.
- Risks for infants exposed to substance use in utero include prematurity, IUGR, low birth weight, congenital infections, impaired neurobehavioral outcomes, birth defects, stillbirth, and neonatal abstinence syndrome (NAS).

Specific Substance Risk Factors

- Marijuana: long-term brain development issues (behavior and learning)
- Cocaine: placental abruption, intraventricular hemorrhage (IVH), and cardiovascular disorders
- Amphetamines: cleft lip, cardiovascular disorders, biliary atresia, and cerebral hemorrhages
- Benzodiazepines: hypotonia
- Narcotics/opioids: birth defects

NEONATAL ABSTINENCE SYNDROME

Signs and Symptoms

- Sleep and wake cycle disturbances
- Alterations in tone or movement (e.g., hypertonicity, jitteriness, tremors, seizures)
- Autonomic dysfunction: feeding difficulties (gagging, uncoordinated suck-swallow), fever, frequent yawning, gastrointestinal (GI) problems (vomiting, loose stools), mottling, nasal stuffiness, sweating, sneezing, and tachypnea
- Sensory processing difficulties: easy overstimulation, irritability, high-pitched cry, hyperarousal, and sensitivity

Finnegan Neonatal Abstinence Scoring

- The Finnegan Neonatal Abstinence Scoring is a standardized scoring system used to assess and identify neonatal withdrawal symptoms.
- It is used to determine if medication is necessary and to assess the need for ongoing treatment.
- Scores should reflect the infant's behavior for the entire period since the last score was given.
- The Finnegan Neonatal Abstinence Scoring tool can be found online: http://www.academyofneonatalnursing.org/NAS/FinneganNASTool.pdf.

Pharmacologic Treatment

- Pharmacologic therapy is used for severe symptoms.
- Medication is typically initiated for Finnegan scores of 8 or higher.
- Table 2.1 lists the medications used for NAS.

Nonpharmacologic Treatment

- Breastfeeding: opioid substitution therapy not contraindicated in breastfeeding
- Nonoscillating waterbed
- Parental rooming-in
- Quiet, dimly lit room
- Skin-to-skin contact
- Swaddling

Nursing Interventions

- Careful assessment is needed in infants born to patients who are suspected of substance use.
- Screening should be done per hospital protocol.
- Infants with expected exposure should remain in the hospital for 5 days to monitor for withdrawal.
- Maintain a dark, quiet, calm environment for infants experiencing withdrawal.
- Monitor carefully for central nervous system (CNS) disturbances, especially seizures.
- Monitor skin closely for signs of breakdown, especially in the diaper area.

TABLE 2.1 Pharmacologic Treatment for Neonatal Abstinence Syndrome

OPIOID TREATMENT	NONOPIOID TREATMENT
Morphine	Clonidine
Methadone	Phenobarbital
Buprenorphine	

Screening for Substance Use

- Maternal and infant urine
- Meconium
- Cord blood
- Maternal plasma
- Negative results not assumed to rule out substance abuse as positive results vary based on last maternal exposure and type of substance
- Infant to be monitored for withdrawal if substance abuse suspected

MATERNAL PHARMACOLOGIC TREATMENT FOR OPIOID USE

- Pregnant patients are less likely to overdose if prescribed opioid agonists. Receiving treatment is also linked to better prenatal care and support for patients.
- NAS still occurs in infants whose mothers receive treatment, but it is less severe than without treatment.
- Methadone stabilizes fetal levels of opioids.
- With buprenorphine, studies show shorter neonatal treatment time and lower amount of morphine used for NAS treatment.

SMOKING

Tobacco exposure in utero has been associated with the following:

- Nearly 50% increased risk of stillbirth
- Increased risk of premature rupture of membranes
- 1.5 to 3.5 times increased risk of low birth weight
- Up to 3.5 times the risk of placental abruption
- Approximately double the risk of preterm birth
- Small increase in risk of miscarriage
- Possible increase in congenital malformations
- Double the risk of sudden unexpected infant death

[⚙] **ALERT!**

Studies of neonates born to patients who smoke have reported increased signs of stress, irritability, and hypertonicity compared with those born to patients who do not smoke.

FETAL ALCOHOL SPECTRUM DISORDERS

- Alcohol is a teratogen, and prenatal exposure may adversely impact the developing fetus.
- Risks include IUGR, spontaneous abortion, and stillbirth.
- Fetal alcohol spectrum disorders (FASD) are among the most devastating effects of alcohol exposure to the fetus.

Signs and Symptoms

- Characteristic dysmorphic features
- Cognitive, behavioral, emotional, and adaptive functioning deficits
- Cognitive impairments: CNS impairment, congenital anomalies, and pre- and postnatal growth restriction
- No known treatment to reverse alcohol-induced damage to the infant

INTRAPARTUM COMPLICATIONS

- *Intrapartum* is the time period from the onset of labor through the delivery of the placenta. ▶

INTRAPARTUM COMPLICATIONS (*continued*)

- Intrapartum complications are those that occur during labor and delivery and can affect both the pregnant patient and the baby.
- Neonatal morbidity and mortality rates increase significantly in the presence of intrapartum complications.

Risk Factors

- Maternal age older than 35 years or younger than 20 years
- Existing maternal health conditions
- Maternal obesity
- Multiple births (twins and higher order multiples)
- Maternal substance use (cigarettes, alcohol, drugs)
- Complicated obstetric history
- Late or no prenatal care

ANTEPARTUM BLEEDING

- *Antepartum bleeding* is defined as bleeding from the genital tract any time between 20 weeks' gestation and the onset of labor.
- The most common causes of antepartum bleeding are conditions of abnormal implantation of the placenta (placenta previa, accreta, increta, and percreta), placental abruption, and uterine rupture.

Signs and Symptoms

- Placenta previa usually presents as painless vaginal bleeding in the second or third trimester.
- Placental abruption presents as vaginal bleeding, abdominal pain, increased uterine tone, and premature labor with signs of fetal distress.
- Uterine rupture presents as abdominal pain, uterine tenderness, hypovolemic shock, and fetal distress.

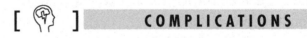

COMPLICATIONS

Neonatal complications from antepartum bleeding include hypoxia secondary to hypoperfusion, premature delivery, IUGR, intrauterine death, and birth asphyxia. Preventing these complications requires rapid identification of maternal complications and, in some cases, prompt delivery in the setting of fetal distress and deterioration.

Treatment

- All management interventions are directed toward stabilizing the pregnant patient and the fetus and aiming for a normal delivery.
- Initial management includes assessment of maternal and fetal conditions for evidence of compromise: Monitor vital signs (VS); assess maternal blood loss and provide fluid resuscitation; perform abdominal exam to assess pain, rigidity, and fetal presentation, size, and movement; and determine the placenta's position and condition, cervical length, and fetal well-being via ultrasound.

Medications

- Administer corticosteroids for fetal lung maturity if less than 34 weeks' gestation.
- Administer magnesium sulfate for fetal neuroprotection if delivery is imminent (**contraindicated during active bleeding**). If less than 34 weeks' gestation, administer tocolytics unless there is active bleeding.
- In case of maternal or fetal acute decompensation, immediate delivery is warranted.

HYPERTENSIVE DISORDERS OF PREGNANCY

Overview

Maternal hypertensive disorders (Table 2.2) result in placental insufficiency, which exposes the fetus to chronic hypoxia and can lead to premature delivery, fetal growth restriction, and fetal demise.

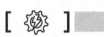

COMPLICATIONS

Eclampsia is the development of seizures or altered level of consciousness (LOC) in the setting of preeclampsia and is an emergency.

HEMOLYSIS, ELEVATED LIVER ENZYMES, AND LOW PLATELETS (HELLP)

Hemolysis, elevated liver enzymes, and low platelets, also known as HELLP syndrome, is a life-threatening complication and is a progression of severe preeclampsia.

Signs and Symptoms

- The most common symptoms of HELLP syndrome include shoulder, epigastric, or right upper quadrant (RUQ) pain, as well as nausea, vomiting, and malaise.
- Less common symptoms include headache and vision changes.

Labs and Diagnostics

Diagnosis of HELLP syndrome is based on laboratory criteria:

- Hemolysis
- Elevated lactate dehydrogenase (LDH; greater than or equal to 600 IU/L) ▶

[⚡]   ALERT!

The most effective treatment for preeclampsia is delivery; however, other interventions may be attempted first depending on the gestational age of the fetus. Immediate delivery is warranted with any maternal or fetal deterioration such as eclampsia.

[🧠]   COMPLICATIONS

Fetal complications of HELLP (hemolysis, elevated liver enzymes, and low platelets) syndrome include preterm delivery, IUGR, respiratory distress syndrome, thrombocytopenia, and perinatal death.

TABLE 2.2	Classification of Hypertensive Disorders of Pregnancy		
DISORDER	**DEFINITION**	**ONSET**	**SIGNS/SYMPTOMS**
Chronic hypertension	BP greater than 140/90 mmHg	Prior to pregnancy or less than 20 weeks' gestation	Usually asymptomatic
Gestational hypertension	BP greater than 140/90 mmHg on two separate occasions at least 4 hours apart	Greater than 20 weeks' gestation	Usually asymptomatic
Preeclampsia	BP greater than 140/90 mmHg on two separate occasions at least 6 hours apart and proteinuria	Greater than 20 weeks' gestation	Proteinuria greater than 5 g/24 hr, thrombocytopenia, new-onset headaches, vision impairment, and signs of systemic organ involvement such as liver or kidney dysfunction or pulmonary edema
Eclampsia	BP greater than 160/110 mmHg and development of seizures or altered LOC in the setting of preeclampsia	Greater than 20 weeks' gestation	Altered LOC, seizures, and worsening signs of systemic organ involvement

BP, blood pressure; LOC, level of consciousness.

Labs and Diagnostics (*continued*)

- Elevated aspartate aminotransferase (AST; greater than or equal to 70 IU/L)
- Thrombocytopenia (less than 100,000/L)

Treatment

- Treatment and management of HELLP syndrome are based on maternal–fetal conditions and gestational age.
- The recommended treatment for patients who are 24 to 34 weeks' gestation include continuous maternal–fetal monitoring, in addition to maternal blood pressure control using labetalol, nifedipine, or hydralazine, administration of magnesium sulfate for maternal seizure prophylaxis and fetal neuroprotection (Appendix 2.1), as well as steroid administration (betamethasone or dexamethasone) for fetal lung maturity and improvement of maternal laboratory values, specifically platelet count.
- Prompt delivery is the only effective treatment for HELLP syndrome.
- Candidates for prompt delivery include those with pregnancy of greater than 34 weeks' gestation or less than the limit of viability, placental abruption, or fetal demise.

PRETERM LABOR

- Preterm labor occurs between 20 and 37 weeks' gestation.
- Preterm labor is categorized as either early preterm (prior to 33 weeks' gestation) or late preterm (between 34 and 36 weeks' gestation).
- Neonatal adverse effects of preterm labor vary largely depending on the gestational age at birth.
- Improvements in obstetric and neonatal care have decreased the incidence of preterm birth.

Risks

- Stress
- Infection
- Placental complications
- Preterm premature rupture of membranes (PPROM)
- IUGR
- Fetal anomalies
- History of preterm births
- Substance use
- Maternal age
- Environmental factors

Treatment

- Management of preterm labor is dependent on gestational age.
- Tocolytics are considered for use between 22 and 34 weeks' gestation to inhibit labor (Appendix 2.2).
- Tocolytics are contraindicated in preeclampsia, intrauterine fetal demise, lethal fetal anomaly, chorioamnionitis, hemorrhage, and maternal cardiac disease.

[🧠]   **COMPLICATIONS**

Neonatal complications of preterm birth include bronchopulmonary dysplasia, intraventricular hemorrhage, retinopathy of prematurity, poor weight gain, necrotizing enterocolitis, feeding difficulties, and poor neurodevelopmental outcomes. The risk of these complications increases as gestational age decreases.

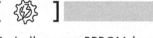

[⚙]   **ALERT!**

Typically, once PPROM has occurred, pregnancy cannot be prolonged enough for further fetal growth and maturation. Interventions to reduce neonatal morbidity and mortality should include administration of magnesium sulfate in early preterm labor for fetal neuroprotection, administration of antenatal steroids for fetal lung maturation, and administration of appropriate antibiotics for group B strep prophylaxis.

RESOURCES

American College of Obstetricians and Gynecologists' Committee on Practice Bulletins. (2020). Gestational hypertension and preeclampsia. *Obstetrics & Gynecology, 135*(6), 237–260. https://doi.org/10.1097/aog .0000000000003891

American College and Obstetricians and Gynecologists. (2021). *Preeclampsia and High Blood Pressure During Pregnancy.* https://www.acog.org/womens-health/faqs/preeclampsia-and-high blood-pressure -during-pregnancy?utm_source = redirect&utm_medium = web&utm_campaign = otn

Bansal, R., Goyal, M. K., & Modi, M. (2018). Management of myasthenia gravis during pregnancy. *Indian Journal of Pharmacology, 50*(6), 302–308. https://doi.org/10.4103/ijp.IJP_452_17

Barrett, P. M., McCarthy, F. P., Kublickiene, K., Cormican, S., Judge, C., Evans, M., Kublickas, M., Perry, I. J., Stenvinkel, P., & Khashan, A. S. (2020). Adverse pregnancy outcomes and long-term maternal kidney disease: A systematic review and meta-analysis. *JAMA Network Open. 3*(2), e1920964. https://doi.org/10.1001/jamanetworkopen.2019.20964

Bossung, V., Fortmann, M. I., Fusch, C., Rausch, T., Herting, E., Swoboda, I., Rody, A., Härtel, C., Göpel, W., & Humberg, A. (2020). *Neonatal outcome after preeclampsia and hellp syndrome: A population-based cohort study in Germany.* Frontiers. Retrieved January 16, 2022, from https://www.frontiersin.org/articles/10.3389/fped .2020.579293/full

Centers for Disease Control and Prevention. (2021). *Chlamydia.* U.S. Department of Health and Human Services, Centers for Disease Control and Prevention. https://www.cdc.gov/std/chlamydia/stdfact-chlamydia-detailed.htm.

Chollat, C., Sentilhes, L., & Marret, S. (2018). Fetal neuroprotection by magnesium sulfate: From translational research to clinical application. *Frontiers in Neurology, 9*, 247. https://doi.org/10.3389/fneur.2018.00247

Ely, D. M., Driscoll, A. K., & Mathews, T. J. (2018). *Infant mortality by age at death in the United States, 2016.* (NCHS Data Brief, no 326). U.S. Department of Health and Human Services, Centers for Disease Control and Prevention. https://www.cdc.gov/nchs/data/databriefs/db326-h.pdf

Eunice Kennedy Shriver National Institute of Child Health and Human Development. (n.d.). *Phenylketonuria.* Eunice Kennedy Shriver National Institute of Child Health and Human Development, U.S. Department of Health and Human Services. https://www.nichd.nih.gov/health/topics/newborn/conditioninfo/purpose

Hamel, J., & Ciafaloni, E. (2018). An update: Myasthenia gravis and pregnancy. *Neurologic Clinics. 36*(2), 355–365. https://doi.org/10.1016/j.ncl.2018.01.005. PMID: 29655454.

Huget-Penner, S., & Feig, D. S. (2020). Maternal thyroid disease and its effects on the fetus and perinatal outcomes. *Prenatal Diagnosis. 40*, 1077– 1084. https://doi.org/10.1002/pd.5684

Intrapartum. (n.d.) *Medical dictionary for the health professions and nursing.* Retrieved January 17, 2022 from https:// medical-dictionary.thefreedictionary.com/intrapartum

Jansson, L. M., & Patrick, S. W. (2019). Neonatal abstinence syndrome. *Pediatric Clinics of North America, 66*(2), 353–367. https://doi.org/10.1016/j.pcl.2018.12.006

Khalid, F., & Tonismae, T. (2021). HELLP syndrome. *StatPearls.* Retrieved January 17, 2022 from https://www.ncbi .nlm.nih.gov/books/NBK560615

Lam, M., & Dierking, E. (2017). Intensive care unit issues in eclampsia and HELLP syndrome. *International Journal of Critical Illness and Injury Science, 7*(3), 136–141. https://doi.org/10.4103/IJCIIS.IJCIIS_33_17

Mattina, C. (2020). *Heart disease in pregnant women raises risk of maternal, neonatal complications.* AJMC. https:// www.ajmc.com/view/heart-disease-in-pregnant-women-raises-risk-of-maternal-neonatal-complications

Mayo Clinic. (2020a). *Preeclampsia.* https://www.mayoclinic.org/diseases conditions/preeclampsia /diagnosis-treatment/drc-20355751

Mayo Clinic. (2020b). *Pregnancy Week by Week.* https://www.mayoclinic.org/healthy lifestyle /pregnancy-week-by-week/in-depth/high-risk-pregnancy/art-20047012

Morgan, J. A., Zafar, N., & Cooper, D. B. (2021). Group B streptococcus and pregnancy. *StatPearls.* Retrieved January 17, 2022 from https://www.ncbi.nlm.nih.gov/books/NBK482443

Moroni, G., & Ponticelli, C. (2016). Pregnancy in women with systemic lupus erythematosus (SLE). *European Journal of Internal Medicine, 32*, 7–12. https://doi.org/ 10.1016/j.ejim.2016.04.005. Epub 2016 Apr 30. PMID: 27142327.

NIDA. (2017). *Treating opioid use disorder during pregnancy.* Retrieved from https://nida.nih.gov/publications/treating-opioid-use-disorder-during-pregnancy on 2022, February 20

NIDA. (2021). *What are the effects of maternal cocaine use?.* Retrieved from https://nida.nih.gov/publications/research-reports/cocaine/what-are-effects-maternal-cocaine-use on 2022, February 11

Prescribers' Digital Reference. (n.d.a). *Ampicillin* [Drug Information]. PDR Search. https://www.pdr.net/drug-summary/Ampicillin-for-Injection-ampicillin-677.5656#14

Prescribers' Digital Reference. (n.d.b). *Gentamicin* [Drug Information]. PDR Search. https://www.pdr.net/drug-summary/Garamycin-Ophthalmic-Solution-gentamicinsulfate2963.56#11

Prescribers' Digital Reference. (n.d.c). *Hydralazine* [Drug Information]. PDR Search. https://www.pdr.net/drug-summary/Hydralazine-Hydrochloride-Tablets hydralazinehydrochloride-738#10

Prescribers' Digital Reference. (n.d.d). *Indomethacin* [Drug Information]. PDR Search. https://www.pdr.net/drug-summary/Tivorbex-indomethacin-3466#12

Prescribers' Digital Reference. (n.d.e). *Labetalol* [Drug Information]. PDR Search. https://www.pdr.net/drug-summary/Labetalol-Hydrochloride-Injection-labetalol-hydrochloride1568.5751#13

Prescribers' Digital Reference. (n.d.f). *Nifedipine* [Drug Information]. PDR Search. https://www.pdr.net/drug-summary/Nifedipine-nifedipine-1481.8352#14

Prescribers' Digital Reference. (n.d.g). *Penicillin* [Drug Information]. PDR Search. https://www.pdr.net/drug-summary/Penicillin-G-Potassium-penicillin-G-potassium-1150#14

Prescribers' Digital Reference. (n.d.h). *Terbutaline* [Drug Information]. PDR Search. https://www.pdr.net/drug-summary/Terbutaline-Sulfate-Tablets-terbutaline-sulfate-1659#4

Prescribers' Digital Reference. (n.d.i). *Vancomycin* [Drug Information]. PDR Search. https://www.pdr.net/drug-summary/Vancocin-vancomycin-hydrochloride-802#14

Pennell, P. B., & McElrath, T. (n.d.). *Risks associated with epilepsy during pregnancy and postpartum period.* UpToDate. Retrieved January 18, 2022, from https://www.uptodate.com/contents/risks-associated-with-epilepsy-during-pregnancy-and-postpartum-period#!

Popova, S., Dozet, D., Shield, K., Rehm, J., & Burd, L. (2021). Alcohol's Impact on the Fetus. *Nutrients, 13*(10), 3452. https://doi.org/10.3390/nu13103452

Ramsey, P. S., & Shenken, R. S. *Obesity in pregnancy: Complications and maternal management.* UpToDate. Retrieved January 18, 2022, from https://www.uptodate.com/contents/obesity-in-pregnancy-complications-and-maternal-management

Rodriguez, D. (2022). *UpToDate.* Retrieved January 16, 2022, from https://www.uptodate.com/contents/cigarette-and-tobacco-products-in-pregnancy-impact-on-pregnancy-and-the-neonate#

Shyken, J. M., Babbar, S., Babbar, S., & Forinash, A. (2019). Benzodiazepines in pregnancy. *Clinical Obstetrics and Gynecology, 62*(1), 156–167. https://doi.org/ 10.1097/GRF.0000000000000417. PMID: 30628916.

Spiegel, E., Shoham-Vardi, I., Goldbart, A., Sergienko, R., & Sheiner E. (2018). Maternal asthma is an independent risk factor for long-term respiratory morbidity of the offspring. *American Journal of Perinatology. 35*(11), 1065–1070. https://doi.org/10.1055/s-0038-1639507. Epub 2018 Mar 29. PMID: 29597240.

Suman, V., & Luther, E. E. (2021). Preterm labor. *StatPearls.* Retrieved January 17, 2022 from https://www.ncbi.nlm.nih.gov/books/NBK536939/?report=classic

Thornburg, K. L., & Valent, A. M. (2018). The maternal nutritional milieu and neonatal outcomes: Connecting the dots. *The Journal of Pediatrics, 195,* 9–11. https://doi.org/10.1016/j.jpeds.2017.12.047

Trikha, A., & Singh, P. M. (2018). Management of major obstetric haemorrhage. *Indian Journal of Anaesthesia, 62*(9), 698–703. https://doi.org/10.4103/ija.IJA_448_18

Varytė, G., Zakarevičienė, J., Ramašauskaitė, D., Laužikienė, D., & Arlauskienė, A. (2020). Pregnancy and multiple sclerosis: An update on the disease modifying treatment strategy and a review of pregnancy's impact on disease activity. *Medicina (Kaunas, Lithuania), 56*(2), 49. https://doi.org/10.3390/medicina56020049

Vijayan, V., & Naeem, F. (2021). Management of infants born to mothers with HIV infection. *American Family Physician.* Retrieved February 11, 2022 from https://www.aafp.org/afp/2021/0700/p58.html.

APPENDIX 2.1 MEDICATIONS FOR HYPERTENSION IN PREGNANCY

INDICATIONS	MECHANISM OF ACTION	CONTRAINDICATIONS, PRECAUTIONS, AND ADVERSE EFFECTS
Anticonvulsant (magnesium sulfate)		
• Seizure prophylaxis in preeclampsia/eclampsia • Fetal neuroprotective effects	• Decreases peripheral vascular resistance • Relaxes smooth muscle	• Medication is contraindicated in patients with myasthenia gravis. • Administer with precaution in patients with renal disease. • Maternal adverse effects include flushing, lethargy, nausea/vomiting, dizziness, blurred vision, muscle weakness, loss of deep tendon reflexes, and cardiac arrest. • Neonatal adverse effects include hypotonia and respiratory depression.
Beta blocker (labetalol)		
• Hypertension	• Blocks alpha-1 receptors in vascular smooth muscle, reducing systemic vascular resistance	• Medication is contraindicated in patients with asthma, COPD, AV block, and hypotension. • Maternal adverse effects include dizziness, hypotension, bradycardia, and headache. • Neonatal adverse effects include hypotension, bradycardia, hypoglycemia, and respiratory depression.
Calcium channel blocker (nifedipine)		
• Hypertension	• Decreases intracellular calcium inhibiting the contractile process of smooth muscle cells, resulting in decreased systemic BP	• Medication is contraindicated in patients with coronary artery disease and cardiac lesions. Do not administer for BP less than 90/50 mmHg. • Maternal adverse effects include dizziness, flushing, hypotension, bradycardia, headache, wheezing or SOB, nausea, and muscle cramps.
Vasodilator (hydralazine)		
• Hypertension	• Peripheral vasodilator resulting in decreased arterial BP	• Medication is contraindicated in patients with coronary artery disease, rheumatic heart disease, and acute stroke or cerebral vascular accidents. • Maternal adverse effects include chest pain, tachycardia, palpitations, hypotension, nausea, headache, and dizziness.

AV, atrioventricular; BP, blood pressure; COPD, chronic obstructive pulmonary disease; SOB, shortness of breath.

APPENDIX 2.2 MEDICATIONS FOR PRETERM LABOR

INDICATIONS	MECHANISM OF ACTION	CONTRAINDICATIONS, PRECAUTIONS, AND ADVERSE EFFECTS
Beta-adrenergic receptor agonist (terbutaline)		
• Preterm labor	• Stimulates beta-2 receptors, causing uterine relaxation	• Medication is contraindicated in cardiac disease, diabetes, and prolonged tocolysis. • Maternal adverse effects include tachycardia, hyperglycemia, cardiac arrhythmias, pulmonary edema, and myocardial ischemia. • Neonatal adverse effects include tachycardia and hypoglycemia.
Calcium channel blocker (nifedipine)		
• Preterm labor	• Decreases intracellular calcium inhibiting the contractile process of smooth muscle cells	• Medication is contraindicated in patients with coronary artery disease and cardiac lesions. Do not administer for BP less than 90/50 mmHg. • Maternal adverse effects include dizziness, flushing, hypotension, bradycardia, headache, wheezing or SOB, nausea, and muscle cramps.
COX inhibitor/NSAID (ibuprofen, indomethacin, ketorolac)		
• Preterm labor	• Blocks production of prostaglandin; prostaglandin causes uterine contractions	• Medication is contraindicated in patients with bleeding or platelet disorders. • Adverse effects include bleeding, nausea, vomiting, and dizziness.
Magnesium sulfate		
• Fetal neuroprotection	• Prevents excitotoxic calcium-induced injury • Reduces oxidative stress and production of proinflammatory cytokines • Normalizes cerebral blood flow	• Medication is contraindicated in patients with myasthenia gravis. • Administer with caution in patients with renal disease. • Maternal adverse effects include flushing, lethargy, nausea/vomiting, dizziness, blurred vision, muscle weakness, loss of deep tendon reflexes, and cardiac arrest. • Neonatal adverse effects include hypotonia and respiratory depression.

BP, blood pressure; COX, cyclooxygenase; NSAID, nonsteroidal anti-inflammatory drug; SOB, shortness of breath.

3 ADAPTATION TO EXTRAUTERINE LIFE

GESTATIONAL AGE AND GROWTH ASSESSMENT

Overview
- A detailed examination of all newborns should be completed after birth.
- The newborn should be assessed for gestational age by combining neurologic and physical exams.
- This assessment will be used to determine a pattern of fetal growth and maturity.

Physical Assessment
- Observe before touching.
- Auscultate before palpating.
- Palpate gently.

Ballard Score
- There are six physical characteristics and six neuromuscular maturity criteria (Figure 3.1).
- This evaluation of physical and neuromuscular maturity is widely accepted across hospitals.
- Reliability is maximized if performed by 12 hours of life.
- The sum of the scores for physical maturity and neuromuscular maturity correlates to weeks of gestation.

NEUROMUSCULAR MATURITY

Complete the following assessments with the infant in supine position and the head midline:

Posture
- Arms and legs extension versus flexion
- Hips and knees flexion versus abduction

Square Window
- Square window assesses wrist flexibility or resistance. The angle decreases as gestational age increases.

Arm Recoil
- Tests one arm at a time to avoid Moro reflex
- Tests for passive flexor tone of the biceps

Popliteal Angle
- Assesses maturation of passive flexor tone above the knee joint

Scarf Sign
- Tests passive tone of the posterior shoulder girdle flexor muscles

Score
Neuromuscular ___   Physical ___   Total ___

Neuromuscular maturity sign	Score							Record score here
	−1	0	1	2	3	4	5	
Posture								
Square window (wrist)	>90°	90°	60°	45°	30°	0°		
Arm recoil		180°	140°–180°	110°–140°	90°–110°	<90°		
Popliteal angle	180°	160°	140°	120°	100°	90°	<90°	
Scarf sign								
Heel to ear								
			Total neuromuscular maturity score					

Maturity rating

Score	Weeks
−10	20
−5	22
0	24
5	26
10	28
15	30
20	32
25	34
30	36
35	38
40	40
45	42
50	44

Physical maturity sign	Score							Record score here
	−1	0	1	2	3	4	5	
Skin	Sticky, friable, transparent	Gelatinous, red, translucent	Smooth, pink, visible veins	Superficial peeling and/or rash; few veins	Cracking pale areas, rare veins	Parchment, deep cracking, no vessels	Leathery, cracked, wrinkled	
Lanugo	None	Sparse	Abundant	Thinning	Bald areas	Mostly bald		
Plantar surface	Heel-toe 40–50 mm: −1 <40 mm: −2	>50 mm no crease	Faint red marks	Anterior transverse crease only	Creases ant. 2/3	Creases over entire sole		
Breast	Imperceptible	Barely perceptible	Flat areola no bud	Stipple areola 1–2 mm bud	Raised areola 3–4 mm bud	Full areola 5–10 mm bud		
Eye-ear	Lids fused loosely: −1 tightly: −2	Lids open pinna flat stays folded	Sl. curved pinna; soft; slow recoil	Well-curved pinna; soft but ready recoil	Formed and firm instant recoil	Thick cartilage, ear stiff		
Genitals (male)	Scrotum flat, smooth	Scrotum empty, faint rugae	Testes in upper canal, rare rugae	Testes descending, few rugae	Testes down, good rugae	Testes pendulous, deep rugae		
Genitals (female)	Clitoris prominent and labia flat	Prominent clitoris and small labia minora	Prominent clitoris and enlarging minora	Majora and minora equally prominent	Majora large, minora small	Majora cover clitoris and minora		
					Total physical maturity score			

FIGURE 3.1 Ballard Score.

Source: Adapted from Ballard, J. L., Khoury, J. C., Wedig, K., Wang, L., Eilers-Walsman, B. L., & Lipp, R. (1991). New Ballard score, expanded to include extremely premature infants. *Journal of Pediatrics*, 119(3), 417–423. https://doi.org/10.1016/s0022-3476(05)82056-6.

Heel-to-Ear

- Tests for passive flexion or resistance to extension of the posterior hip flexor muscles

Reflexes

- Babinski reflex
- Moro reflex ▶

Reflexes (*continued*)
- Step reflex
- Sucking

PHYSICAL MATURITY
Skin
- The skin is the largest organ in the body; infants have a large surface area.
- The skin is somewhat transparent and the thin outer layer of the epidermis begins to develop at 21 weeks of gestation.
- Physical maturity of the skin ranges from sticky and transparent to leathery, cracked, and wrinkled.

Lanugo
- Lanugo is the fine, soft, unpigmented hair present in the fetus and newborn.
- It helps bind vernix caseosa to the skin of a fetus.
- The hair starts on the scalp, eyebrow, nose, and forehead.
- Lanugo proceeds in a cephalocaudal direction head to toe.
- The fetus typically sheds lanugo at about 33 to 36 weeks of gestation and it is absorbed into the amniotic fluid.
- The presence of lanugo in a neonate may indicate prematurity. However, lanugo remains in 30% of full-term newborns and will shed in the first few weeks of life. The amount and location of lanugo vary based on ethnicity and hormonal and metabolic factors.

Plantar Surface
- Creases should cover the entire foot.
- Foot crease begins to appear on the ball of the foot between 28 and 30 weeks' gestation.
- Foot length is measured from the tip of the great toe to the back of the heel in very premature infants who have not developed a foot crease yet.

Eyes
- Eyelids
- Red reflex test: performed using an otoscope; light projected into both eyes simultaneously
- Normal red reflex test: symmetry in both eyes without opacities, white spots, or dark
- Abnormal red reflex test: warrants urgent referral to an ophthalmologist

Ears
- Position: Low-set ears are often a sign of a congenital anomaly.
- Shape
- Size
- Cartilage: Content increases as the infant matures. Fold the pinna toward the face and release; evaluate how fast it folds back. In extremely premature infants, the pinna will remain folded.

[ ]   **NURSING PEARLS**

Neuromuscular exams may be too stressful for preterm and ill infants. They should only be performed if indicated and by a skilled NICU provider once the neonate is stabilized and able to tolerate the exam.

[ ]   **NURSING PEARLS**

Both the popliteal angle and the heel-to-toe neuromuscular maturity assessment components are unreliable if the infant was frank breech in utero.

Genitals

Male

- Testes begin to descend between 28 and 30 weeks of gestation.
- Testes are palpated in the lower inguinal canals by weeks 33 to 34.
- Testes are normally completely descended by 40 weeks of gestation with rugae present.

Female

- As fetus matures: less prominent clitoris, labia minora prominent
- Extremely preterm: labia flat, clitoris very prominent

NEWBORN CLASSIFICATION

After the gestational age of the neonate has been determined, the gestational age is plotted by the neonate's weight, length, and occipitalfrontal circumference (OFC) on growth charts (Table 3.1).

- Knowledge of gestational age and appropriate growth patterns helps identify potential risks to the neonate.
- An intrauterine growth restriction (IUGR) neonate has not grown at the expected in-utero rate for weight, length, or OFC. IUGR is typically a result of a pathophysiologic process in the pregnancy. Symmetry involves the head, length, and weight. Asymmetry involves just the infant's weight.
- Low birth weight is less than 2,500 grams.
- Very low birth weight is less than 1,500 grams.
- Extremely low birth weight is less than 1,000 grams.

[📝]   **POP QUIZ 3.1**

What class of infants are typically born to patients with diabetes and what is the most common cause?

NEONATAL MANAGEMENT IN THE DELIVERY ROOM

Overview

- A fetus must transition from using the placenta for respiratory function with fluid-filled lungs to establishing adequate lung inflation and ventilation after birth with air-filled lungs.
- The primary goal of neonatal care at birth is to facilitate a safe transition to extrauterine life.
- Table 3.2 shows oxygen saturation over time.

TABLE 3.1 Newborn Classification

NEWBORN CLASSIFICATION	WEIGHT
Appropriate for gestational age	10th and 90th percentile
Small for gestational age	Below 10th percentile
Large for gestational age	Above 90th percentile

Source: Data from Tappero, E. P., & Honeyfield, M. E. (2019). *Physical assessment of the newborn: A comprehensive approach to the art of Physical Examination. Sixth edition.* Retrieved February 3, 2022.

TABLE 3.2 Target Oxygen Saturation Over Time After Birth	
TIME POST BIRTH	TARGET OXYGEN SATURATION (%)
1 min	60–65
2 min	65–70
3 min	70–75
4 min	75–80
5 min	80–85
10 min	85–95

Source: Data from Neonatal Resuscitation. nationalcprassociation.com.

CORD CLAMPING

- Cord milking is not recommended in infants under 28 weeks of gestation.
- Delayed cord clamping for longer than 30 seconds is reasonable in preterm and term infants who do not require resuscitation at birth.

RESUSCITATION

- A pre-resuscitation team briefing should be initiated when anticipating a high-risk birth to identify potential interventions and assign roles and responsibilities.
- Resuscitation is indicated in infants who are bradycardic, apneic, or hypoxic, and/or unresponsive or minimally responsive.
- Resuscitation is required when the usual means of stimulating the infant post delivery fail. Drying the infant generally provides adequate stimulation to encourage spontaneous respiration in the neonate.
- Standardized risk factor assessment tools should be used to assess perinatal risk before every birth.

Preparing for Resuscitation

- A standardized equipment check should be performed prior to every birth. Checking the function of equipment and supplies is vital.
- Every birth should be attended by at least one person who can perform the initial steps of newborn resuscitation and is able to initiate positive pressure ventilation (PPV).

Resuscitation Equipment

- Cord clamp
- Hat
- personal protective equipment (PPE)
- Suction device
- Stethoscope
- Radiant warmer
- Warm linen
- Airway and breathing management
- Circulation management
- Emergency medications
- Thermal management

[ ]   **NURSING PEARLS**

The most common reason for the heart rate to remain low is that lung inflation has not been successful. Cardiac compromise is almost always the result of respiratory failure and can only be effectively treated if there is effective ventilation.

ABCs of Resuscitation

- Airway: Position the head in neutral position. Clear the airway and assess for adequate ventilation.
- Breathing: Assess aeration breaths and ventilation as lung fluid in the alveoli is replaced with air/oxygen. Initiate positive pressure ventilation as necessary.
- Circulation: If the heart remains less than 60 beats per minute even after the lungs have been aerated, begin chest compressions.
- Drugs: If the heart rate still does not respond even after adequate lung inflation and chest compressions, consider medications such as epinephrine.

Apgar Score

- This is a quick assessment of newborn well-being immediately following birth.
- Assess the infant at delivery, 5 minutes post delivery, and every additional 5 minutes until resuscitation is complete using the Apgar scale (Table 3.3), with values of 0, 1, or 2.

Performing Resuscitation

Indications for resuscitation include:

- Bradycardia (less than 100 beats per minute)
- Cyanosis
- Depressed or absent ventilatory rate
- Flaccidity
- No spontaneous movement

Initial Steps of Resuscitation

- Provide warmth.
- Position the neonate.
- Clear the airway.
- Dry, stimulate, and reposition.
- Evaluate breathing, heart rate, color, and tone.

[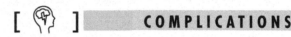]   **COMPLICATIONS**

An Apgar score of 4 to 6 indicates a moderately depressed infant, and a score of 3 or less indicates a severely depressed infant, which requires further evaluation.

[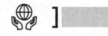]   **NURSING PEARLS**

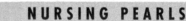

Questions to ask immediately after delivery:
- Amniotic fluid clear?
- Breathing or crying?
- Good muscle tone?
- Term gestation?

If the answer is no to any of the questions, further evaluation is needed and possible resuscitation.

	TABLE 3.3 Apgar Score					
SCORE	0	1	2	1 MINUTE	5 MINUTES
Color	Blue, pale	Pink body, blue extremities	Pink		
Heart rate	Absent	Less than 100 beats per minute	Greater than 100 beats per minute		
Muscle tone	Limp	Some flexion	Good flexion		
Reflex/irritability	Absent	Some motion	Good motion		
Respiratory effort	Absent	Weak cry	Strong cry		
				Total:	

BAG-AND-MASK VENTILATION

PPV is recommended in infants who do not breathe within the first 60 seconds of life, are gasping, or are persistently bradycardic (heart rate less than 100 per minute) despite appropriate actions.

- PPV delivered at a rate of 40 to 60 per minute
- Inspiratory time of 1 second or less
- Infant's neck remains in neutral position

Self-Inflating Bags

- Bag spontaneously filled with oxygen with a simple squeeze
- Cannot deliver continuous positive airway pressure (CPAP)
- Do not require a compressed gas source
- Remain inflated on their own
- Require a tight seal

Flow-Inflating Bags

- Can administer CPAP
- Can be regulated with a valve
- Require a compressed gas source
- Require a tight seal

T-Piece Resuscitators

- Can administer CPAP
- Require a compressed gas source
- Require a tight seal

ENDOTRACHEAL INTUBATION

- Consider endotracheal intubation if bag-and-mask ventilation fails.
- Table 3.4 shows the sizes and placement.
- Endotracheal tube (ETT) placement is visually assessed during intubation and usually confirmed by rapid response in heart rate with ventilation via the ETT.
- The infant's head is kept in the sniffing position.
- The laryngoscope is held in the left hand.
- Carbon dioxide (CO_2) detector is used to confirm placement.

CHEST COMPRESSIONS

- Begin chest compressions if heart rate remains less than 60 per minute despite adequate ventilation with PPV for 30 seconds. ▶

 NURSING PEARLS

It is vital that each step of neonatal resuscitation be performed sequentially, as subsequent resuscitative efforts are dependent upon the success of previous steps. For example, the mouth must be suctioned before the nose as infants are obligate nose-breathers; if the nares are suctioned first, this may trigger a gasp which may cause the infant to aspirate secretions which have yet to be cleared.

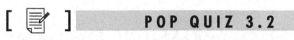 **POP QUIZ 3.2**

An infant is noted to have a heart rate of 80 beats minute at delivery after they are warmed and stimulated. What should the nurse do next?

 NURSING PEARLS

Laryngoscope blade sizes:
- Very preterm: 00
- Preterm: 0
- Term: 1

TABLE 3.4 Endotracheal Tube Sizing and Placement		
WEIGHT	**ETT SIZE**	**ETT PLACEMENT**
<1 kg	2.5	6
1-2 kg	3.0	7
2-3 kg	3.5	8
>3 kg	4.0	9

ETT, endotracheal tube.

CHEST COMPRESSIONS (*continued*)

- Intubate and attach EKG leads if not already completed. FiO_2 concentration should be 100% at this time.
- Use two thumb-encircling hand technique. This technique is associated with improved blood pressure. Provide 30 inflations and 90 compressions per minute (3:1 ratio for 120 total events per minute).
- Check the infant's heart rate after 60 seconds of compressions.
- Continue chest compressions until heart rate is greater than 60 beats per minute.
- If heart rate remains less than 60 beats per minute, administer medications (Appendix 3.1).

[📝] **POP QUIZ 3.3**

PPV is initiated in a gasping infant with a heart rate of 65. It has been 60 seconds. How does the nurse know when to stop ventilating?

EMERGENCY SITUATIONS

Conditions in the Delivery Room

- Asphyxia
- Congenital diaphragmatic hernia: needs surgical repair and infant will need to be intubated
- Congenital heart malformations
- Hydrops fetalis
- Impaired respiratory drive due to maternal opioid use; naloxone is administered
- Meconium aspiration syndrome
- Neural tube defects
- Oral/pharyngeal airway anomalies
- *Pleural effusion*: buildup of excess fluid between the layers of the pleural space outside the lungs
- *Pneumothorax*: presence of air in the pleural space between the chest wall and outside of the lungs, causes significant respiratory distress
- *Pulmonary hypoplasia*: unformed lungs during fetal development

Procedures in the Delivery Room

- Needle aspiration/thoracostomy: catheter placed to evacuate air in the pleural space in the event of a pneumothorax
- Thoracentesis or thoracostomy to remove fluid in the event of pleural effusion
- Umbilical catheterization for medication administration

[🧠] **COMPLICATIONS**

Common complications during resuscitation include:
- Improper mask seal and poor head positioning
- Improper tracheal tube placement
- Mucus-plugged tracheal tube

EXTRAUTERINE TRANSITION

Successful transition to extrauterine life consists of:
- Alveolar fluid clearance
- Circulatory changes increasing pulmonary systemic pressure
- Closure of right to left shunt
- Lung expansion

Healthcare providers can assist with extrauterine transition by:
- Drying and stimulating
- Clearing the airway as needed
- Providing warmth
- Observing the infant every 30 to 60 minutes

TRANSITIONAL PERIOD

Most fetuses transition to extrauterine life without difficulty. The transition period includes:
- Shift from maternally dependent oxygenation to continuous respiration
- Change from fetal circulation with increase in pulmonary blood flow and closure of right to left shunting
- Independent glucose homeostasis
- Independent thermoregulation
- Ability to tolerate oral feedings

Routine Care in the Transitional Period
Benefits of Kangaroo Care (Skin-To-Skin)
- Bonding
- Calming the infant
- Decreased pain
- Immune boost
- Improved initiation of breastfeeding
- Reduced risk of maternal hemorrhage
- Temperature regulation
- Regulates vital signs (VS) and improves oxygen saturation
- Reduces cortisol following painful procedures

Monitor
- Blood glucose
- Blood pressure
- Central nervous system
- Electrolytes: intravenous (IV) administered if necessary
- Feeding difficulties
- Infection
- Metabolic acidosis
- Pulmonary function
- Renal function
- Temperature

Administer

Administer the following after obtaining parental consent:

- Erythromycin
- Hepatitis B
- Vitamin K

EXAMINATION OF THE NEWBORN

- A complete examination should be performed within the first 24 hours.
- The examination detects congenital malformations or disease.
- The infant should be examined immediately for respiration, circulation, temperature, neurologic status, and anything that may necessitate emergency treatment.
- The purpose of examination of the newborn is to assess the transition from intrauterine to extrauterine life.

Observation Examination

Observation examination is completed without touching the infant.

- General condition: Observe the infant's general appearance, including sex determination, detection of birth defects, fetal nutrition, color, skin, and symmetry.
- Crying: Assess for type of cry. Facial palsies and asymmetrical crying facies are most obvious when the infant is crying.
- Respirations: Visually count the respiratory rate by watching the rise and fall of the infant's chest. Assess for symmetrical respirations and any signs of respiratory distress.
- Anomalies: Perform a head-to-toe visual assessment for any anomalies.
- Resting posture: Assess the infant's posture while they are calm and relaxed for any abnormalities.

Quiet Examination

- Observe before touching.
- Visually count respiratory rate.
- Auscultate the heart, lungs, and bowel sounds before palpating.
- Palpate gently.
- Provide a calm, quiet environment.

Head-to-Toe Examination

Assess the infant from head to toe in sequence.

- Head: symmetry, molding, fontanelles, swelling
- Neck: full range of motion, clavicles
- Eyes: symmetry, slanting, pupils, opacities ▶

[🧠] **COMPLICATIONS**

Abnormal transition includes:

- Abnormal neurologic behavior (lethargy, excessive irritability, tremors, hypotonia)
- Bradycardia or prolonged apnea
- Persistent cyanosis or pallor
- Persistent signs of respiratory distress (grunting, flaring, retracting, tachypnea); excessive secretions with inability to clear airway
- Temperature instability

[🌐] **NURSING PEARLS**

The respiratory count should be conducted over a full minute to account for the variable breathing rate in the neonate.

Head-to-Toe Examination (*continued*)

- Mouth: palates for clefts
- Ears: low-lying, patency
- Nose: patency, shape
- Upper extremities: symmetrical movement
- Genitalia: abnormalities; males: check for descended testes, hypospadias, or hydroceles
- Rectum: assess for a patent anus
- Lower extremities: abnormalities, symmetrical movement
- Back: check for any openings in the spine
- Skin: birth marks, overall appearance
- Reflexes: tone and response
- Measurements: length, head and chest circumference, weight

RESOURCES

American Heart Association. (2016). *Textbook of neonatal resuscitation.* (7th edition). American Academy of Pediatrics.

Chen, C.-M. (2018). A new formula for estimating endotracheal tube insertion depth in neonates. *Pediatrics & Neonatology*, 59(3), 225–226. https://doi.org/10.1016/j.pedneo.2018.04.007

Kieran, E. A., & O' Donnell, C. P. F. (2014). Variation in size of laryngoscope blades used in preterm newborns. *Archives of Disease in Childhood - Fetal and Neonatal Edition* 99(3)F250. https://doi.org/10.1136/archdischild-2013-305880

Mckee-Garret, T. M. (2021). *UpToDate*. Retrieved February 4, 2022, from https://www.uptodate.com/contents/assessment-of-the-newborn-infant?source=history

Neonatal crash CART Supply & Equipment Checklist / broselow™. (n.d.). Retrieved February 1, 2022 from https://www.acls.net/neonatal-crash-cart

Neonatal resuscitation. cpr.heart.org. (n.d.). Retrieved February 1, 2022, from https://cpr.heart.org/en/resuscitation-science/cpr-and-ecc-guidelines/neonatal-resuscitation

NRP study guide. National CPR Association. (n.d.). Retrieved February 4, 2022, from https://www.nationalcprassociation.com/nrp-study-guide/

Resuscitation of the baby at birth I - alsg. (n.d.). Retrieved February 1, 2022, from https://www.alsg.org/fileadmin/_temp_/Specific/App_I_Newborn.pdf

Tappero, E. P., & Honeyfield, M. E. (2019). *Physical assessment of the newborn: A comprehensive approach to the art of Physical Examination. Sixth edition*. Retrieved February 3, 2022.

APPENDIX 3.1 MEDICATIONS FOR NEONATAL RESUSCITATION

INDICATIONS	MECHANISM OF ACTION	CONTRAINDICATIONS, PRECAUTIONS, AND ADVERSE EFFECTS
Alpha- and beta-adrenergic agonist (epinephrine)		
• Asystole or severe bradycardia	• Increases coronary artery perfusion, enhances oxygen delivery in resuscitation • Sympathomimetic catecholamine	• Intravascular is the preferred method. • Medication may be given every 3–5 minutes as needed. • Medication may cause tachycardia and CNS effects.

(continued)

APPENDIX 3.1 MEDICATIONS FOR NEONATAL RESUSCITATION (*continued*)

INDICATIONS	MECHANISM OF ACTION	CONTRAINDICATIONS, PRECAUTIONS, AND ADVERSE EFFECTS
Volume expander (normal saline, Ringer's lactate, O-negative blood)		
• Hypotension due to intravascular volume loss	• Increases volume of fluid in the circulatory system	• Give IV over 5–10 minutes, slower in premature infants.
Opioid antagonist (naloxone)		
• Narcotic depression due to maternal narcotic use	• Blocks opioid effects in the body	• Do not mix with bicarbonate. • May repeat medication three times.

CNS, central nervous system; IV, intravenous.

NEONATAL PHARMACOLOGY

PRINCIPLES OF NEONATAL PHARMACOLOGY

■ Neonatal medication dosing is based on age, body weight (in kilograms), and body surface area.
■ Routes of medications include oral, optic, nasal, enteral, parenteral, and rectal.

Pharmacodynamics and Pharmacokinetics

■ The accurate determination of a safe and effective dose of a drug being prescribed to a neonate is dependent on understanding the pharmacokinetics (PK) and pharmacodynamics (PD) of that particular drug, as well as the clinical characteristics of the patient being treated.
■ There is great variability in PK and PD in the neonate due to rapid changes in physiology and the effect of various disease states.
■ The two most important parameters of the PK of drugs are volume of distribution and clearance.

Absorption

■ Composition of milk (formula, hydrolysate, or human milk) could influence gastric emptying.
■ Congenital defects involving bowel disease may alter the development of intestinal transporters, further influencing the variability of drugs' absorption.
■ With the nonintravenous route, absorption depends on various patient-related factors, such as the functional maturation processes of the organs and systems.
■ Orally, absorption depends on gastric emptying, gastric pH, intestinal motility, intestinal metabolism, and permeability.

Clearance (Elimination)

■ Drug excretion is usually via renal or hepatic routes.
■ Glomerular filtration rate (GFR) is highly dependent on postnatal age.
■ GFR is responsible for the elimination of water-soluble drugs and drug metabolites.
■ Low GFR delays drug clearance and prolongs the drug's half-life. These effects are more pronounced in preterm infants.

Half-Life

■ Half-life studies should be performed instead of single peak and trough studies.
■ The time interval between sampling should be sufficient to allow the drug concentration to decrease by one-half.
■ Two or three blood samples should be drawn to ensure the greatest accuracy.

Distribution

■ Neonates have a proportionally higher amount of body water per kilogram of body weight. ▶

[⚡]  **ALERT!**

Avoid sampling blood too close to the time of administration or at a time when the concentration of the drug may be too low to chemically detect. Generally, 2 to 3 hours postadministration is best.

Distribution (*continued*)

- Preterm neonates have an even higher value when compared with term neonates.
- Larger extracellular and total body water spaces in neonates result in lower plasma concentrations for drugs when administered by weight.
- Distinguishing neonatal characteristics has a deep impact on the distribution volume of both lipophilic and hydrophilic compounds.
- The protein binding of drugs influences their distribution.
- Neonates have lower concentrations of most plasma-binding proteins.

CATEGORIES OF DRUGS

Antimicrobial

- Consider starting antibiotics in any infant with suspected infection or sepsis.
- Obtain blood culture, complete blood count with differential, and C-reactive protein.
- Obtain cerebrospinal fluid in suspected meningitis.
- Common medications include antibacterial, antifungal, and antiviral medications, such as ampicillin, ceftazidime, cefotaxime, gentamicin, and vancomycin.

Cardiovascular

Common medications include:

- Antiarrhythmic drugs: adenosine, digoxin, propranolol, and procainamide
- Prostaglandin E: used in infants suspected of having ductal-dependent congenital cardiac defects and ductal-dependent pulmonary blood flow
- Drugs for closure of significant patent ductus arteriosus (PDA): ibuprofen and indomethacin
- Inotropic agents: dobutamine, dopamine, and epinephrine

Diuretics

- Diuretics are frequently used in the treatment of respiratory distress syndrome and bronchopulmonary dysplasia and for removing excess extracellular fluid. Diuretics include furosemide, hydrochlorothiazide, and spironolactone.

Nervous System Drugs

- Analgosedatives: These are used for management of postoperative pain, paralyzation, and sedation in ventilated infants and bronchopulmonary dysplasia. Examples include chloral hydrate, fentanyl, lorazepam, methadone, midazolam, morphine, propofol, and remifentanil.
- Antiepileptics: These are used to treat seizures. Examples include diazepam, levetiracetam, lorazepam, phenobarbital, and phenytoin.

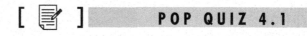

[🧠]   **COMPLICATIONS**

The presence of a PDA or sepsis has been associated with a further increase in the distribution volume in preterm neonates, especially of water-soluble compounds.

[📝]   **POP QUIZ 4.1**

A patient was prescribed vancomycin for a methicillin-resistant *Staphylococcus aureus* infection. The nurse accidentally infuses the medication over 10 minutes instead of 60 minutes. What symptoms might the infant experience?

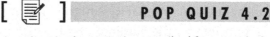

[📝]   **POP QUIZ 4.2**

A patient in the NICU is prescribed furosemide for excess fluid retention. What does the nurse need to monitor when the patient starts diuresis?

METHODS OF ADMINISTRATION

"Six Rights" of Drug Administration

Medication administration errors and adverse effects of medications can be prevented by performing the six rights of medication checks prior to administration. Always evaluate the patient's response to the medication. Assess the six rights of medication administration:

- Right documentation
- Right dose
- Right drug
- Right patient
- Right route

Oral Administration

- Oral medications can be given PO or via gastric tube.
- Use caution when administering oral medications in the infant's cheek to prevent choking.
- If administering medication in the bottle, consider placing the medication in 10 to 15 mL to ensure the infant receives all the medication.

Intramuscular Administration

- Choose the correct needle size based on age, site, and type of injection.
- Anterolateral thigh is the preferred injection site.
- Insert the needle at a 90° angle.
- Attempt to reduce pain during the injection.

Intravenous Administration

- This is used for short-term and intermittent medications.
- Always check compatibility with other intravenous (IV) medications.
- Flush IV lines before and after medication administration.

Intravenous Routes

- Peripheral IV
- Central lines such as implanted ports: subclavian and internal jugular
- Peripherally inserted central catheter (PICC): inserted in a vein in the arm or leg threaded to the superior vena cava
- Umbilical artery catheter (UAC): inserted through an umbilical artery, into the anterior division of the internal iliac artery, common iliac artery, and into the aorta; appropriate placement of the tip is either in a low (L3–L4) or high (T6–T10) position
- Umbilical venous catheter (UVC): inserted through the umbilical vein, into the inferior vena cava, below the right atrium; placement confirmed by x-ray or ultrasound

[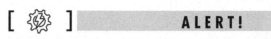] **ALERT!**

Additional rights have been added to include right assessment, right indication, right evaluation, patients' right to education, and patients' right to refusal.

[ ] **NURSING PEARLS**

The right dose is an important check in neonatal patients due to dosing based on weight.

[ ] **NURSING PEARLS**

When giving infants oral medications, gently stroking the infant's cheek can help to open their mouth.

[⚙] **ALERT!**

Observe both legs for evidence of blanching, cyanosis, or mottling in infants with UAC. If a "blue leg" (vasospasm) develops, the catheter should be removed or carefully observed for a short period of time to allow for resolution of the impaired circulation.

Intravenous Routes (continued)

- Precautions: Assess for infiltration and phlebitis. The site should be assessed every hour. Transparent dressings should be used to view the insertion site. Prevent central line-associated bloodstream infections with routine dressing changes and sterile protocol for access.

Complications of Intravenous Therapy

- Edema
- Effusion
- Infection
- Infiltration
- Leakage
- Occlusion
- Phlebitis

FLUID AND ELECTROLYTE MANAGEMENT

Overview

- Careful fluid and electrolyte management is essential for the well-being of neonates. Improper fluid balance can result in hypovolemia, metabolic issues, and renal failure. Excess fluid administration may result in edema, altered pulmonary function, as well as PDA and congestive heart failure (CHF).

Intake Versus Output

- Strict recording of enteral fluid intake and IV fluids is necessary for fluid and electrolyte management.
- Urine output should be measured by weighing diapers.
- Record all intake and output in milliliters in a 24-hour period. Subtract the input from the output. Note if it is positive or negative input and output (I&O).

Normal Physiologic Loss of Fluid

- Neonates may lose up to 5% to 10% of their body weight post birth.
- Check serum electrolytes and glucose prior to initiating IV fluids, and every 24 to 48 hours during the process.
- The neonate has an excess of total body fluid at birth. Extracellular water must be redistributed and excreted.
- The nongrowing neonate requires 60 to 75 kcal/kg/d. Fluid losses are closely related to caloric expenditure.

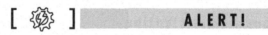

[⚡]   **ALERT!**

Phototherapy may increase insensible water loss; fluid intake may need to be increased by 10 to 20 mL/kg/d while receiving phototherapy.

Difficulties Maintaining Balance

- Fluid balance is difficult to maintain in the preterm neonate due to increases in insensible water loss, reduced renal function, and low birth weight.

Insensible Water Loss

- This occurs via the skin and mucous membrane (two-thirds) and respiratory tract (one-third).
- Large surface area of a neonate leads to excess insensible water loss.

Increased By

- Ambient temperature outside neutral thermal environment (hyperthermia)
- Increased minute ventilation
- Increased skin blood flow (phototherapy, radiant heat) ▶

Increased By (continued)
- Lower birth weight
- Younger gestation

Decreased By
- Heat shields (double-walled incubators)
- Increased humidity

ELECTROLYTE IMBALANCES AND INTRAVENOUS TREATMENT

- Neonates can experience various electrolyte imbalances throughout the course of their hospital stay.
- Treatment for electrolyte imbalances is administered via central lines and peripheral intravenous line (PIV) as well as via nasogastric feeding tube (NGT).

Intravenous Therapy

- Indications include resuscitation, antibiotics, short-term IV fluids, nothing by mouth (NPO), and parenteral nutrition.

HYPERCALCEMIA

- Serum calcium levels over 12 mg/dL

Causes

- Abnormal renal function
- Excess calcium
- Excess vitamin D
- Phosphate deprivation
- Prolonged feeding of incorrectly prepared formula
- Maternal hypoparathyroidism

Signs and Symptoms

- Constipation
- Dehydration
- Feeding intolerance
- Gastroesophageal reflux (GER)
- Hypertension
- Lethargy
- Nausea/vomiting
- Seizures

Treatment

- IV normal saline and furosemide
- Corticosteroids
- Calcitonin

HYPOCALCEMIA

- Serum calcium levels lower than 7 mg/dL

Causes

- Elevated serum phosphate
- Ingestion of cow's milk or formula with too high of a phosphate load
- Maternal diabetes
- Perinatal asphyxia
- Prematurity

Signs and Symptoms

- Apnea
- Hypotonia
- Hypotension
- Jitteriness
- Poor feeding
- Seizures
- Tachycardia
- Tachypnea

Treatment

- IV 10% calcium gluconate

HYPERKALEMIA

- Normal potassium level: 3 to 6 mmol/L
- Required potassium: 2 to 3 mmol/kg/d

Causes

- Metabolic acidosis
- Renal impairment
- Hypovolemia

Signs and Symptoms

- Arrhythmias: prolonged PR interval, peaked T-waves, disappearing P-waves, and ventricular tachycardia
- Cardiac arrest
- Weakness
- Paralysis

Treatment

- 6 mmol/L: Monitor.
- 7 mmol/L: Give glucose infusion. If it persists, give salbutamol.
- Arrhythmia: Give calcium gluconate.

HYPOKALEMIA

- Serum potassium level below lower level limits of normal
- Common in diuretic therapy

Causes

- Vomiting/diarrhea
- Renal impairment ▶

Causes (*continued*)

- Diuretics
- Hypomagnesaemia
- Hypernatremia
- Alkalosis

Signs and Symptoms

- Muscle weakness
- Cardiac dysrhythmias
- Wide flat T-waves
- ST depression
- Prolonged PR segment
- Prolonged QT/QRS
- Arrhythmia

Treatment

- Give potassium chloride supplement.
- Oral potassium is well-absorbed in the gastrointestinal tract.

OTHER ELECTROLYTE IMBALANCES

- Hyponatremia
- Hypomagnesaemia
- Metabolic acidosis

Signs and Symptoms

- Hyponatremia: vomiting, weakness, and seizures
- Hypomagnesemia: seizures
- Metabolic acidosis: vomiting, seizures, irregular breathing, and hypotonia

Treatment

- Hyponatremia: sodium chloride
- Hypomagnesemia: magnesium sulfate
- Metabolic acidosis: sodium bicarbonate

CLINICAL SYNDROMES

- Asphyxiated neonates: Decrease fluid intake for the first 48 to 72 hours. Monitor serum sodium and weight.
- Extreme prematurity: Large insensible water loss is due to thin immature skin barrier. Fluid requirement may be decreased in the first week of life. Sodium and potassium should be added after the first 48 hours.
- Infants of diabetic patients: Assess risk of hypoglycemia and administer IV glucose. Monitor for hyponatremia.
- Postoperative abdominal surgery: Fluid requirements may be two to three times higher. Monitor blood pressure and urine output. Isotonic saline may be needed due to third spacing.
- Shock: Restrict fluids in the immediate postnatal period. Hypovolemia gives 10 to 20 mL/kg of normal saline over 20 to 30 minutes.

TOTAL PARENTERAL NUTRITION

Total parenteral nutrition (TPN) is used in neonates where enteral nutrition is not expected to be achieved within 3 to 5 days or if NPO for more than 3 days (feeding intolerance, necrotizing enterocolitis).

- Improves growth
- Prevents essential fatty acid deficiency
- Promotes positive nitrogen balance
- Prevents catabolism
- Administered via UVC, peripherally, or PICC

Components

Table 4.1 shows the components of TPN.

Complications

- Electrolyte disturbances
- Glucose intolerance
- Hypermagnesemia
- Hypertriglyceridemia
- Hypo/hyperglycemia
- Parenteral nutrition-associated liver disease (PNALD): A complication of long-term (over 14 days) TPN use, PNALD is characterized by inflammation-causing cholestasis and fatty liver disease resulting in fibrosis and leading to cirrhosis.

[📝]   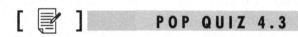 **POP QUIZ 4.3**

Phenytoin oral suspension 100 mg TID per feeding tube is ordered and supplied in a 5-mL bottle, which contains 125 mg/mL. How many milliliters per dose should be administered?

DOSAGE CALCULATIONS

Tables 4.2, 4.3, and 4.4 show aspects of dosage calculations.

- Dosage calculations based on weight: weight (in kg) × dosage ordered (per kg) = y (required dose)
- Flow rate for infusion pump: volume (mL) = flow rate mL/hr

TABLE 4.1 Components of Total Parenteral Nutrition	
MIXTURE	**VALUE**
Glucose	6–9 g/kg/d
Amino acids	1.5–2 g/kg/d
Acetate	Varies
Calcium	0.8–1 mmol/kg/d
Phosphate	1 mmol/kg/d
Multivitamins	1 mL/kg
Sodium and potassium	Varies per infant
Magnesium	Varies per infant
Trace elements	Varies
Lipids	1–2 g/kg/d

TABLE 4.2 Conversions	
Milligram to gram	1,000 mg = 1 g
Microgram to milligram	1,000 mcg = 1 mg
Pounds to kilogram	2.2 lb. = 1 kg
Centimeter to inch	2.54 cm = 1 in.
Milliliter to liter	1,000 mL = 1 L
Milliliter (cc) to ounces	30 mL (cc) = 1 oz.

TABLE 4.3 IV Rate Calculations

DROP FACTOR CONSTANT	RATE
IV drip rate in drops per minute = volume to be infused (mL) over 1 hour / drop factor constant	Determine rate per hour = multiply rate per hour by drip rate / 60 (minutes) (converts rate per hour to rate per minute)

IV, intravenous.

TABLE 4.4 Calculation Methods

RATIO PROPORTION	FORMULA METHOD
mg = mg 1 mL "x" mL Cross-multiply and solve for "x"	(dose desired) x 1 mL = "x mL" (dose on hand) "Desired over have"

Reducing Medication Error

- Barcode medication administration
- Computer provider order entry
- Dedicated neonatal pharmacists
- Redundant safety checks
- Six rights of medication administration
- Smart pump technology
- Staff education

COMMON NEONATAL MEDICATIONS

Common medications in the NICU are shown in Appendix 4.1.

RESOURCES

De Rose, D. U., Cairoli, S., Dionisi, M., Santisi, A., Massenzi, L., Goffredo, B. M., Dionisi-Vici, C., Dotta, A., & Auriti, C. (2020). Therapeutic drug monitoring is a feasible tool to personalize drug administration in neonates using new techniques: An overview on the pharmacokinetics and pharmacodynamics in neonatal age. *International Journal of Molecular Sciences*, 21(16), 5898. MDPI AG. http://doi.org/10.3390/ijms21165898

Donovan, M. D., Boylan, G. B., Murray, D. M., Cryan, J. F., & Griffin, B. T. (2015). Treating disorders of the neonatal central nervous system: Pharmacokinetic and pharmacodynamic considerations with a focus on Antiepileptics. *British Journal of Clinical Pharmacology, 81*(1), 62–77. https://doi.org/10.1111/bcp.12753

Gkentzi, D., & Dimitriou, G. (2019). Antimicrobial stewardship in the neonatal intensive care unit: An update. *Current Pediatric Reviews, 15*(1), 47–52. https://doi.org/10.2174/1573396315666190118101953

Guignard, J. P., & Iacobelli, S. (2021). Use of diuretics in the neonatal period. *Pediatric Nephrology 36*, 2687–2695. https://doi.org/10.1007/s00467-021-04921-3

Herting, E., Härtel, C., & Göpel, W. (2019). Less Invasive Surfactant Administration (LISA): Chances and limitations. *Archives of Disease in Childhood-Fetal and Neonatal Edition. 104*(6), F655–F659. https://doi.org/10.1136/archdischild-2018-316557. Epub 2019 Jul 11. PMID: 31296694; PMCID: PMC6855838.

Linakis, M. W., Roberts, J. K., Lala, A. C. Spigarelli, M. G., Medlicott, N. J., Reith, D. M., Ward, R. M., & Sherwin, C. M. (2016). Challenges associated with route of administration in neonatal drug delivery. *Clinical Pharmacokinetics. 55*(2), 185–196. https://doi.org/10.1007/s40262-015-0313-z

Medication safety in the NICU - nann.org. NAAN.org. (n.d.). Retrieved February 9, 2022, from http://nann.org/uploads/About/PositionPDFS/FINAL%202021_Medication%20Safety%20in%20th e%20NICU.pdf

Pacifici, G. M. (2015). Clinical pharmacology of fentanyl in preterm infants. A review. *Pediatrics & Neonatology, 56*(3), 143–148. https://doi.org/10.1016/j.pedneo.2014.06.002

Rostas, S. E., & McPherson, C. (2019). Caffeine therapy in preterm infants: The dose (and timing) make the medicine. *Neonatal Network. 38*(6), 365–374. https://doi.org/10.1891/0730-0832.38.6.365. PMID: 31712401.

van den Anker, J., Reed, M. D., Allegaert, K., & Kearns, G. L. (2018). Developmental changes in pharmacokinetics and pharmacodynamics. *The Journal of Clinical Pharmacology, 58*, S10–S25. https://doi.org/10.1002/jcph.1284

APPENDIX 4.1 COMMON MEDICATIONS IN THE NICU

INDICATIONS	MECHANISM OF ACTION	CONTRAINDICATIONS, PRECAUTIONS, AND ADVERSE EFFECTS
Narcotic analgesics (morphine, fentanyl)		
• Pain • Sedation	• Stimulate opiate receptors in the CNS • Act as an agonist binding to opioid receptors	• Use caution in unventilated patients as it may cause respiratory depression. • It may cause hypotension. • It may cause physical dependence. • Fentanyl may cause chest wall rigidity and respiratory depression.
Antiepileptics (phenobarbital, phenytoin)		
• Antiseizure management	• Depress CNS	• This can cause respiratory arrest. • This may cause hypotension. • This may cause sedation.
Antimicrobials (ampicillin, gentamicin, vancomycin, cefotaxime)		
• Infection • Sepsis	• Bind to penicillin-binding proteins to inhibit bacterial cell wall synthesis	• These help to monitor renal and hepatic function. • Use caution not to infuse rapidly with vancomycin as "red man/red neck" syndrome may occur.

(continued)

APPENDIX 4.1 COMMON MEDICATIONS IN THE NICU (*continued*)

INDICATIONS	MECHANISM OF ACTION	CONTRAINDICATIONS, PRECAUTIONS, AND ADVERSE EFFECTS
Lung surfactants (calfactant, poractant)		
• Prevents respiratory distress syndrome	• Absorb rapidly to the surface of alveolar air; modify surface tension in the lung	• Intubate infants to administer or use LISA method. • Infants may experience apnea, bradycardia, or airway obstruction.
CNS stimulants (caffeine citrate)		
• Apnea of prematurity	• Mechanism of action not well-known; hypothesized to stimulate respiratory center and increase minute ventilation	• It helps to monitor for tachycardia and jitteriness. • Use caution in infants who have seizure disorders; may cause seizures.
Diuretics (furosemide, hydrochlorothiazide, spironolactone)		
• Excessive extracellular fluid (edema) • Chronic lung disease • Bronchopulmonary dysplasia	• Inhibit NaCl active reabsorption	• Monitor for hypoglycemia. • Monitor for hypovolemia, hyponatremia, and hypokalemia.
Alpha- and beta-adrenergic agonists (epinephrine)		
• Asystole or severe bradycardia	• Sympathomimetic catecholamine • Increase coronary artery perfusion and enhance oxygen delivery in resuscitation	• Intravascular is the preferred method. • May be given every 3–5 minutes as needed. • May cause tachycardia and CNS effects.

CNS, central nervous system; LISA, less invasive surfactant administration; NaCl, sodium chloride.

5 RESPIRATORY SYSTEM

DEVELOPMENT OF THE RESPIRATORY SYSTEM

Overview

- The development of the respiratory system begins at 22 days' gestation and continues through birth and early childhood.
- As breathing organs, lungs are unnecessary for intrauterine existence as the placenta serves as the sole gas exchange surface. However, they must be developed enough to be functional at birth.
- Survival of premature neonates is directly related to the stage of lung development they reached at the time of birth.

[🧠] **COMPLICATIONS**

Respiratory complications of preterm delivery include respiratory distress syndrome, chronic lung disease/bronchopulmonary dysplasia, increased rates of hospitalizations due to respiratory illness prior to 1 year of age, and higher rates of respiratory diseases into adulthood, such as asthma, coughing, and wheezing.

Stages of Lung Development

The five stages of lung development are the embryonic, pseudoglandular, canalicular, saccular, and alveolar stages.

- Embryonic stage (3–6 weeks' gestation): The larynx, trachea, lobes of the lungs, and major bronchi are formed.
- Pseudoglandular stage (5–17 weeks' gestation): The respiratory tree, as far as the terminal bronchioles, is formed.
- Canalicular stage (16–25 weeks' gestation): Existing terminal bronchioles grow and elongate into further respiratory bronchioles and alveolar ducts, forming the gas exchange portion of the lungs. Respiration becomes possible at this stage; therefore, babies born at this stage may survive if provided with intensive care.
- Saccular stage (24 weeks' gestation to birth): Saccules that will develop into alveoli are formed. Pulmonary surfactant production begins at 24 weeks' gestation.
- Alveolar stage (36 weeks' gestation to early childhood): The alveoli form and mature.

Surfactant Production

- *Pulmonary surfactant* is a mixture of phospholipids and proteins that reduces surface tension at the air–liquid interface of the alveoli.
- Reduced surface tension prevents the alveoli from collapsing at the end of exhalation.
- Surfactant is produced by the type II pneumocytes of the lungs. ▶

[🤲] **NURSING PEARLS**

Fetal hyperinsulinemia secondary to maternal diabetes disrupts the production of surfactant, leading to surfactant deficiency and respiratory distress syndrome at birth.

Surfactant Production (*continued*)

■ Production of surfactant starts at 24 weeks' gestation; however, there are no adequate amounts of surfactant to prevent atelectasis until 32 weeks' gestation. Morbidity and mortality in infants born after 32 weeks' gestation are much lower than in infants born at 24 weeks' gestation.

■ Surfactant deficiency due to either inadequate surfactant production or inactivation of surfactant causes neonatal respiratory distress syndrome (RDS).

■ Risk factors for RDS due to surfactant deficiency include preterm delivery, low birth weight, male sex, maternal diabetes, perinatal hypoxia and ischemia, and delivery via Cesarean section in the absence of labor.

ASSESSMENT OF RESPIRATORY SYSTEM

Overview

■ The newborn respiratory exam is a priority as the newborn is transitioning from intrauterine to extrauterine circulation.

■ An abnormal newborn respiratory exam may be due to sepsis, retained fetal lung fluid, meconium aspiration, pulmonary pathology, cardiac disease, metabolic disorders, or cold stress.

Respiratory Examination

■ A focused respiratory exam should include auscultation, observation and inspection, and assessment of work of breathing.

■ A normal newborn respiratory rate is 30 to 60 breaths per minute and varies based on activity level such as sleeping, feeding, or crying.

■ Normal breath sounds are clear and equal bilaterally.

■ Abnormal findings include crackles, wheezes, stridor, rhonchi, or grunting. Grunting is a physiologic response to end-expiratory alveolar collapse and helps maintain functional residual capacity and oxygenation.

■ The color of the skin and mucus membranes should be noted. Acrocyanosis is a normal finding in newborns immediately after birth and may persist for 24 to 48 hours. Cyanosis and pallor are abnormal findings.

■ The shape of the chest wall should be symmetrical with a 1:2 ratio of the anteroposterior diameter to transverse diameter.

Respiration Examination

Respiration should be observed to provide critical information on the newborn's status. The following should be noted:

■ Rate: number of respirations per minute

■ Rhythm: regular, irregular, or periodic, with periodic breathing in newborns a normal finding

■ Depth: deep or shallow

■ Quality: unlabored or labored with retractions and accessory muscle use

Nonrespiratory Examination

It is important for the nurse to observe for nonrespiratory signs and symptoms that may present with respiratory distress in the newborn.

■ Neurologic exam: hypotonia, hypothermia, and lethargy

■ Cardiac exam: murmur, weak or bounding pulses, and edema

■ Abdominal exam: abnormal shape such as scaphoid abdomen, which possibly indicates a congenital diaphragmatic hernia

■ Other pertinent findings: poor feeding and poor weight gain

Laboratory Data

Blood Gases

- Arterial blood gases (ABG) measure the partial pressure of hydrogen (pH), the partial pressure of carbon dioxide ($PaCO_2$), the bicarbonate level (HCO_3), and the partial pressure of oxygen (PaO_2). Expected values are shown in Table 5.1.

Complete Blood Count

Complete blood count (CBC) is a comprehensive blood panel that evaluates several types of blood cells, including erythrocytes (red blood cells [RBCs]), leukocytes (white blood cells [WBCs]), and platelets. Indications for obtaining a CBC are as follows:

- Anemia (low RBC count, low hemoglobin, low hematocrit): The normal range for hemoglobin is 14 to 24 g/dL. The normal range for hematocrit is 45% to 65%.
- Thrombocytopenia (low platelet count): The normal value is 150,000 to 450,000 mm^3. Thrombocytopenia is a late sign of infection.
- Sepsis: There is no established norm for total WBC count. The general range is 5,000 to 30,000 mm^3. Both low and high WBC counts may be concerning for infection.

Pulse Oximetry

- Pulse oximetry provides a measurement of oxygen saturation in the blood.
- It is the saturation of the hemoglobin molecule with oxygen at the capillary bed using a light absorption sensor through a noninvasive probe that can be placed on the newborn's fingertip, toe, foot, or earlobe.
- Normal oxygen saturation is 93% to 100%.
- Pulse oximetry should be measured using preductal oxygen saturation immediately after birth.

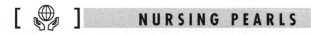

[⊕]   NURSING PEARLS

A mnemonic to help remember acid–base imbalances is ROME: Respiratory Opposite, Metabolic Equal. In respiratory imbalances, the affected values are inverse of each other (pH and partial pressure of carbon dioxide). In metabolic imbalances, the affected values are equal or in the same direction (pH and bicarbonate level).

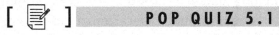

[📝]   POP QUIZ 5.1

The nurse is caring for a newborn with the following arterial blood gas results: pH 7.23, carbon dioxide 52, and bicarbonate level 17. How should the nurse interpret these results?

TABLE 5.1 Arterial Blood Gas Acid–Base Imbalances Without Compensation

IMBALANCE	PH	PACO$_2$ (MMHG)	HCO$_3$ (MEQ/L)
Normal values	7.35–7.45	35–45	21–28
Metabolic acidosis	Low	Normal	Low
Metabolic alkalosis	High	Normal	High
Respiratory acidosis	Low	High	Normal
Respiratory alkalosis	High	Low	Normal

HCO$_3$, bicarbonate; PaCO$_2$, partial pressure of carbon dioxide.

PATHOPHYSIOLOGY: RESPIRATORY DISORDERS

Overview

- Neonatal respiratory diseases are breathing disorders that affect both preterm and term newborns.
- There are several cardiopulmonary adaptations that need to occur at birth to achieve a normal transition to extrauterine life.
- In utero, the fetus receives oxygen via gas exchange in the placenta instead of the lungs; pulmonary vascular resistance is high in utero.
- At birth, several events trigger a decrease in pulmonary vascular resistance, including umbilical cord clamping and air entering the lungs with the first breath. These events cause a decrease in pulmonary vascular resistance while simultaneously increasing blood flow to the lungs. If pulmonary vasoconstriction occurs, pulmonary vascular resistance remains elevated, leading to respiratory disease.
- Fetal lung reabsorption is triggered by labor; the thoracic squeeze during vaginal birth also plays a small role in lung fluid reabsorption. Delivery occurring before the onset of labor or via Cesarean section may delay the reabsorption of fetal lung fluid, leading to respiratory disease.
- Adequate surfactant production at the time of delivery significantly impacts the newborn's respiratory status.

Risk Factors for Respiratory Diseases

- Cesarean section
- Maternal complications
- Meconium aspiration
- Prematurity
- Structural lung or cardiac disorders

COMMON NEONATAL RESPIRATORY DISEASES

RESPIRATORY DISTRESS SYNDROME

Overview

- *Neonatal RDS* is a common cause of respiratory distress in newborns, primarily preterm neonates, and often presents immediately after delivery.

Signs and Symptoms

- Cyanosis
- Grunting
- Nasal flaring
- Retractions
- Tachypnea

Treatment

- Administer antenatal corticosteroids before 34 weeks' gestation to significantly lower the incidence of RDS.
- Monitor oxygenation and ventilation using continuous pulse oximetry and serial ABG analyses. ▶

[🧠]   **COMPLICATIONS**

Complications of neonatal respiratory distress syndrome include both acute and chronic complications. Acute complications include pneumothorax, pulmonary interstitial emphysema, intraventricular hemorrhage, and patent ductus arteriosus (PDA). Chronic complications include bronchopulmonary dysplasia and neurodevelopmental delays such as cerebral palsy.

[📝]   **POP QUIZ 5.2**

A term large for gestational age (LGA) newborn of a patient with diabetes was delivered via Cesarean section and had Apgar scores of 8 and 9. Initial vital signs (VS) were stable. At 2 hours of age, the newborn had increased work of breathing and a pulse oximetry reading of 85% on room air. Blood gas results revealed mild respiratory acidosis and hypoxemia. What immediate interventions should the nurse anticipate implementing for this newborn?

Treatment (*continued*)

- Provide supplemental oxygen.
- Administer exogenous surfactant (Appendix 5.1).

PERSISTENT PULMONARY HYPERTENSION

Overview

- Most newborns are born with elevated pulmonary pressures, patent foramen ovale (PFO), and patent ductus arteriosus (PDA) immediately at birth.
- Shortly after birth, pulmonary vascular resistance should decrease. However, in some newborns, this does not occur, leading to persistent pulmonary hypertension (PPHN).
- PPHN is a syndrome characterized by markedly elevated pulmonary pressures with a right to left shunt that causes hypoxemia.
- Risk factors for PPHN include birth asphyxia, meconium aspiration syndrome (MAS), RDS, congenital diaphragmatic hernia, pulmonary hypoplasia, pneumonia, sepsis, and being the newborn of a patient with diabetes, asthma, or obesity.

Signs and Symptoms

- Cyanosis
- Desaturations
- Hypotension and other signs of shock
- Loud, single second heart sound (H2) with a harsh murmur due to tricuspid regurgitation
- Low Apgar scores
- Preductal–postductal saturation gradient of 10% or greater
- Respiratory distress and hypoxemia
- Tachypnea

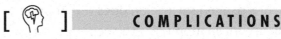

COMPLICATIONS

Although most infants with persistent pulmonary hypertension survive, about 25% experience neurologic deficits and hearing difficulties.

Treatment

- Mechanical or high-frequency oscillatory ventilation
- Extracorporeal membrane oxygenation (ECMO) if optimal ventilator support fails
- Exogenous surfactant administration if lung disease is present (Appendix 5.1)
- Inhaled nitric oxide (iNO) and supplemental oxygen
- Inotropic support such as dopamine (first-line), dobutamine, or milrinone (Appendix 5.1)
- Induced paralysis and sedation
- Correction of hypoglycemia, hypocalcemia, and acidosis

COMPLICATIONS

Complications of pneumothorax include pneumoperitoneum, pneumopericardium, pulmonary edema, empyema, respiratory failure or arrest, and cardiac arrest.

ALERT!

Any accumulation of air in the pleural space can compromise lung function, placing the patient at risk of adverse events. Treatment requires early identification and evacuation of invading air from the pleural space.

PNEUMOTHORAX

Overview

- *Pneumothorax* is an accumulation of air between the visceral or the parietal space and the lung.
- The most common causes include air trapping as seen in RDS, MAS, positive pressure ventilation (PPV), and birth trauma.

Signs and Symptoms

- Asymmetrical chest movement
- Cyanosis
- Diminished breath sounds on the affected side
- Increased oxygen and/or respiratory support needs
- Increased work of breathing
- Irritability/restlessness
- Sudden deterioration with bradycardia, oxygen desaturation, and/or hypotension
- Transillumination of the chest: can be used in emergencies or while waiting for an x-ray and will show hyperluminescence on the affected side

Treatment

Treatments to assist with draining air around the lung:

- Needle aspiration
- Chest tube insertion
- Thoracentesis
- Supplemental oxygen: Titrate to maintain oxygen saturation greater than 90%. Notify the provider if the patient's oxygen saturation does not improve despite increasing supplemental oxygen. Prepare for rapid sequence intubation (RSI) to secure the airway and better ventilate the patient.
- Medications as ordered (Appendix 5.1): Medications include analgesics and antibiotics if indicated.

Nursing Interventions

- Assess and maintain chest tube integrity. Assess for air leak. Attach to low wall suction or water seal as ordered. Change chest tube dressing per facility protocol. Maintain clean, dry, and occlusive chest tube dressings. Monitor chest tube output volume, color, and consistency. Notify the provider of any rapid increase in drainage amount.
- Prepare for needle decompression if tension pneumothorax is suspected.
- Prepare for possible thoracentesis, if indicated.
- Titrate oxygen as needed.
- Promote hemodynamic stability. Administer blood transfusion, medications, and intravenous (IV) fluids if indicated.

[⚡]   **ALERT!**

Alert the provider if absence of breath sounds is noted on assessment, especially in the context of vital sign (VS) changes or increasing oxygen demand. These findings require immediate intervention.

[⚡]   **ALERT!**

Tension pneumothorax is a life-threatening emergency due to the buildup of air in the thoracic cavity, which can lead to tracheal deviation, mediastinal shift, and profound hypotension. If tension pneumothorax is suspected, immediate intervention is needed via needle decompression to the affected lung or rapid chest tube insertion. Intervention should not be delayed to obtain an x-ray first.

[⚡]   **ALERT!**

A small pneumothorax in a minimally symptomatic patient may be spontaneously reabsorbed. In these patients, close monitoring of symptoms and serial chest x-rays may be performed to evaluate the size and progression.

TRANSIENT TACHYPNEA OF THE NEWBORN

Overview

- *Transient tachypnea of the newborn (TTN)* is a self-limiting condition that presents shortly after birth and is caused by delayed clearance of fetal lung fluid. ▶

Overview (*continued*)

- Symptoms typically resolve in 2 to 3 days.
- Risk factors for TTN include delivery before 39 weeks' gestation, Cesarean section without labor, gestational diabetes, maternal asthma, small or large for gestational age, male sex, and perinatal asphyxia.

Signs and Symptoms

- Crackles or diminished breath sounds
- Cyanosis
- Grunting
- Nasal flaring
- Retractions
- Tachypnea

Treatment

- Oxygen supplementation
- Respiratory support (nasal cannula, continuous positive airway pressure [CPAP])
- Antibiotic therapy
- IV therapy or gastric feeding tube for nutritional support

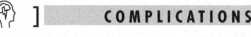

COMPLICATIONS

Complications of transient tachypnea of the newborn are rare but include pneumothoraces, persistent pulmonary hypertension due to elevated pulmonary pressures from retained fetal lung fluid, and the development of asthma later in life.

MECONIUM ASPIRATION SYNDROME

Overview

- *MAS* is a respiratory distress that occurs when the newborn passes meconium prior to or during delivery, resulting in aspiration of meconium-stained amniotic fluid.
- Aspiration of meconium inactivates surfactant, causes airway obstruction, and triggers an inflammatory process.
- Intrauterine hypoxia or infection can cause early fetal meconium passage.

Signs and Symptoms

- Limp or depressed at birth
- Meconium-stained amniotic fluid
- Respiratory distress at birth
- Signs of postmaturity: vernix, peeling or flaky skin, and long nails

Treatment

- Supplemental oxygen
- Ventilator support
- Nitric oxide
- Surfactant administration (Appendix 5.1)

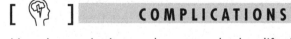

COMPLICATIONS

Meconium aspiration syndrome may lead to life-threatening conditions such as persistent pulmonary hypertension or air leak syndromes. Long-term complications may include neurodevelopmental delays and asthma.

NEONATAL PNEUMONIA

Overview

- *Pneumonia* is inflammation of the lungs secondary to a bacterial, viral, or fungal infection or an aspiration that may lead to alveolar consolidation.
- Pneumonia may either be the result of a primary disease process or a complication of another respiratory illness. ▶

Overview (*continued*)

- Neonates are at risk of early-onset neonatal pneumonia caused by bacterial pathogens present in the birth canal, including organisms such as group B streptococci, *Klebsiella*, *Escherichia coli*, and *Listeria monocytogenes*.
- *Streptococcus pneumonia*, *Streptococcus pyogenes*, and *Staphylococcus aureus* can cause late-onset neonatal pneumonia.

Signs and Symptoms

- Abnormal breath sounds
- Fever
- Hypoxemia
- Increased work of breathing
- Lethargy
- Poor feeding
- Tachycardia
- Tachypnea

[ ]   **COMPLICATIONS**

Untreated pneumonia can progress to sepsis, empyema, lung abscess, multiple organ dysfunction syndrome, and respiratory failure. Timely diagnosis and treatment can prevent progression to any of these complications.

Treatment

- Provide oxygen supplementation and ventilator support.
- Support adequate hydration and nutrition via IV or gastric feeding tube.
- Identify the cause and treat it with appropriate antibiotics.
- Administer antipyretics as needed.

[ ]   **ALERT!**

Do not start broad-spectrum antibiotics until cultures have been collected. Beginning antibiotics before drawing or collecting cultures can yield inconclusive or inaccurate results, making identification of the causative agent difficult.

APNEA

Overview

- Apnea is defined as the cessation of breathing that lasts for at least 20 seconds or is accompanied by bradycardia and/or oxygen desaturation.
- If apnea occurs in newborns less than 37 weeks' gestation, it is considered apnea of prematurity.

Types of Apnea

- Central apnea: A depressed respiratory control center leads to no respiratory effort. Causes include central nervous system (CNS) infections (meningitis), seizures, head trauma from delivery or birth, exposure to toxins, inborn errors of metabolism, electrolyte imbalances, and congenital anomalies.

[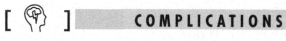]   **COMPLICATIONS**

Apnea may cause sudden deterioration with bradycardia, hypoxia, and cyanosis. These findings require rapid interventions, including infant stimulation, oxygen supplementation, airway clearance, bag/mask ventilation, and/or resuscitation.

- Obstructive apnea: An obstruction in the airway makes respiratory effort ineffective. Causes include infections (pneumonia), obstructive sleep apnea, vocal cord paralysis, and congenital airway anomalies (Pierre Robin syndrome).
- Mixed: A period of central apnea is followed by obstructive apnea. Mixed is the most common type in preterm infants. Causes include gastroesophageal reflux, pertussis, and bronchiolitis.

Signs and Symptoms

- Absent breath sounds or no chest movement for 20 seconds or more
- Bradycardia
- Cyanosis
- Oxygen desaturation

Treatment

- Provide immediate resuscitation and stabilization.
- Initiate CPAP therapy or other modes of respiratory support.
- Administer caffeine citrate to preterm infants (Appendix 5.1).
- Administer antibiotics if ordered.

COMPLICATIONS OF RESPIRATORY DISEASE

- Complications of respiratory disease range from acute to chronic.
- The gestational age of the newborn at birth significantly impacts respiratory health.
- The incidence of respiratory complications increases as gestational age decreases.

ACUTE COMPLICATIONS OF RESPIRATORY DISEASE

Central Nervous System: Intraventricular Hemorrhage

- May lead to seizures
- May be triggered by stressful events such as intubation, surfactant administration, and chest tube insertion
- More likely to occur in infants with respiratory disease

Cardiac

- Hypotension
- Pneumomediastinum
- PDA and PFO in the setting of increased pulmonary pressures post birth

Pulmonary Hemorrhage

- This is an acute event that occurs when there is fresh blood in the upper respiratory tract.
- Pulmonary edema is typically the cause. Perinatal depression leads to cardiac failure, increased pulmonary vascular resistance, and pulmonary edema. If pulmonary capillaries are under stress, they may break and leak fluid into the lungs. A PDA with a left to right shunt increases blood flow to the lungs, leading to pulmonary edema.
- It presents as a rapid decompensation with the presence of pink-tinged or bloody secretions in the airway.
- Morbidity and mortality rates are high.

Infection

Neonatal infections that may contribute to respiratory disease include:
- Congenital infections (HIV, cytomegalovirus [CMV], herpes simplex virus [HSV], toxoplasmosis)
- Guillain-Barré syndrome (GBS) sepsis
- Meningitis (*Listeria*, *E. coli*, GBS)
- Neonatal pneumonia

CHRONIC COMPLICATIONS OF RESPIRATORY DISEASE

- Chronic complications from respiratory disease may develop due to high ventilator settings and subsequent barotrauma, oxygen supplementation, prematurity, and periods of oxygen deprivation.

Long-Term Neurologic Complications

- Cerebral palsy and neurologic impairments: Causes and links include birth asphyxia and postnatal steroid therapy in neonates for treatment or prevention of bronchopulmonary dysplasia (BPD).
- Hearing loss: Hearing loss is linked to antibiotic therapy.
- Blindness: See retinopathy of prematurity in Chapter 12, "Head, Eyes, Ears, Nose, and Throat."

CHRONIC LUNG DISEASE/BRONCHOPULMONARY DYSPLASIA

Overview

- Chronic lung disease (CLD)/BPD is a form of newborn lung disease in which long-term ventilator support and oxygen therapy damage the lungs and airways, causing dysplasia in the alveoli.
- The majority of newborns with BPD are born prematurely; the incidence of BPD increases as gestational age at birth decreases.

Signs and Symptoms

- Cyanosis
- Nasal flaring
- Oxygen requirement past 36 weeks' corrected gestation
- Retractions
- Tachypnea
- Wheezing

Treatment

- Mechanical ventilation via endotracheal tube (ETT) or tracheostomy tube
- Oxygen therapy
- Optimal nutritional support
- Medications: bronchodilators, steroids, diuretics, and pulmonary vasodilators (see Appendix 5.1)

NURSING INTERVENTIONS FOR RESPIRATORY DISEASES

- Monitor airway for secretions and suction as needed.
- Continuously monitor oxygen saturation, blood pressure, and perfusion.
- Titrate supplemental oxygen to maintain oxygen saturation within appropriate parameters.
- Initiate and maintain IV access.
- Maintain optimal fluid and electrolyte balances.
- Collect labs and cultures.
- Administer medications as ordered.
- Assess response to paralytics and sedatives, if needed.
- Maintain a quiet and low-stimulation environment with minimal handling of the newborn.
- Minimize invasive procedures such as suctioning.
- Maintain a neutral thermal environment.
- Provide therapeutic and developmental positioning. ▶

NURSING INTERVENTIONS FOR RESPIRATORY DISEASES (*continued*)

■ Respond to apneic events and provide stimulation, supplemental oxygen, and bag/mask ventilation if needed.
■ Document all apneic events.

DIAGNOSTIC PROCEDURES

Laboratory Data

■ ABG to show respiratory and metabolic acidosis
■ CBC, blood and urine cultures, C-reactive protein (CRP), and/or lactate to rule out infection/sepsis
■ Cerebrospinal fluid (CSF) culture via lumbar puncture to rule out meningitis

X-Ray

■ Plays a critical role in diagnosing, categorizing, and managing neonatal respiratory diseases
■ RDS: ground-glass reticulogranular appearance with air bronchograms and low lung volumes
■ PPHN: may be normal, but can reveal cardiomegaly and decreased pulmonary blood flow
■ Pneumothorax: accumulation of air in the pleural space
■ TTN: hyperinflation or fluid in fissures
■ MAS: streaky densities bilaterally, hyperinflation, and atelectasis
■ Pneumonia: diffuse alveolar densities and air bronchograms

Electroencephalogram/Head Ultrasound

■ EEG may be used to rule out seizures as the cause of apnea in a term infant.
■ Head ultrasound may reveal intraventricular hemorrhage (IVH) in infants with respiratory disease. IVH may be either the cause or a complication of respiratory disease.

Echocardiogram

■ May be used to rule out structural heart defects (see Chapter 6, Cardiovascular System and Circulation) or in the presence of suspected PPHN

COMMON PROCEDURES

Supplemental Oxygen

■ Oxygen therapy increases the oxygen concentration the lungs are receiving, thereby increasing systemic oxygen delivery.
■ High-flow devices include a high-flow nasal cannula, CPAP, nasal intermittent positive pressure ventilation (NIPPV), and mechanical ventilation.
■ Low-flow devices include low-flow nasal cannula.

Continuous Positive Airway Pressure

■ CPAP is a noninvasive mode of providing respiratory support to a spontaneously breathing neonate. Early and effective CPAP decrease the need for mechanical ventilation and the risks associated with intubation.
■ CPAP delivers constant positive pressure to the airway, which maintains functional residual capacity and prevents alveolar collapse. The goal of CPAP is to prevent atelectasis and improve oxygenation.

INDICATIONS FOR CONTINUOUS POSITIVE AIRWAY PRESSURE

- Increased work of breathing (tachypnea, nasal flaring, grunting, retractions, cyanosis) as seen in the following conditions:
  - Apnea of prematurity
  - Atelectasis
  - Lower airway disorders such as tracheomalacia
  - Recent extubation
  - RDS
  - TTN
  - Respiratory acidosis on blood gas

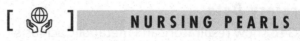

NURSING PEARLS

Because continuous positive airway pressure is noninvasive, it often leads to gastric distention. An orogastric tube should be placed to allow air to vent from the stomach and minimize the effects of gastric distention such as feeding intolerance.

NURSING PEARLS

To estimate the length of the endotracheal tube (ETT), use the "7-8-9" rule: oral ETT length = weight (kg) + 6 cm. For example, if a newborn weighs 2 kg, the ETT should be secured at 8 cm.

Intubation

- Intubation is indicated in infants who have bradycardia; are apneic, hypoxic, unresponsive, or minimally responsive; and/or are not responding to current less invasive respiratory interventions.
- Other indications include upper airway obstruction, such as in Pierre Robin syndrome, and respiratory distress due to diaphragmatic hernia or meconium aspiration, where CPAP may be contraindicated.

NURSING RESPONSIBILITIES

- Before, during, and after intubation: Continuously monitor cardiorespiratory, oxygen saturation, and blood pressure; auscultate breath sounds in all lung fields; and support thermoregulation during the procedure.
- Assist with gathering equipment and supplies for intubation: These include appropriately sized ETT (Table 5.2), Miller blade and pediatric laryngoscope, appropriately sized suction catheter attached to the working suction canister, appropriately sized and cut adhesive tape for ETT securement, end-tidal CO_2 detector NeoPuff checked for appropriate settings, correct-sized face mask, and stethoscope.
- Administer medications for analgesia and sedation as ordered.
- Provide airway support: Position the neonate in the optimal position for intubation—supine on a flat surface, head midline. Ensure gastric contents are aspirated prior to the procedure to prevent aspiration. Assist with securing the ETT once successfully placed; Table 5.3 shows the recommended ETT length. If intubation attempt fails, maintain mask ventilation via NeoPuff until next attempt.
- Confirm ETT position.

TABLE 5.2 Recommended Uncuffed ETT Size	
TUBE SIZE (INTERNAL DIAMETER IN MM)	INFANT WEIGHT (KG)
2.5	<1
3.0	1–2
3.5	2–3.5
4.0	>3.5

ETT, endotracheal tube.

Modes of Ventilation

- The two primary modes of ventilation used in neonates are conventional mechanical ventilation and high-frequency ventilation.
- Conventional mechanical ventilation is more commonly used.

TYPES OF CONVENTIONAL MECHANICAL VENTILATION

- Assist-control ventilation: The ventilator provides mandatory breaths at a set rate (control breaths) while also supporting the patient's spontaneous breaths above the set rate (assist breaths).
- Pressure support ventilation: There is no set rate; all breaths are initiated by the patient and are pressure-limited.
- Synchronized intermittent mandatory ventilation (SIMV): The ventilator only provides mandatory breaths at a set rate but attempts to synchronize breaths with the patient's spontaneous breaths; spontaneous breaths above the set rate are not supported. SIMV may be combined with pressure support ventilation to allow the patient's spontaneous breaths above the set rate to be supported.
- Volume-targeted ventilation: The desired tidal volume to be delivered to the patient is set, and the peak inspiratory pressure (PIP) required to deliver it varies. Tidal volume is calculated with a weight-based approach, typically 4 to 6 mL/kg.

TYPES OF HIGH-FREQUENCY VENTILATION

High-frequency ventilation delivers small tidal volumes at a very rapid rate while maintaining set mean airway pressure.

- High-frequency oscillatory ventilation (HFOV): A piston within the ventilator creates oscillations around a constant mean airway pressure, which creates small tidal volumes; the frequencies are typically 480 to 900 breaths per minute (8–15 Hz). Expiration in HFOV is an active process, whereas in conventional ventilation expiration is passive.
- High-frequency jet ventilation (HFJV): A pinch valve releases short jets of gas in the inspiratory circuit and produces small volume pulses of gas at a high rate; it is used in conjunction with a conventional ventilator to provide positive end-expiratory pressure (PEEP). Expiration in HFJV is passive.

Inhaled Nitric Oxide

- iNO is a medication used as rescue therapy for hypoxic respiratory failure or PPHN. It reduces the need for ECMO therapy.
- iNO is a potent and direct pulmonary vasodilator; thus, there is a low risk of systemic vasodilation and subsequent hypotension.
- iNO results in improved oxygenation and pulmonary circulation. ▶

TABLE 5.3 Recommended ETT Length	
WEIGHT (KG)	ETT LENGTH (CM)
<1	6.5–7
1–2	7–8
2–3	8–9
3–4	9–10

ETT, endotracheal tube.

Inhaled Nitric Oxide (*continued*)

- Therapy should be initiated at 20 ppm, then gradually weaned over the course of 14 days to prevent pulmonary vasospasm.

Chest Tube Insertion

Indications for a thoracostomy chest tube include:

- Hemothorax: *Hemothorax* is collection of blood in the pleural space.
- Pneumothorax: *Pneumothorax* is accumulation of air between the visceral or the parietal space and the lung. The accumulation of air can cause the lung to collapse. A tension pneumothorax is when air enters the pleural space on inhalation but cannot exit during expiration. It can be spontaneous or caused by trauma. A pleural effusion is a collection of fluid (serous fluid, or pus) in the pleural space.

Nursing Responsibilities

- Assist with placement: Administer pain or sedation medication as ordered. Monitor vital signs (VS) and airway, breathing, and circulation.
- Manage chest tubes. A wet system allows suction of up to 20 cm of water. A dry system allows suction of up to 40 cm of water.
- Set up chest tube drainage system.
- Attach to the level of suction, or gravity, as ordered.
- If the chest tube is dislodged from the patient's chest, cover the site with sterile gauze, tape on three sides, and notify the provider.
- If the chest tube drainage system has disconnected, place tubing from the patient into a bottle of sterile water.
- Monitor the water seal chamber for signs of an air leak or excessive bubbling.
- Monitor for subcutaneous emphysema (air crackling around the chest tube insertion site).
- Monitor drainage in the drainage collection chamber. Note the amount, color, and consistency.
- Monitor dressing. Maintain clean, dry, and intact dressing at the insertion site.
- Keep the drainage system below the level of the patient's chest.
- Avoid clamping tubing.
- Do not attach the drainage system to a moveable part of the crib or bed.
- Do not milk or strip tubing.
- Ensure tubing is free of dependent loops.
- Assist with removal: Administer pain or sedation medication as ordered. Gather sterile occlusive dressing and apply according to policy.

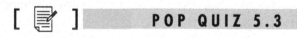

[📝]   **POP QUIZ 5.3**

The nurse is preparing to administer a dose of caffeine citrate to a preterm infant. The infant is tachycardic with a heart rate of 192 beats per minute. What action should the nurse take next?

Suctioning

- Suction is the primary intervention to clear secretions and mucus plugs from the nose, mouth, nasopharynx, or artificial airways such as ETT or tracheostomy tube.
- Set suction pressure to 60 to 80 mmHg.
- Use an appropriately sized suction catheter for the age or size of an artificial airway.
- Instill catheter to premeasured length, not until meeting resistance.
- Do not apply suction on insertion.
- Apply intermittent suction and gentle catheter rotation as the catheter is removed.
- Monitor pulse oximetry while suctioning.
- To help prevent hypoxia during suctioning, hyperventilate with oxygen or increase FiO_2 and limit suction passes.

RESOURCES

Bamat, N., & Eichenwald, E. (2022). Overview of mechanical ventilation in neonates. *UpToDate*. Retrieved Feb. 4, 2022. https://www.uptodate.com/contents/overview-of-mechanical-ventilation-in-neonates#H3215372643

Boyd, K. (2021). What is Retinopathy of Prematurity (ROP)? *American academy of ophthalmology*. https://www.aao.org/eye-health/diseases/what-is-retinopathy-prematurity

Cincinnati Children's. (2019). *Bronchopulmonary Dysplasia (BPD)/Chronic lung disease of prematurity*. https://www.cincinnatichildrens.org/health/b/bronchopulmonary-dysplasia

Cousins, M., Hart, K., Gallacher, D., & Palomino, M. (2018). Long-term respiratory outcomes following preterm birth. *Revista Medica Clinica Las Condes. 29*(1), 87–97. https://doi.org/10.1016/j.rmclc.2018.02.002

Ebeledike C., Ahmad T., & Martin, S. (2021). Pediatric pneumonia (Nursing). *StatPearls*. Retrieved February 3, 2022 from https://www.ncbi.nlm.nih.gov/books/NBK568682

Jha K., Nassar G., & Makker K. (2021). Transient Tachypnea of the Newborn. *StatPearls*. Retrieved Feb 3, 2022 from https://www.ncbi.nlm.nih.gov/books/NBK537354/

Kayton, A., Timoney, P., Vargo, L., & Perez, J. (2018). A review of oxygen physiology and appropriate management of oxygen levels in premature neonates. *Advances in Neonatal Care, 18(2)*, 98–104. https://doi.org/10.1097/ANC.0000000000000434

Kondamudi, N., Krata, L., & Wilt, A. (2021). Infant Apnea. *StatPearls*. Retrieved February 4, 2022 from https://www.ncbi.nlm.nih.gov/books/NBK441969

Nkadi, P. O., Merritt, T. A., & Pillers, D. A. (2009). An overview of pulmonary surfactant in the neonate: Genetics, metabolism, and the role of surfactant in health and disease. *Molecular Genetics and Metabolism*, 97(2), 95–101. https://doi.org/10.1016/j.ymgme.2009.01.015

Prescribers' Digital Reference. (n.d.-a). *Atrovent* [Drug Information]. PDR Search. https://www.pdr.net/drug-summary/Atrovent-HFA-ipratropium-bromide-1743.318#5

Prescribers' Digital Reference. (n.d.-b) *Caffeine Citrate* [Drug Information]. PDR Search. https://www.pdr.net/drug-summary/Caffeine-Citrate-caffeine-citrate-3724.3725#14

Prescribers' Digital Reference. (n.d.-c). *Dexamethasone* [Drug Information]. PDR Search. https://www.pdr.net/drug-summary/Dexamethasone-Sodium-Phosphate-Injection--USP 10-mg-mL-dexamethasone-sodium-phosphate-1725#5

Prescribers' Digital Reference. (n.d.-d). *Sildenafil* [Drug Information]. PDR Search. https://www.pdr.net/drug-summary/Viagra-sildenafil-citrate-471#11

Rehman, S., & Bacha, D. (2021). Embryology, Pulmonary. *StatPearls*. Retrieved January 30, 2022 from https://www.ncbi.nlm.nih.gov/books/NBK544372

Sayad E., & Silva-Carmona M. (2021). Meconium Aspiration. *StatPearls*. Retrieved February 3, 2022 from https://www.ncbi.nlm.nih.gov/books/NBK557425

Seattle Children's Hospital. (2021). *Neonatal Pulmonary Hemorrhage*. https://www.seattlechildrens.org/globalassets/documents/healthcare professionals/neonatal-briefs/pulmonary-hemorrhage.pdf

Tauber, K. (2019). Persistent Pulmonary Hypertension of the Newborn (PPHN). Retrieved February 3, 2022 from https://emedicine.medscape.com/article/898437-overview#a1

The Royal Children's Hospital Melbourne. (2020). *Continuous Positive Airway Pressure (CPAP) - Care in the Newborn Intensive Care Unit (Butterfly Ward*. https://www.rch.org.au/rchcpg/hospital_clinical_guideline_index/Continuous_Positive_Airway_Pressure_(CPAP)__Care_in_the_Newborn_Intensive_Care_Unit_(Butterfly_Ward)/#:~:text = Continuous%20Positive%20Airway%20Pressure%20(CPAP)%20is%20a%20means%20of%20providing,or%20failure%20of%20lung%20function

Walker, V. (2018). Newborn evaluation. *Avery's Diseases of the Newborn* (10th Edition), 289–311. https://doi.org/10.1016/B978-0-323-40139-5.00025-5

Yadav, S., Lee, B., & Kamity, R. (2021). Neonatal respiratory distress syndrome. *StatPearls*. Retrieved January 30, 2022 from https://www.ncbi.nlm.nih.gov/books/NBK560779

APPENDIX 5.1 RESPIRATORY MEDICATIONS

INDICATIONS	MECHANISM OF ACTION	CONTRAINDICATIONS, PRECAUTIONS, AND ADVERSE EFFECTS
Beta-2 agonists/bronchodilators (e.g., albuterol, ipratropium)		
• Reverse and prevent airway obstruction related to CLD/BPD	• Relax airway smooth muscle and decrease obstruction and inflammation, resulting in improved airway clearance	• Use caution in patients with cardiac disease, hyperthyroidism, and hypertension. • Adverse effects include bronchospasm, restlessness, arrhythmia, and tachycardia.
Corticosteroids (e.g., prednisone, dexamethasone, methylprednisolone)		
• Prevention of extubation failure • Prevention of CLD/BPD	• Inhibit steps in the inflammatory pathway to prevent inflammation of the lungs and reduce mucus production	• Patients receiving corticosteroids for an extended time or in high doses are at increased risk of immunosuppression, making them more prone to infection. • Adverse effects include osteopenia, irritability, diaphoresis, and bronchospasm. • Long-term use of steroids is associated with poor neurodevelopmental outcomes such as cerebral palsy.
Diuretics: loop (furosemide)		
• Pulmonary hypertension, fluid overload, heart failure, and hypertension	• Secretion of electrolytes and water by preventing resorption and increasing urine output	• Medication is contraindicated in cross sensitivity with sulfonamides (thiazide diuretics). • Use caution in hypokalemia, digoxin therapy, cardiac disease, and arrhythmia.
Diuretics: aldosterone antagonists (e.g., spironolactone)		
• Fluid overload, pulmonary hypertension, heart failure, and hypertension	• Inhibit sodium potassium change in the distal tubules, increasing urine output without loss of potassium	• Medication is contraindicated in anuria, renal failure, and hyperkalemia. • Use caution in liver failure. • Adverse effects include arrhythmias, hyperkalemia, and hyponatremia.
Diuretics: thiazide (hydrochlorothiazide)		
• Fluid overload, pulmonary hypertension, heart failure, and hypertension	• Increase water excretion by inhibiting reabsorption of sodium and chloride at the distal tubule	• Medication is contraindicated in anuria and renal failure. • Use caution in hepatic disease, hypotension, and hypovolemia. • Adverse effects include photosensitivity, hypokalemia, and hyperglycemia.
Inotropic support (dopamine, milrinone)		
• Increased cardiac output • Increased blood pressure	• Stimulates adrenergic and dopaminergic receptors • Produces cardiac stimulation	• Medication is contraindicated in pheochromocytoma, tachyarrhythmias, and ventricular fibrillation. • Precautions need to be taken in case of arrhythmias, extravasation, heart conditions, electrolyte imbalance, and shock. • Adverse effects include sloughing and necrosis of the IV site. Monitor closely. • Adverse effects also include restlessness, cardiac rhythm changes, vomiting, increased work of breathing, polyuria, and increased intraocular pressure.

(continued)

APPENDIX 5.1 RESPIRATORY MEDICATIONS (*continued*)

INDICATIONS	MECHANISM OF ACTION	CONTRAINDICATIONS, PRECAUTIONS, AND ADVERSE EFFECTS
Methylxanthines (caffeine citrate)		
• Apnea of prematurity • Extubation facilitation	• Stimulate the respiratory center	• Administer IV caffeine slowly over a period of at least 10 minutes. • Use cautiously in patients with cardiac disease. • Monitor for signs of NEC such as abdominal distention, emesis, bloody stool, and lethargy. • Adverse effects include tachycardia, hyperthermia, hypo/hyperglycemia, and irritability.
Neuromuscular blocking agents (vecuronium, rocuronium)		
• Rapid sequence intubation, induced paralysis in infants with PPHN	• Intermediate-acting neuromuscular blockade used with general anesthesia to facilitate rapid sequence intubation as well as mechanical ventilation maintenance	• Administer following sedation for RSI. • If giving continuously through infusion, be sure patient is adequately sedated. • Electrolyte imbalances may increase sensitivity to NMBAs. Be sure to replace electrolytes as needed based on lab draws prior to administration. • NMBAs stimulate histamine release and may exacerbate asthma or respiratory disorders.
Phosphodiesterase inhibitors (sildenafil)		
• For treatment of PPHN and weaning of iNO	• Block PDE enzymes, causing blood vessels to relax and vasodilate	• Delay sildenafil use in preterm neonates until retinal blood vessel development is complete. • Adverse effects include visual impairment, hypotension, flushing, and nasal congestion.
Sedation (midazolam, propofol)		
• Given prior to RSI as well as for ventilator synchrony	• Acts on GABA receptors to produce muscle relaxation and produce sedative effect	• Only give in a controlled setting with proper monitoring and resuscitative equipment available. • Sedation may cause hypoventilation. Use with caution in already compromised respiratory patients.
Surfactant replacement (poractant alfa, calfactant, lucinactant, beractant)		
• For prevention and treatment of RDS in preterm neonates • For treatment of respiratory disease in term infants requiring mechanical ventilation and oxygen therapy	• Reduces surface tension at the air–liquid interface of the alveoli, preventing alveolar collapse	• During administration, bradycardia, oxygen desaturation, and/or ETT blockage may occur. Ensure bag/mask and suction are set up prior to administration. • Adverse effects include pulmonary hemorrhage, intraventricular hemorrhage, and pneumothorax.

BPD, bronchopulmonary dysplasia; CLD, chronic lung disease; ETT, endotracheal tube; GABA, gamma-aminobutyric acid; iNO, inhaled nitric oxide; IV, intravenous; NEC, necrotizing enterocolitis; NMBA, neuromuscular blocking agents; PDE, phosphodiesterase; PPHN, persistent pulmonary hypertension; RDS, respiratory distress syndrome; RSI, rapid sequence intubation.

6 CARDIOVASCULAR SYSTEM AND CIRCULATION

DEVELOPMENT OF THE CARDIOVASCULAR SYSTEM

Overview

- The cardiovascular system is the first system to develop in the growing fetus.
- The heart begins beating around day 22 of gestation via the primitive heart tube.
- By the end of 4 weeks' gestation, there is active fetal blood circulation.
- Intrauterine fetal life is sustained in a relatively hypoxic environment; survival in this hypoxic environment is dependent on the placenta as a means for gas exchange and nutrient delivery to the fetus and fetal cardiac shunts diverting blood from the lungs.

[🧠] **COMPLICATIONS**

Any disruption in early fetal cardiovascular development can have adverse and long-lasting effects on the neonate's transition to extrauterine life.

FETAL CIRCULATION

- Fetal circulation uses three shunts to bypass the fetal lungs and liver. Ductus venosus is the shunt between the liver and the inferior vena cava. Ductus arteriosus is the shunt between the pulmonary artery and aorta. Foramen ovale is the shunt between the right and left atria.
- Blood flow pathway from pregnant patient to fetus: Oxygen and nutrients are transferred across the placenta, and then into the fetus through the umbilical vein. Oxygen-rich blood flows through the umbilical vein toward the fetal liver. Blood passes through the ductus venosus, the first fetal shunt. This allows a small amount of blood to be delivered to the liver. The majority of the blood bypasses the liver and flows into the inferior vena cava.
- From the inferior vena cava, blood flows into the right atrium. Most of this blood flows through the foramen ovale into the left atrium.
- From the left atrium, blood flows to the left ventricle, aorta, heart muscle, brain, rest of the body.
- Blood returns from the body containing carbon dioxide (CO_2) and waste products and flows into the right atrium. From the right atrium, blood flows to the right ventricle, pulmonary artery, ductus arteriosus, and descending aorta. The ductus arteriosus allows blood to bypass the lungs.
- Pathway of blood flow from fetus to placenta: From the descending aorta, blood flows through the two umbilical arteries into the placenta, where gas and nutrient exchange occurs.

CIRCULATION CHANGES AT BIRTH

- At birth, the three fetal shunts are no longer needed.
- With the first breath, pressure and oxygen enter the lungs, triggering a decrease in pulmonary vascular resistance.
- Clamping the umbilical cord causes an increase in systemic vascular resistance. ▶

CIRCULATION CHANGES AT BIRTH (*continued*)

- Oxygen signals an increase in calcium channel activity in the smooth muscle of the ductus arteriosus, causing constriction and closure of the shunt.
- The increased systemic resistance creates higher pressure in the left atrium than in the right, causing the foramen ovale to close.
- The ductus venosus constricts and closes after the umbilical cord is clamped, and eventually becomes a ligament.

RISK FACTORS ASSOCIATED WITH CONGENITAL HEART DEFECTS

There are several risk factors associated with congenital heart defects (CHD). These include:

- Prematurity
- Multifetal pregnancy
- Use of assisted reproductive technology
- Family history of CHD
- Maternal drug and substance use
- Maternal infections and conditions
- Chromosomal anomalies

Maternal Medications

- Angiotensin-converting enzyme (ACE) inhibitors
- Lithium
- Nonsteroidal anti-inflammatory drugs (NSAIDs)
- Phenytoin
- Retinoic acid
- Selective serotonin reuptake inhibitors (SSRIs)
- Thalidomide

Maternal Substance Use

- Smoking
- Alcohol

Infections

- Cytomegalovirus
- Influenza
- Rubella

Maternal Conditions

- Diabetes
- Epilepsy
- Hypertension
- Lupus
- Maternal age >40
- Mood disorders
- Obesity
- Phenylketonuria (PKU)
- Preeclampsia ▶

Maternal Conditions (*continued*)
- Systemic connective tissue disorders
- Thyroid disorders

Chromosomal
- Coloboma, heart defects, atresia choanae, growth retardation, genital abnormalities, and ear abnormalities (CHARGE) syndrome
- Cri-du-chat syndrome
- DiGeorge syndrome (22q11)
- Marfan syndrome
- Noonan syndrome
- Trisomy 13 and 18
- Trisomy 21 (Down syndrome)
- Turner syndrome
- Vertebral defects, anal atresia, cardiac defects, tracheo-esophageal fistula, renal anomalies, and limb abnormalities (VACTERL) syndrome
- Williams syndrome
- Wolf-Hirschhorn syndrome

ASSESSMENT OF THE CARDIOVASCULAR SYSTEM

AUSCULTATION AND PALPATION

Upon inspection, the nurse should evaluate the neonate's:
- Capillary refill (less than 3 seconds)
- Chest wall for precordial activity or abnormal shape
- Level of alertness
- Respiratory effort
- Skin color
- Auscultation using a pediatric stethoscope should occur while the neonate is quiet and at rest to accurately evaluate heart sounds and identify any murmurs or abnormal heart sounds.
- During palpation, the nurse should assess upper and lower extremity peripheral pulses, including rate, rhythm, and intensity; check for a thrill; and palpate the abdomen to assess liver size and location.

HEART SOUNDS AND MURMURS

The four heart sounds are S1, S2, S3 and S4.
- S3 and S4 are rarely heard in a newborn.
- S1 is the sound of ventricular systole and is best auscultated at the left lower sternal border, or the apex. Displaced point of maximal impulse may indicate cardiac structural abnormality or ventricular enlargement.
- S2 is the sound of ventricular diastole and is best auscultated at the upper left sternal border or pulmonic area. Abnormal S2 or wide fixed split S2 may be present in CHD.
- A murmur is an abnormal swishing sound of the heart caused by turbulent blood flow.

Murmur Intensity
- Grade 1: barely audible
- Grade 2: soft, but audible ▶

Murmur Intensity (*continued*)

- Grade 3: moderately loud, no thrill
- Grade 4: loud, thrill present
- Grade 5: loud, audible with stethoscope barely on the chest
- Grade 6: loud, audible without stethoscope touching the chest

Additional Murmur Characterization

- Location
- Quality: harsh, musical, sweet/soft
- Timing: diastolic (early-diastolic, mid-diastolic, or presystolic) or systolic (occur between S1 and S2)
- Transmission

Innocent Murmurs

- The majority of murmurs are common findings in newborns and infants and originate from normal flow patterns, rather than structural defects. These murmurs are known as innocent murmurs.

Structural Defects

Murmurs that are associated with structural heart disease have the following characteristics:

- Associated with a systolic click
- Diastolic
- Grade 3 or higher
- Harsh quality
- Holosystolic (regurgitant)

CYANOSIS

It is important to differentiate normal versus abnormal cyanosis in the immediate newborn period.

- Acrocyanosis is a bluish discoloration around the mouth and in the extremities (hands and feet) caused by peripheral vasoconstriction and is a normal finding in the first 48 hours of life.
- Central cyanosis is a bluish discoloration of the mouth, torso, and head and may be present in the first 5 to 10 minutes of life as the newborn's oxygen saturation increases to 85% to 95%. Persistent central cyanosis is abnormal and should be investigated and treated immediately.

[🌐] **NURSING PEARLS**

Innocent murmurs can be characterized by the "Seven S's":
- Sensitive (changes with the child's position or respiration)
- Short duration (not holosystolic)
- Single (no associated clicks or gallops)
- Small (limited to a small area, nonradiating)
- Soft (low amplitude)
- Sweet (not harsh sounding)
- Systolic (occurs only during systole)

DIAGNOSTIC PROCEDURES

Arterial Blood Gases

- Please see Chapter 5, Respiratory System, for acid–base imbalances.

Four-Extremity Blood Pressure

- Measuring blood pressure in the upper and lower extremities simultaneously is known as four-extremity blood pressure. ▶

Four-Extremity Blood Pressure (*continued*)

- It helps assist with a diagnosis of coarctation of the aorta. The narrowing causes increased pressure proximal to the defect (the head and upper extremities) and decreased pressure distal to the defect (the lower extremities). A pressure gradient of >15 mmHg between upper and lower extremities is indicative of coarctation of the aorta.

Chest X-ray

Classic radiologic signs of specific CHD include:

- Boot-shaped heart: tetralogy of Fallot (TOF)
- Egg on a string: transposition of the great arteries (TGA)
- Figure of three: coarctation of the aorta
- Snowman: total anomalous pulmonary venous return (TAPVR)
- Wall to wall heart: Ebstein anomaly

Electrocardiogram

An *EKG* is a graphical representation of the electrical activity of the heart. EKGs are ordered on pediatric patients to:

- Assess a baseline rhythm before any intervention
- Assess a change in rhythm or dysrhythmias seen on a monitor
- Assess the heart after procedure or surgery
- Diagnose structural or conductive heart abnormalities
- Evaluate the effectiveness of prescribed heart medications
- Monitor a patient with syncope

Electrocardiogram Strips

EKG strips have several components that are used to help interpret rhythms:

- Small squares: 0.04 seconds
- Large squares: 0.20 seconds
- P wave: atrial depolarization
- ST wave: atrial repolarization
- PR interval: atrial depolarization and conduction through the atrioventricular (AV) node and Purkinje system
- QRS: ventricular depolarization
- T wave: ventricular repolarization
- QT interval: ventricular repolarization

Echocardiogram

- A noninvasive procedure to assess the overall structure and function of the heart
- Uses ultrasound (high-frequency sound waves) technology to create a graphical outline of the heart's movement
- The gold standard for diagnosing heart defects

Computed Tomography

- Intravenous (IV) contrast dye may be used.
- Contrast may be contraindicated in patients with heart disease, kidney disease, or thyroid disease.
- The patient needs to be able to tolerate a supine position.

Magnetic Resonance Imaging

- MRI may use IV contrast dye.
- Contrast may be contraindicated in patients with heart disease, kidney disease, or thyroid disease.

Cardiac Catheterization

- The main purpose of cardiac catheterization is to collect hemodynamic data and/or to confirm a heart disease diagnosis.
- A cardiac catheterization can detect heart defects, measure pressures within the heart chambers and great vessels, and measure cardiac output.
- It is an invasive procedure, usually performed in a cardiac catheterization lab, where a flexible catheter is inserted into an artery or vein, usually through either the femoral or radial arteries.
- During a cardiac catheterization, other procedures, such as closing heart defects (ventricular septal defect [VSD], atrial septal defect [ASD], patent ductus arteriosus [PDA]), can also be performed by a cardiologist, interventional radiologist, or other qualified provider.

Nursing Interventions

- Assess affected extremity for color, temperature, and capillary refill.
- Assess the family's understanding of the procedure.
- Assess pressure dressing according to protocol.
- Keep patient in bed in a supine position for 6 hours following catheterization, keeping extremity straight.
- Monitor IV fluids and encourage PO as soon as appropriate.
- Monitor for bleeding at the insertion site.
- Palpate the distal pulses of extremity used.
- Provide warmth to the opposite extremity.

Patient Education

- Apply pressure to the site if bleeding occurs.
- Learn what to look for in the hands/feet of extremity used for the procedure: Temperature should be warm, and color should not change. When a nail bed is compressed until it is pale, it should rapidly return to its usual color.

[ ]   **COMPLICATIONS**

There are several major complications that can happen with cardiac catheterization:

- Arrhythmias
- Atrial thrombosis
- AV fistula
- Bleeding
- Death
- Embolism
- Infection
- Myocardial infarction
- Perforation of the heart or great vessels
- Pseudoaneurysm
- Radiation exposure
- Retroperitoneal extension
- Stroke
- Thrombosis at the catheter insertion site

- Notify the provider of concerning changes, such as bleeding at the site, or pale or cool extremity.
- Remove the pressure dressing after 24 hours or according to the provider recommendation.

Critical Congenital Heart Defect Screening

- Critical congenital heart defect (CCHD) screening is a required screening that can identify newborns with heart defects before signs and symptoms are present and before the infant is discharged from the hospital.
- Oxygen saturation is measured on the right hand (preductal saturation) and the right or left foot (postductal saturation) simultaneously.
- Infant should be at least 24 hours old before screening is completed. ▶

Critical Congenital Heart Defect Screening (*continued*)

- A passed screening includes oxygen saturation greater than 95% in the right hand or foot and less than or equal to a 3% difference in oxygen saturations between the right hand and foot.
- A failed screening includes any oxygen saturation less than 90% in the initial screen or repeat screens, oxygen saturation between 90% and 95% in the hand and foot on three screens each separated by 1 hour, and/or a less than 3% difference in oxygen saturation between the hand and foot on three screens each separated by 1 hour.
- Any infant who fails the screening should be evaluated for causes of hypoxemia and receive an echocardiogram.

RESPIRATORY DISTRESS

- Respiratory distress is typically present with CHD due to changes in pulmonary blood flow and congestive heart failure (CHF).

Signs and Symptoms

- Tachypnea
- Retractions
- Nasal flaring
- Increased work of breathing
- Rales and crackles, which may be present on auscultation from pulmonary congestion

DIMINISHED CARDIAC OUTPUT

- Cardiac output is the volume of blood pumped per minute (L/min) and is determined by four factors: afterload, contractility, heart rate, and preload.
- The presence of shunts, obstructive lesions, ventricular hypoplasia, and abnormal arterial or venous connections as seen in CHD negatively affect cardiac output.
- Signs of reduced cardiac output include abnormal heart sounds such as S3 or S4, dysrhythmias, hypotension, tachycardia, decreased urine output, and decreased oxygen saturation.

ABNORMAL CARDIAC RHYTHM

- See Cardiac Dysrhythmias section.

CONGESTIVE HEART FAILURE

- CHF occurs when the infant's heart cannot effectively pump enough blood to meet the demands of the body.
- The main cause of neonatal CHF is cardiac structural defects that cause increased pulmonary blood flow.

Signs and Symptoms

- Poor weight gain
- Difficulty feeding
- Tachypnea
- Tachycardia ▶

Signs and Symptoms (*continued*)

- Excessive sleepiness
- Hepatomegaly
- Edema

PATHOPHYSIOLOGY: CARDIOVASCULAR DISORDERS

Overview

- *CHDs*, or malformations, are the most common type of birth defect.
- Many are diagnosed in utero.
- Defects can be in structure or function, involving the wall of the heart, the valves of the heart, and/or the arteries and veins surrounding the heart.
- Defects can also affect blood flow, causing the blood to flow in the wrong direction, flow to the wrong place, or flow too slowly.

Cyanotic Heart Defects

- Hypoplastic left heart syndrome (HLHS)
- Pulmonary atresia
- TOF
- TGA

Acyanotic Heart Defects

- ASD
- Atrioventricular septal defect (AVSD)
- Aortic valve stenosis
- Coarctation of the aorta
- Pulmonary valve stenosis
- PDA
- VSD

Signs and Symptoms of Cardiovascular Disorders

- CHF: difficulty feeding, edema, hepatomegaly, lethargy/excessive sleepiness, poor weight gain, tachycardia, and tachypnea
- Cyanosis or pallor
- Diaphoresis
- Irritability
- Murmur
- Oxygen desaturation
- Respiratory distress
- Thrill on auscultation
- Weak or bounding pulses

Nursing Interventions for Cardiovascular Disorders

- Administer medications as ordered.
- Assess peripheral pulses and capillary refill. ▶

[🧠]   **COMPLICATIONS**

Patients with congenital heart defects are at an increased risk of developing bacterial endocarditis. Frequently, prophylactic antibiotics are prescribed prior to dental visits or procedures.

[⚡]   **ALERT!**

Families with children who have heart defects must learn CPR before leaving the hospital.

Nursing Interventions for Cardiovascular Disorders (*continued*)

- Educate the family about symptoms of heart failure.
- Evaluate activity tolerance.
- Explain the condition to the family using diagrams and answer questions.
- Implement a high-calorie, small-volume feeding regimen to maximize calories and minimize effort during feeds; educate families on home feeding management.
- Monitor for color changes (cyanosis).
- Monitor EKG for changes.
- Monitor pulse oximetry and CO_2.
- Monitor strict input/output (I/O).
- Monitor vital signs (VS), temperature, and heart sounds.
- Postoperative care: Administer medications for blood pressure support and cardiac function (Appendix 6.1). Assess for infection at the surgical site. Monitor for arrhythmias. Monitor for pain.
- Provide emotional support to the patient and the family.
- Review the need for vaccination against respiratory syncytial virus (RSV).
- Stabilize and prepare the infant for surgery when necessary.
- Titrate supplemental oxygen to maintain saturations within the desired range.
- Weigh daily.

Patient Education for Cardiovascular Disorders

- Air travel may be restricted.
- All respiratory infections should be treated promptly.
- Attend follow-up appointments.
- Avoid sick contacts and visitors.
- Family members should seek support groups to help them face challenges and connect with other families going through similar experiences.
- Follow recommendations for the proper activity level for the infant; the patient may need more rest periods than other infants their age.
- Follow strict infection prevention guidelines, such as proper hand hygiene.
- Learn about cardiac defect and signs of problems: blue cast to lips or fingernails, cyanosis, dyspnea, fatigue, jugular vein distention, noisy breathing, palpitations, and syncope.
- Monitor the child's weight and report a loss/failure to gain to the physician.
- Patient may require more surgeries as they get older.
- Prophylactic antibiotics may be needed before medical and dental procedures.
- Recognize the importance of immunizations for a child with a heart defect.

[🧠]   **COMPLICATIONS**

Persistent patent ductus arteriosus may lead to heart failure, renal dysfunction, necrotizing enterocolitis (NEC), intraventricular hemorrhage (IVH), and poor nutrition and growth.

[⚡]   **ALERT!**

Multiple complex congenital heart defects require the patent ductus arteriosus (PDA) to remain open to supply oxygenated blood to the body for perfusion. To do this, the patient is administered prostaglandin E1 (Appendix 6.1) to reopen or keep open the ductus arteriosus.

PATENT DUCTUS ARTERIOSUS

- The ductus arteriosus is a normal fetal artery that connects the aorta and the pulmonary artery and is necessary during intrauterine life for directing blood away from the lungs. ▶

PATENT DUCTUS ARTERIOSUS (*continued*)

- The ductus arteriosus typically closes within the first 72 hours of life; failure to close within this time frame is known as PDA. It is common in preterm infants and rare in term infants.
- In the presence of a PDA, blood is shunted from the aorta into the pulmonary artery and lungs.

Signs and Symptoms

- Depend on the size of the PDA and the degree of left-to-right shunting
- Can be asymptomatic
- Bounding peripheral pulses
- Wide pulse pressure
- Unexplained metabolic acidosis
- Poor growth
- Increased work of breathing
- Tachycardia

Treatment

- There are three levels of treatment intervention available for PDA: fluid restriction, medication management, and surgical closure.

Fluid Restriction

- Most conservative approach to PDA treatment
- Allows for spontaneous closure while monitoring the infant closely for worsening signs and symptoms
- May decrease the volume of circulating blood and prevent pulmonary edema, improving respiratory function
- May include use of diuretics if clinically indicated

Medication Management

- Appendix 6.1
- IV ibuprofen
- IV indomethacin

Surgical Closure

- Transcatheter device closure with a coil
- Surgical closure with stitches or clips (PDA ligation)

VENTRICULAR SEPTAL DEFECT

- VSD is a hole or opening between the right and left ventricles of the heart, or the ventricular septum, which results in increased pulmonary blood flow.
- VSD can vary in size, from a small pinhole to absence of the septum.
- Blood in the left ventricle (high pressure) will flow through the VSD into the right ventricle (lower pressure), creating a left-to-right shunt, which causes right ventricular hypertrophy.
- The effects and treatment depend on the size and pulmonary vascular resistance.

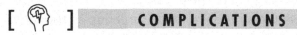

COMPLICATIONS

Complications associated with a ventricular septal defect include pulmonary hypertension, heart failure, arrhythmias, stroke, endocarditis, aortic regurgitation, subaortic stenosis, left-to-right shunting at the atrial level, and right ventricle obstruction.

Treatment

- Mild or small VSD may close spontaneously.
- Medication management (Appendix 6.1) includes diuretics and inotropes for heart failure.
- Surgical closure requires cardiopulmonary bypass.
- Transcatheter closure is reserved for patients who cannot tolerate bypass.

COARCTATION OF THE AORTA

- Coarctation of the aorta is an obstructive heart defect characterized by narrowing of the aorta, most often at or near the ductus arteriosus.
- The narrowing causes increased pressure proximal to the defect (the head and upper extremities) and decreased pressure distal to the defect (the lower extremities). Discrepancies in four-extremity blood pressures are an indication of this heart defect. It usually presents after the PDA closes in an infant.
- The obstruction causes the left ventricle to be overloaded.
- Usually, it occurs in addition to another heart abnormality, including ASD, bicuspid aortic valve, congenital mitral valve stenosis, PDA, subaortic stenosis, or VSD.

[COMPLICATIONS]

If left untreated, coarctation of the aorta can lead to heart failure or death in infants. It can also lead to an aneurysm in the brain or the aorta. Hypertension is the most common long-term complication.

Signs and Symptoms

- Hypertension in the upper extremities
- Hypotension, or lower blood pressure, in the lower extremities
- Bounding pulses in the arms
- Weak or absent pulses in the lower extremities
- Absent or delayed femoral pulse
- Cyanotic lower extremities
- Diaphoresis
- Preductal pulse ox saturation higher than postductal

Treatment

Medication to palliate symptoms until the coarctation is corrected (Appendix 6.1):

- Dopamine
- Furosemide
- Nifedipine
- Prostaglandin E1

Surgical Management

- Angioplasty or stent placement for mild cases
- Removal or widening of narrowed part of the aorta

Nursing Interventions

- Administer hypertension medication if blood pressure remains high.
- Monitor four-extremity blood pressures.
- Monitor upper and lower bilateral pulses, using Doppler if needed. Notify provider of absent pulses.

Patient Education

- Even with treatment, the coarctation can return. Recognize the signs and symptoms of a recoarctation.
- Prevent prolonged crying after surgery.

CRITICAL AORTIC STENOSIS

- Critical aortic stenosis is a very severe narrowing of the aortic valve, causing left ventricular outflow obstruction.
- The heart is unable to pump enough blood to meet the needs of the body.
- It requires immediate treatment after birth.

Treatment

Medication Management

- Prostaglandin E1 (see Appendix 6.1)

Surgical management

- Balloon valvuloplasty via cardiac catheterization, which may be the only intervention needed, but often used as temporary means to delay open heart surgery

Surgical Repair

- Valve replacement and valvotomy

[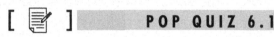]   **NURSING PEARLS**

Recoarctation refers to stenosis after surgery or angioplasty. Symptoms include resting hypertension, headaches, and trouble walking or standing with pain and numbness.

[ ]   **POP QUIZ 6.1**

A laboring patient had a prenatal ultrasound that showed coarctation of the aorta in the fetus. What abnormal assessment findings should the nurse expect after delivery? What nursing interventions should be done to care for this baby after delivery?

[🧠]   **COMPLICATIONS**

Critical aortic stenosis results in left ventricular hypertrophy. Over time and without treatment, this may lead to left-sided heart failure, shock, arrhythmias, and may be fatal.

CRITICAL PULMONARY STENOSIS

- *Critical pulmonary stenosis* is a severe narrowing of the pulmonary valve.
- Blood flow from the right ventricle to the pulmonary artery and lungs is limited.
- The ductus arteriosus must remain open, or patent, for the blood to flow to the lungs.
- This typically occurs as a part of other CHDs.

Treatment

Medication Management

- Prostaglandin E1 (see Appendix 6.1)

Surgical Management

- Cardiac catheterization, which is used to assess abnormalities and perform interventions such as balloon dilation

Surgical Repair

- Create or widen the pulmonary valve.
- Balloon or stent is used to keep the ductus arteriosus open.

[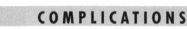]   **COMPLICATIONS**

Without prompt treatment, critical pulmonary stenosis causes right-sided heart failure and arrhythmias.

ATRIOVENTRICULAR SEPTAL DEFECT

- *AVSD* is characterized by a group of CHDs involving the AV septum and AV valves.
- This heart defect (along with VSD, PDA, and TOF) is common in children with trisomy 21. ▶

ATRIOVENTRICULAR SEPTAL DEFECT (*continued*)

- Complete AVSD: Blood flows freely between all four chambers. There is one valve instead of two.
- Partial AVSD: There is a hole in the atrial or ventricle septum near the center of the heart. Both valves are usually present but may leak and cause blood backflow. Due to lack of symptoms, it may not be diagnosed until later in life.

Treatment

Medication Management

- ACE inhibitors, beta blockers, diuretics, and inotropic agent (see Appendix 6.1)

Surgical Management

- Surgery is the definitive treatment. Timing is determined by the severity of the AV defect. If the defect is complete, surgery will be done early in infancy.

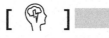 **COMPLICATIONS**

Complications of atrioventricular septal defect include arrhythmias, congestive heart failure, and pulmonary hypertension.

EBSTEIN ANOMALY

- *Ebstein anomaly* is an abnormality in the tricuspid valve which separates the right atrium and the right ventricle.
- During right ventricular contraction, the tricuspid valve allows blood to leak backwards into the right atrium, resulting in right atrial hypertrophy.

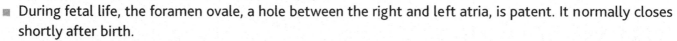 **COMPLICATIONS**

Ebstein anomaly may lead to congestive heart failure, heart block, arrhythmias, and blood clots.

- During fetal life, the foramen ovale, a hole between the right and left atria, is patent. It normally closes shortly after birth.
- The high pressure in the right atrium forces the foramen ovale to remain open, or patent (patent foramen ovale [PFO]).
- The PFO allows unoxygenated blood from the right atrium to flow into the left atrium and subsequently to the rest of the body.

Treatment

- Depends on the severity of the abnormality and degree of symptoms
- Oxygen supplementation and respiratory support

Medical Management

- Diuretics for heart failure (see Appendix 6.1)

Surgical Management

- Closure of the PFO, surgical repair of the valve, and valve replacement

PERSISTENT PULMONARY HYPERTENSION

- See Chapter 5, Respiratory System.

TRANSPOSITION OF THE GREAT ARTERIES

- *TGA* is a CHD in which the pulmonary artery and aorta are switched or transposed. ▶

TRANSPOSITION OF THE GREAT ARTERIES (*continued*)

- Unoxygenated blood returns to the right side of the heart from the body, and instead of going into the lungs it flows into the aorta and back out to the body.
- Oxygenated blood from the lungs enters the left side of the heart, and instead of flowing out to the body it returns to the lungs via the pulmonary artery.
- Other defects such as VSD, ASD, and PDA are typically present, which allow mixing of blood so that some oxygenated blood is delivered to the body.

Treatment

Medication Management
- Prostaglandin E1 (see Appendix 6.1)

Surgical Repair

Surgical repair is required for all infants with TGA.
- Arterial switch operation: Arteries are switched back to normal positions. This is the most common surgical approach to TGA.
- Atrial switch operation: This is less common as it can lead to complications later in life.

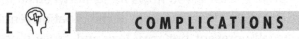

COMPLICATIONS

Complications of untreated transposition of the great arteries (TGA) may include tissue hypoxia and heart failure. Arrhythmias may occur following surgical correction of TGA.

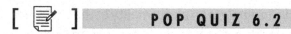

POP QUIZ 6.2

A term infant is admitted to the NICU for cyanosis and is diagnosed with transposition of the great arteries (TGA). The nurse recognizes that the degree of cyanosis depends on what factors?

TETRALOGY OF FALLOT

- *TOF* is a heart defect with decreased pulmonary blood flow.
- Four abnormalities are, together, referred to as TOF: overriding aorta, the aorta that overrides the ventricular septum, to the right above the VSD, pulmonary stenosis, right ventricular hypertrophy, or thickening of the right ventricular wall, and VSD.
- The overriding aorta allows deoxygenated blood from the right ventricle to flow into the aorta and be mixed with the systemic blood flow.
- The right side of the heart develops hypertrophy because it works hard pushing against the obstruction at the pulmonary valve.
- TOF may present along with other deformities but typically presents with no other anomalies.

Risk Factors

- Alcohol use during pregnancy
- Environmental factors
- Genetic predisposition
- Parent with TOF
- Poor nutrition during pregnancy
- Pregnancy past the age of 40 years
- Prematurity
- The presence of trisomy 21 or DiGeorge syndrome
- A viral illness during pregnancy (e.g., rubella)

Signs and Symptoms

■ The main sign of TOF is a TET spell, or a hypercyanotic episode, in which the infant's skin, nails, and lips turn dark blue. These episodes are caused by activities such as stooling or crying and cause a decrease in blood flow to the lungs and decreased amount of oxygen in the blood.

Treatment

Medication Management

■ Appendix 6.1
■ Antibiotic prophylaxis prior to repair
■ Opioid for TET spells
■ Propranolol

Surgical Management

■ Elective repair is usually done within the first year of life. This is dependent on the severity of cyanosis and the development of hypercyanotic spells.

■ Complete repair usually occurs between 6 and 12 months of life. Complete repair includes closure of the VSD, preserving right ventricle function, and relieving right ventricular outflow by removing the obstruction. Procedure requires median sternotomy and the use of cardiopulmonary bypass.

Nursing Interventions

Unrepaired Tetralogy of Fallot

Be prepared to treat TET spells.

■ Position the infant in a knee-chest position.
■ Supply oxygen if needed, although it does not always help oxygenation.
■ Administer an opioid.
■ Administer propranolol (Appendix 6.1).
■ If interventions are not effective, emergency surgery is needed.

Postoperative Tetralogy of Fallot Care

■ Assess and medicate for pain as needed.
■ Initiate sternal precautions. Avoid lifting both arms overhead. Avoid reaching both arms out to the side. Do not allow infants to push with their arms (e.g., tummy time).
■ Monitor for postsurgical complications such as chronic pulmonary regurgitation, pulmonary valve dysfunction, and right ventricular enlargement and dysfunction.
■ Monitor strict I/O.

Patient Education

■ Activity may have to be limited as infants with TOF may tire more easily.
■ Learn how to treat TET spells, such as knee-chest positioning (see Nursing Interventions section). ▶

[ ]   **COMPLICATIONS**

There are several possible complications from tetralogy of Fallot repair, including the following:

• Altered cardiac rhythms
• Anemia
• Blood clots
• Brain abscess
• Coagulation defects
• Death
• Embolism
• Heart failure
• Infection
• Stroke

[⚡]   **ALERT!**

TET spells occur when the infant becomes agitated and can also occur if the infant is in pain, has a fever, is anemic or hypovolemic, or after feeding, prolonged crying, or any activity or exercise. TET spells present with fast, deep breathing, irritability, inconsolability, and progressively worsening cyanosis.

Patient Education (*continued*)

- Learn the "scoop lift," a technique to lift the patient under their bottom instead of under their arms. The "scoop lift" is used because the chest bone takes approximately 6 weeks to heal after surgery.
- The patient may need to have further heart surgery or interventional procedures as they age.

PULMONARY ATRESIA

- *Pulmonary atresia* is a CHD that is normally diagnosed soon after birth.
- Pulmonary atresia is a complete obstruction of the right ventricular outflow tract.
- The pulmonary valve, a heart valve that allows blood to flow out of the right ventricle to go to the lungs, is not completely formed.
- Blood is unable to move from the right ventricle to the pulmonary artery and lungs.
- The ductus arteriosus must remain open, or patent, for the blood to flow to the lungs.
- There are two subcategories of pulmonary atresia: intact ventricular septum and VSD.
- Pulmonary atresia with a VSD is very similar to the TOF. Please refer to that section for more details.
- If left untreated, pulmonary atresia is fatal.

Treatment

Medication Management
- Prostaglandin E1 (see Appendix 6.1)

Surgical Management
- Probable cardiac catheterization to assess abnormalities and perform interventions
- Surgical repair to create or widen the pulmonary valve
- Surgical repair to patch the VSD if necessary
- Surgical repair with balloon or stent to keep the ductus arteriosus open
- Transplant may be necessary.

TOTAL ANOMALOUS PULMONARY VENOUS RETURN

- *TAPVR* is a CHD in which the pulmonary veins do not connect to the left atrium but connect to the right side of the heart.
- Oxygenated blood from the lungs is unable to flow into the left side of the heart.
- Oxygenated blood from the lungs mixes with unoxygenated blood on the right side of the heart, causing cyanosis and hypoxemia.
- The right side of the heart becomes hypertrophied from increased blood volume.
- To survive, babies with TAPVR typically have another heart defect such as an ASD or PDA, which allow mixed blood to get to the left side of the heart and the rest of the body.

POP QUIZ 6.3

An infant is brought to the ED crying. The patient is very cyanotic with an oxygen saturation level of 72%, which improves with knee-chest positioning. Their respirations are fast at 80 breaths per minute and labored. Their parent states that this has been happening for a few weeks, but it is getting worse. The infant has not been eating well and has been more tired than usual. What are these signs and symptoms? What can the nurse do to help this patient?

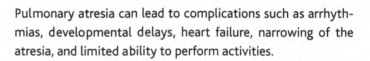

COMPLICATIONS

Pulmonary atresia can lead to complications such as arrhythmias, developmental delays, heart failure, narrowing of the atresia, and limited ability to perform activities.

COMPLICATIONS

Complications of total anomalous pulmonary venous return include shock, pulmonary edema, and pulmonary hypertension.

Treatment
Surgical Repair
Surgical repair is required for all infants with TAPVR.
- Closure of ASD or PDA
- Repairs normal circulation by connecting the pulmonary veins to the left atrium

TRICUSPID ATRESIA

- *Tricuspid atresia* is a CHD in which the tricuspid valve, the valve between the right atrium and the right ventricle, does not form at all.
- Blood returning from the body into the right atrium is unable to go into the right ventricle and to the lungs.
- The right ventricle and main pulmonary artery may be underdeveloped.
- It typically presents with other defects such as ASD, PDA, and VSD to allow blood to bypass the unformed tricuspid valve.

Treatment
Medication Management
- Prostaglandin E1 (see Appendix 6.1)

Surgical Management
- Banding: controls blood flow to the lungs if necessary
- Bidirectional Glenn procedure: connects the pulmonary artery to the superior vena cava, allowing blood returning from the body to bypass the heart and flow directly into the lungs
- Fontan procedure: connects the pulmonary artery to the interior vena cava; probable cardiac catheterization to assess abnormalities and perform interventions
- Septostomy: enlarges the ASD so that more oxygenated blood can get to the body
- Shunt procedure: shunt created between the aorta and pulmonary artery, allowing more blood flow to the lungs

[🧠] **COMPLICATIONS**

Tricuspid atresia may lead to hypoxemia, blood clots, arrhythmias, and liver or kidney disease.

Patient Education
- Surgery is not curative.
- More surgeries may be needed in the future.
- There is possible need for a heart transplant.

TRUNCUS ARTERIOSUS

- *Truncus arteriosus* is a CHD in which a single great vessel leaves the heart, instead of two separate vessels (pulmonary artery and aorta).
- The single vessel sits over the right and left ventricles and receives both unoxygenated and oxygenated blood.
- Too much blood is delivered to the lungs, and the heart must work harder to pump blood to the body.

[🧠] **COMPLICATIONS**

Complications of truncus arteriosus include pulmonary edema and congestive heart failure.

Treatment
Surgical Management
Surgical intervention includes three main repairs:
- Closure of the VSD via a patch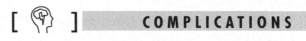

Surgical Management (continued)
- Connecting the pulmonary arteries and the right ventricle using a conduit
- Separation of the pulmonary arteries from the truncus and creation of the aorta from the truncus

Patient Education
- The conduit does not grow, so the infant may need more surgeries to replace it.

HYPOPLASTIC LEFT HEART SYNDROME

- *HLHS* is a severe cardiac defect in which the left ventricle is underdeveloped or hypoplastic (too small) to support systemic circulation, including hypoplasia of the ascending aorta and arch, hypoplasia of the left ventricle, and hypoplasia, or stenosis, of the aortic and/or mitral valves.
- This heart defect has a high mortality rate without intervention.
- HLHS results in a univentricular circulatory system.
- Patients must have a PDA to maintain systemic circulation.
- The severity of the defect depends on the condition of the mitral and aortic valves.
- Due to it being a fatal condition without medical interventions, HLHS has raised many surgical, ethical, social, and economic issues. There is a debate as to whether comfort-only care should be presented as an option to parents.

Treatment
- PDA: balloon PDA to keep open and prostaglandin E1 (Appendix 6.1)

Surgical Management

Three-stage palliative (not curative) surgical care:
- Norwood: completed in the first week of life; creates a neo-aorta, or a single outflow tract from the heart, by fusing the aorta and the pulmonary artery; establishes a source of pulmonary blood flow by placing a stent; dissects atrial septum to allow for adequate mixing of oxygenated and deoxygenated blood
- Glenn: completed between 3 and 6 months of life; original stent removed; superior vena cava anastomosed to pulmonary artery
- Fontan: completed between 2 and 5 years of age; creates a second pathway into the pulmonary artery using the inferior vena cava; relieves cyanosis

Medication Management

Medication management after Norwood procedure (Appendix 6.1):
- ACE inhibitor
- Aspirin
- Digoxin
- Diuretics

[🧠]   **COMPLICATIONS**

Without treatment, hypoplastic left heart syndrome is fatal. With treatment, complications include:
- Additional surgery/transplantation in the future
- Arrhythmias
- Blood clots causing emboli
- Development delays
- Edema, abdomen, legs, feet, lungs
- Excessive fatigue
- Growth retardation

[⚡]   **ALERT!**

If diagnosed at a prenatal visit, choices that are given to the parents are pursuant to additional testing, choice of delivery setting, termination of the pregnancy, and, where possible, prenatal intervention. Postnatal choices discussed are staged palliative surgery, heart transplant, or comfort care only.

Nursing Interventions

- Be mindful and supportive of the stress of coworkers and self when caring for these infants.
- Provide resources for the family, such as chaplain and palliative care team, if appropriate.
- Provide rest periods as needed. Disturb only if necessary.
- Do not allow the baby to cry for long periods.
- Supply oxygen as needed to maintain oxygen saturations within range for each stage of repair.
- Do not hyperoxygenate. These patients will never have oxygen saturations of 100% due to the mixing of oxygenated and unoxygenated blood.

[🌐]   **NURSING PEARLS**

High oxygen saturations may be contraindicated in some cardiac patients due to pulmonary vasodilation. Having high oxygen saturations could potentially be fatal to a patient with hypoplastic left heart syndrome.

CARDIAC DYSRHYTHMIAS

- To understand and identify arrhythmias, a basic understanding of NSR is essential.
- NSR is a regular rhythm at the normal heart rate for age. In infants, NRS is 100 to 180 beats per minute (bpm).
- NSR includes the presence of an upright P wave (indicating depolarization of the atria), a QRS complex (indicating ventricular depolarization and atrial repolarization), and an upright T wave (indicating ventricular repolarization). PR intervals should be between 0.12 and 0.2 seconds. QRS intervals should be less than 0.1 seconds. QT intervals should be under 0.38 seconds. There should be one P wave for every QRS complex.
- Neonatal arrhythmias are classified as either benign or nonbenign.
- Arrhythmias in the newborn period are common and may occur in neonates with or without heart defects.

Benign Dysrhythmias

- Benign neonatal arrhythmias include sinus arrhythmia, premature atrial contraction (PAC), and premature ventricular contraction (PVC). PAC and PVC are the most common benign arrhythmias in neonates. These rhythms require no treatment.
- Sinus arrhythmia is a variation of a normal sinus rhythm with an R-R interval greater than 0.12 seconds. This is a normal finding which requires no treatment. Incidence decreases with age.
- PACs are contractions of the atria that are triggered by the atrial myocardium but have not originated from the sinoatrial node. PACs feature early P waves with normal PR interval and one QRS complex for each P wave. Irregularity of rhythm can sometimes decrease filling times and blood pressure. Early P waves are often caused by electrolyte abnormalities, hypoglycemia, hypoxia, and hyperthyroidism.
- PVCs are contractions of the ventricles that precede atrial contraction and do not originate from the sinoatrial (SA) node; wide and premature QRS complexes without a preceding P wave; and can be caused by cardiomyopathy or other heart disease, metabolic disease, and electrolyte imbalances.

Supraventricular Tachycardia

- Supraventricular tachycardia (SVT) is a tachydysrhythmia characterized by a rapid regular heart rate of 200 to 300 bpm.
- The onset of SVT is typically sudden.
- SVT is the most common tachyarrhythmia in neonates.

Atrial Fibrillation

- P waves will not be seen on the EKG because the atrial rate is so fast and the action potentials produced are of such low amplitude.
- The QRS rate is variable, and the rhythm is irregular.
- In patients with atrial fibrillation (A-fib) with rapid ventricular response (RVR), the ventricles may beat greater than 100 times per minute, resulting in elevated heart rate.
- The irregularity of the atrial contraction causes decreased filling time of the atria. This results in a smaller volume of oxygenated blood being circulated.
- A-fib may be caused by any of the following: congenital heart disease, underlying heart disease, hypertension (systemic or pulmonary), endocrine abnormalities, genetic predisposition, cerebral hemorrhage or stroke, pulmonary embolism, and obstructive sleep apnea.

Atrial Flutter

- Atrial flutter features a P rate up to 500 bpm and a PR interval that is usually not observable.
- This is characterized by "saw-tooth" waves.
- Irregularity and rate of atrial contraction cause decreased filling time of the atria.
- This results in a smaller volume of oxygenated blood being circulated.
- The cause begins with an ectopic beat which depolarizes one segment of the normal conduction pathway.

Ventricular Tachycardia

- Ventricular tachycardia (V-tach) is defined as three or more PVCs in a row at a rate of 120 bpm or faster, with wide QRS complexes and AV disassociation.
- V-tach is a rare arrhythmia in neonates.
- V-tach results in decreased cardiac output and increased myocardial demand.
- It may be caused by myocarditis, cardiac tumor, congenital heart disease, cardiomyopathy, and electrolyte imbalances.
- Common triggering events for V-tach include hypokalemia and hypomagnesemia.

Treatment of Dysrhythmias

- SVT: Treatment of acute SVT includes vagal maneuvers, applying ice to the face, and adenosine. Digoxin or propranolol may be used as maintenance therapy to prevent reoccurrence.
- A-fib: This can be treated with adenosine for acute termination, followed by maintenance antiarrhythmic medication such as digoxin or propranolol.
- Atrial flutter: This can be treated with antiarrhythmic therapy such as digoxin or propranolol. Critical atrial flutter may require cardioversion or transesophageal pacing.
- V-tach: If hemodynamically unstable, V-tach should be treated with cardioversion or lidocaine. Antiarrhythmic medications for prophylaxis include verapamil and beta blockers.

RESOURCES

American Association of Critical Care Nurses. (2017). *Certification and core review for neonatal intensive care nursing*. Elsevier.

Ban, J. (2017). Neonatal arrhythmias: Diagnosis, treatment, and clinical outcome. *Korean Journal of Pediatrics, 60*(11), 344–352. https://doi.org/10.3345/kjp.2017.60.11.344

Centers for Disease Control and Prevention. (2022a). *Congenital heart defects information for healthcare providers*. U.S. Department of Health and Human Services, Centers for Disease Control and Prevention. https://www.cdc.gov/ncbddd/heartdefects/hcp.html

Centers for Disease Control and Prevention. (2022b). *Facts about dextro-Transposition of the Great Arteries (d-TGA)*. U.S. Department of Health and Human Services, Centers for Disease Control and Prevention. https://www.cdc .gov/ncbddd/heartdefects/d-tga.html

Centers for Disease Control and Prevention. (2022c). *Facts about Total Anomalous Pulmonary Venous Return or TAPVR*. U.S. Department of Health and Human Services, Centers for Disease Control and Prevention. https:// www.cdc.gov/ncbddd/heartdefects/tapvr.html#:~:text = Total%20anomalous%20pulmonary%20venous%20 return%20(TAPVR)%20is%20a%20birth%20defect,mixes%20with%20oxygen%2Dpoor%20blood.

Centers for Disease Control and Prevention. (2022d). *Facts about Tricuspid Atresia*. U.S. Department of Health and Human Services, Centers for Disease Control and Prevention. https://www.cdc.gov/ncbddd/heartdefects /tricuspid-atresia.html

Centers for Disease Control and Prevention. (2022e). *Facts about Truncus Arteriosus*. U.S. Department of Health and Human Services, Centers for Disease Control and Prevention. https://www.cdc.gov/ncbddd/heartdefects /truncusarteriosus.html

Cincinnati Children's. (2019). *Ebstein's Anomaly*. https://www.cincinnatichildrens.org/health/e/ebstein

Cincinnati Children's. (2021a). *Aortic (Valve) Stenosis*. https://www.cincinnatichildrens.org/health/a/avs

Cincinnati Children's. (2021b). *Cyanosis*. https://www.cincinnatichildrens.org/health/c/cyanosis

Cincinnati Children's. (2022). *Congestive Heart Failure*. https://www.cincinnatichildrens.org/health/c/chf

Cleveland Clinic. (2019). *Echocardiogram*. https://my.clevelandclinic.org/health/diagnostics/16947-echocardiogram

Dice, J., & Bhatia, J. (2007). Patent ductus arteriosus: An overview. *The Journal of Pediatric Pharmacology and Therapeutics, 12*(3), 138–146. https://doi.org/10.5863/1551-6776-12.3.138.

Frank, J., & Jacobe, K. (2011). Evaluation and management of heart murmurs in children. *American Family Physician*. https://www.aafp.org/afp/2011/1001/p793.html

Mathew, P., & Bordoni, B. (2022). Embryology, heart. *StatPearls*. Retrieved February 11, 2022 from https://www.ncbi .nlm.nih.gov/books/NBK537313/

Prescriber's Digital Reference. *Ibuprofen*. https://www.pdr.net/drug-summary/Ibuprofen -Suspension-ibuprofen-2619#15

Prescriber's Digital Reference. *Indomethacin*. https://www.pdr.net/drug-summary/Indocin -Oral-Suspension-indomethacin-1360#topPage

RadiologyInfo.org For Patients. (2021). *Pediatric CT (Computed Tomography)*. https://www.radiologyinfo.org/en/info /pedia-ct

RadiologyInfo.org For Patients. (2020). *Pediatric MRI*. https://www.radiologyinfo.org/en/info/pediatric-mri

Stanford Children's Health. *Factors that May Lead to a Congenital Heart Defect (CHD)*. https://www.stanfordchildrens .org/en/topic/default?id=factors-contributing-to-congenital-heart-disease-90-P01788#:~:text = Problems%20with%20chromosomes%20that%20lead,will%20have%20a%20heart%20defect.

Stanford Children's Hospital. *Pulmonary Stenosis in Children*. https://www.stanfordchildrens.org/en/topic/default ?id=pulmonary-stenosis-90-P01815

University of Rochester Medical Center. (2022). *Blood Circulation in the Fetus and Newborn*. https://www.urmc .rochester.edu/encyclopedia/content.aspx?ContentTypeID=90&ContentID=P02362

UpToDate. (2022). *Factors Associated with an Increased Risk of Congenital Heart Disease*. Retrieved February 17, 2022. https://www.uptodate.com/contents/image?imageKey=PEDS%2F103088 &topicKey = PEDS%2F101291&source = see_link

APPENDIX 6.1 CARDIOVASCULAR MEDICATIONS

INDICATIONS	MECHANISM OF ACTION	CONTRAINDICATIONS, PRECAUTIONS, AND ADVERSE EFFECTS
ACE inhibitors (enalapril)		
• Treat atrioventricular canal defect • Treat hypertension	• Inhibit ACE	• Medication is contraindicated in pediatric patients with a lowered GFR and contraindicated in patients with hypotension. • Use with caution in children under 6 years old. • Use with caution in patients with risk of hyperkalemia. • Adverse effects include hyperkalemia, myocardial infarction, renal failure, and hypotension.
Adrenergic agonist agents (dopamine)		
• Increase cardiac output • Increase blood pressure	• Stimulate adrenergic and dopaminergic receptors • Produce cardiac stimulation	• Medication is contraindicated in pheochromocytoma, tachyarrhythmias, and ventricular fibrillation. • Use extreme caution if patient is taking MAO inhibitors. • Precautions need to be taken in case of arrhythmias, extravasation, heart conditions, electrolyte imbalance, and shock. • Adverse effects include sloughing and necrosis of the IV site. Monitor closely. • Adverse effects also include anxiety, headache, cardiac rhythm changes, nausea, vomiting, dyspnea, polyuria, and increased intraocular pressure.
Beta blockers (propranolol)		
• Can be used to treat TET spells	• Reduce blood pressure, heart rate, cardiac output, and myocardial contractility	• Medication is contraindicated in patients with severe bradycardia. • Use with caution in patients with pulmonary disease. • Adverse effects include cardiac ischemia if discontinued suddenly, as well as acute MI, nausea/vomiting, and bronchitis.
Calcium channel blockers (nifedipine, verapamil)		
• Treat hypertension	• Relax coronary vascular muscle and produce coronary vasodilation	• Caution must be used in patients with GI strictures, aortic stenosis, heart failure, and hepatic impairment. • Adverse effects include flushing, nausea, heartburn, dizziness, headache, Stevens–Johnson syndrome, and toxic epidermal necrolysis.
COX inhibitors (ibuprofen, indomethacin)		
• Treat hemodynamically significant PDA in premature infants	• Reduce circulating prostaglandins that maintain patency of duct	• Medication is contraindicated in patients with active bleeding, infection, coagulation defects, suspected NEC, and renal dysfunction. • Do not give to patients with ductal-dependent CHD. • Monitor urine output and consider holding further doses if oliguria is present. • Monitor IV site for signs of extravasation. • Adverse effects of ibuprofen include thrombocytopenia and hyperbilirubinemia. • Adverse effects of indomethacin include apnea, renal dysfunction, necrotizing enterocolitis, intracranial hemorrhage, hypoglycemia, and thrombocytopenia.

(continued)

APPENDIX 6.1 CARDIOVASCULAR MEDICATIONS (*continued*)

INDICATIONS	MECHANISM OF ACTION	CONTRAINDICATIONS, PRECAUTIONS, AND ADVERSE EFFECTS
Diuretics (furosemide)		
• Remove excess fluid from the body	• Inhibit the reabsorption of sodium and chloride in the kidneys	• Contraindications include anuria. • Precautions should be used in patients with thyroid impairment, diabetes, urinary stricture, and lupus. • With chronic use, children can develop kidney stones. • Caution is needed if given before surgery, as patient may be volume-depleted and blood pressure may be labile. • Adverse effects include necrotizing angiitis, Stevens–Johnson syndrome, and toxic epidermal necrolysis. • Medication can cause abdominal cramps, nausea/vomiting, constipation, and pancreatitis. • Medication can cause electrolyte imbalances, anemia, headache, vertigo, blurry vision, deafness, tinnitus, and dizziness.
Diuretics (spironolactone)		
• Treat heart failure • Treat hypertension	• Inhibit the action of aldosterone on the distal tubules • Increase NaCl and water excretion while conserving potassium and hydrogen ions	• Medication is contraindicated in patients with hyperkalemia, Addison disease, and renal impairment. • Use with caution in patients with acid–base imbalance, metabolic acidosis, metabolic alkalosis, and respiratory acidosis. • Adverse effects include vasculitis, Stevens–Johnson syndrome, confusion, lethargy, headache, and dizziness.
Inotropic agents (digoxin)		
• Treat HLHS and atrioventricular canal defect	• Increase force and velocity of myocardial contraction • Inhibit the Na-K-ATPase membrane pump	• Medication is contraindicated in patients with bradycardia, cardiomyopathy, thyroid disease, and myocarditis. • Use with caution in patients with renal impairment, hepatic impairment, and patients with electrolyte imbalances such as hypercalcemia, hyperkalemia, hypocalcemia, hypokalemia, and hypomagnesemia. • Monitor for symptoms of digoxin toxicity, including nausea, vomiting, and neurologic changes. • Adverse effects include bradycardia, tachycardia, palpitations, and electrolyte imbalances.
Prostaglandin E1		
• Maintains or reopens the patency of the ductus arteriosus • Used in an infant suspected of having a ductal-dependent congenital cardiac defect and ductal-dependent pulmonary blood flow to prevent hypoxia and metabolic acidosis	• Relaxes the smooth muscle of the ductus arteriosus	• Medication is contraindicated in neonates with respiratory distress syndrome. • Use caution in long-term use as the medication can cause GI obstruction. • Adverse effects include apnea, fever, hypotension, and inhibition of platelets, causing excessive bleeding. • Medication can cause flushing.

ACE, angiotensin-converting enzyme; CHD, congenital heart defect; COX, cyclooxygenase; GFR, glomerular filtration rate; GI, gastrointestinal; HLHS, hypoplastic left heart syndrome; IV, intravenous; MAO, monoamine oxidase; MI, myocardial infarction; NaCl, sodium chloride; NEC, necrotizing enterocolitis; PDA, patent ductus arteriosus.

7 GASTROINTESTINAL SYSTEM

FETAL GASTROINTESTINAL SYSTEM

Fetal growth and development are determined by genetic and environmental factors. Maternal nutritional and metabolic factors influence fetal growth, body composition, and body weight via the placenta. To monitor growth in fetuses with suspected gastrointestinal (GI) anomalies:

- Consult with specialists.
- Determine the best delivery route.
- Perform frequent ultrasounds.
- Know possible premature delivery may be needed in case of severe growth restriction.

Postnatal Growth of Preterm Infants

- Preterm infants have greater nutritional needs to mimic intrauterine fetal development and to provide optimal growth.
- Preterm infants are often growth-restricted.
- An immature GI tract may impede absorption.
- Preterm infants have less efficient gastric emptying and slower intestinal transit.
- Gastric dysmotility usually manifests as increased residuals before feeds, abdominal distention, or constipation.
- The microbiome of a premature infant is dysbiotic. It is highly variable, low in diversity, and harbors potential pathogens. This places the infant at an increased risk of acute and chronic diseases and developmental abnormalities.
- Medical conditions in preterm infants may increase metabolic needs.
- Medical treatments, like corticosteroids, may impede growth.

ASSESSMENT OF GASTROINTESTINAL SYSTEM

Assessment of the GI system includes:

- Auscultation of the bowels: four quadrants
- Palpation: assessment for tenderness, soft, firm, or hard
- Abdominal girth: baseline girth versus distention
- Assess gastric contents: residuals: amount and color
- Monitor stools: frequency, color, and consistency

Abnormal Findings

Abnormal findings/signs of feeding intolerance consist of:

- Abdominal distention
- Abnormal gastric residuals
- Emesis ▶

Abnormal Findings (*continued*)

- Increased abdominal growth
- Visible bowel loops
- Absent bowel sounds

Residuals

Aspiration of Gastric Residuals

- Verifies feeding tube placement
- Prevents aspiration/pneumonia
- Indirect measure of intestinal function
- Influenced by infant position
- Increased in supine or left lateral
- Decreased in prone or right lateral
- Abnormal residuals greater than 2 mL/kg per feed and/or greater than 50% of feeding volume

Refeeding Versus Discarding Residuals

- Residuals are often discarded.
- Hydrochloric acid is lost. Intestinal bacteria may increase and lead to sepsis or necrotizing enterocolitis (NEC). Whenever possible, refeed residual.

Evaluation of Residuals

- Advance when infant appears to be tolerating feeds.
- When to hold feeds: cardiopulmonary instability, discoloration, frank blood in stool, residual volumes above 50% of the feed, and significant abdominal distension
- Acceptable: milk or partially digested milk, mucous, slightly bilious when initiating feeds, and small amount of blood streaks
- Unacceptable: bilious after feeds are already established and coffee grounds

Emesis

- Characterized by color (brown, clear, green/bilious, red/bloody, white, yellow) and consistency (mucousy, partially digested, watery)
- Acute management of emesis: intravenous (IV) hydration, nothing by mouth (NPO), and stomach decompression nasogastric tube/suction

Causes

- Abdominal distension (increased girth compared with the infant's baseline): may be firm to the touch, taut, or discolored
- Bilious
- Congenital obstructive lesions
- Gastroesophageal reflux (GER)
- Infant fails to pass stool longer than 24 hours.
- Infant appears unwell.

 POP QUIZ 7.1

A 32-week infant has a slightly distended abdomen, new-onset frequent bradycardia, and a residual of 15 mL out of feeding of 25 mL 3 hours ago. What should the nurse do next?

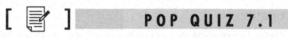 **NURSING PEARLS**

Aspiration and evaluation of gastric residuals are controversial in NICU. Some practitioners prefer to only aspirate residuals when signs of intolerance or necrotizing enterocolitis (NEC) are present.

 **POP QUIZ 7.2**

A 35-week infant presents with a firm distended abdomen and bilious emesis. What steps should the nurse immediately take?

Gastroesophageal Reflux

- Physiologic process secondary to frequent transient lower esophageal sphincter relaxation (TLESR), large-volume liquid diet, and age-specific body positioning; usually resolves with maturation
- Common signs of GER: apnea, desaturation, bradycardia clustered around feeding times, discomfort post feeds, feeding intolerance/aversion, frequent regurgitation, irritability, and poor weight gain
- Diagnosis usually made by clinical assessment of signs and symptoms and trial of nonpharmacologic or pharmacologic treatment rather than through definitive tests
- Pharmacologic agents to be used sparingly

Abdominal Distention

- Change in circumference
- Increase in abdominal size/girth from baseline
- Absence of bowel sounds
- Absence of stool in over 24 hours
- Dilated bowel loops
- Discoloration of the abdomen
- Firm abdomen

Diarrhea

- *Diarrhea* is defined by three or more watery or loose stools per day. The stools may contain mucous, blood, or be foul-smelling.
- Neonates with immediate postnatal diarrhea should be evaluated for anatomic abnormalities, congenital infection, and NEC.
- Causes can be bacterial, feeding intolerance/milk allergy, or viral.
- The skin should be protected from breakdown. See Chapter 11, Integumentary System.
- There is a risk of dehydration.

Rectal Bleeding

- Bleeding in the lower bowel/anus
- Treatment depending on the underlying cause
- Visual examination and imaging/endoscopy
- Anal fissure: bright red blood in stool, usually visible with examination, and can be painful; for treatment, soften stools
- More severe causes: Hirschsprung disease, intussusception, malrotation/volvulus, milk protein allergy, and NEC

Apnea/Bradycardia

- Infants with GI disorders are prone to apnea/bradycardia due to abdominal distention, GER, and pressure on the diaphragm.
- Supportive measures include decompression and respiratory support (can include intubation).
- Treat the underlying issue.

Poor Growth

- Infants may be dependent on total parenteral nutrition (TPN) or tube feedings.
- Infants with GI disorders are at risk of poor growth in utero and postnatally.

Signs Requiring Immediate Intervention

- Bilious vomiting
- Cardiopulmonary compromise ▶

Signs Requiring Immediate Intervention (*continued*)

- Frank blood in stool
- Marked abdominal distension
- Sudden severe/projectile vomiting

PATHOPHYSIOLOGY: GASTROINTESTINAL SYSTEM DISORDERS

There are various GI system disorders in the neonate, ranging from the esophagus to the rectum. Careful assessment and support are required until surgical intervention is possible.

OMPHALOCELE

- *Omphalocele* is central herniation of organs through the widened umbilical ring.
- Contents may include bladder, gonads, intestine, liver, and/or spleen.
- It is covered by a thin translucent membrane.
- It may lead to intrauterine growth restriction (IUGR).
- It is typically seen on prenatal ultrasound. Screen for other congenital anomalies.

Treatment

- Protect the exposed bowel by placing the infant's bowels in a bowel bag.
- Decompress the stomach with the orogastric tube.
- Perform surgery: delayed closure (utilize temporary silo, perform serial reduction of bowel contents).

NECROTIZING ENTEROCOLITIS

- NEC causes intestinal inflammation.
- Inflammation may lead to intestinal perforation and necrosis.

Signs and Symptoms

Physical findings include:

- Absence of bowel sounds
- Abdominal distension
- Bilious vomiting
- Bloody stools
- Bradycardia/apnea
- Erythema/edema of the abdominal wall
- Gastric retention
- Hypotension
- Hypothermia
- Ileus
- Visible/palpable loops of bowel

Treatment

- Antibiotics
- Gastric decompression
- IV fluids
- Withholding feeds ▶

Treatment (*continued*)

- Indications for surgery: air in the portal vein, bowel ischemia, clinical deterioration, and free peritoneal gas
- Increased risk of morbidity/mortality with necrosis

DIAPHRAGMATIC HERNIA

- Diaphragmatic hernia is hole in the diaphragm. Organ contents in the abdomen can move upwards into the infant's chest.
- It may prevent the lungs from developing completely, leading to respiratory difficulties.
- It is usually seen on ultrasound prenatally.
- It is confirmed by x-ray post birth.

Signs and Symptoms

- Abnormal chest development
- Concave abdomen
- Respiratory distress: cyanosis and tachypnea

Treatment

- Surgery is required.

MALROTATION AND VOLVULUS

- Anatomic abnormality allows the midgut to twist clockwise around the superior mesenteric vessels to obstruct or infarct the small and large intestines.
- Unless treated in a timely manner, bowel strangulation leads to loss of extensive bowel and short gut syndrome.
- Most midgut rotations develop volvulus within the first week of life.
- Bilious emesis is the first symptom.

Treatment

Surgical intervention is required.

- Bowel resection
- Ladd procedure
- Laparotomy

ESOPHAGEAL ATRESIA

Esophageal atresia is a birth defect of the esophagus connecting the mouth to the stomach. There are four types:

- Type A: The upper and lower parts of the esophagus do not connect and have closed ends.
- Type B: The upper part of the esophagus is attached to the trachea and the lower part has a closed end. This is very rare.
- Type C: The upper part of the esophagus has a closed end and the lower part is attached to the trachea. This is the most common type.
- Type D: The upper and lower parts are not connected to each other, but each part is connected separately to the trachea. This is the rarest and severe. ▶

ESOPHAGEAL ATRESIA (*continued*)

- It is diagnosed post birth when the neonate chokes or vomits, or when a nasogastric (NG) tube is unable to be passed down into the stomach.
- X-ray will confirm that the tube stops in the upper esophagus.
- Surgical intervention is necessary.

DUODENAL ATRESIA

- This is a congenital obstruction of the second portion of the duodenum.
- It is associated with polyhydramnios in pregnancy.
- Infants present with bilious vomiting and minimal abdominal distension.
- Diagnosis is confirmed with contrast radiography and laparoscopy.
- Management includes correcting electrolyte abnormalities, use of NG tube, and withholding feeds.

Treatment

- Surgery is required.

JEJUNOILEAL ATRESIA

- There are four types: apple-peel, interrupted, membranous, and multiple.
- The symptoms are identical regardless of the type of lesion.
- Infant presents with abdominal distension and bilious vomiting in the first 24 hours of life.
- Management includes stomach decompression, IV fluids, and correcting electrolyte disturbances.

Treatment

- Surgery is required.

MECONIUM ILEUS

- Large amount of meconium with swallowed air and "ground-glass sign" on x-ray
- Retention of thick, tenacious meconium in the bowel during fetal life
- Often seen in infants with cystic fibrosis

Signs and Symptoms

- Bilious emesis
- Bowel distension from swallowed air postnatally
- Results in bowel obstruction
- Thickened bowel loops

Treatment

- Uncomplicated meconium ileus: can be successfully treated with gastrografin enema with IV fluids or laparotomy if enema is not successful
- Complicated meconium ileus: requires bowel resection for perforation or obstruction related to kinking of the bowel
- Immediate surgery
- Temporary enterostomy

[📝]   **POP QUIZ 7.3**

A 36-week infant presents with consistent bilious emesis; an x-ray is obtained and shows a classic "double bubble" sign. Which disorder could this finding indicate?

HIRSCHSPRUNG DISEASE

- Congenital condition consisting of missing nerve cells (ganglions) in the muscles of the colon

Signs and Symptoms

- Backed-up stool
- Bowel obstruction
- Inability to pass meconium
- Ineffective peristalsis
- Abdominal distension
- Delayed passage of meconium
- Hirschsprung-associated enterocolitis
- Sepsis
- Toxic megacolon
- Poor weight gain/slow growth
- Vomiting

Diagnosis

- Suction biopsy of rectum
- X-ray/contrast enema

Treatment

Surgery is required.
- "Pull through" procedure
- Temporary colostomy

ANORECTAL MALFORMATIONS

- *Anorectal malformations* are birth defects in the anus or rectum that affect the normal passage of stool.
- Complications include perforation and sepsis.
- Malformations include abnormal passage between the rectum and the perineum, urethra, bladder, or vagina; fistula; and imperforate anus (complete blockage).

Signs and Symptoms

- Anal opening outside of normal location
- Anus that is tighter or more narrow than normal
- No visible anus
- Bloating
- Intestinal obstruction
- Vomiting

Treatment

Surgery is required.
- Temporary colostomy

PYLORIC STENOSIS

- *Pyloric stenosis* is defined by thickening or swelling of the pylorus. Pylorus is the muscle between the stomach and the intestines. ▶

PYLORIC STENOSIS (*continued*)

- Enlargement of the pylorus causes stenosis of the opening from the stomach to the intestines and blocks stomach contents from moving into the intestine.
- It causes severe and forceful vomiting: nonbilious, projectile, and may result in dehydration.
- Palpation may reveal a mass in the upper central abdominal region. The enlarged pylorus is referred to as the "olive."
- Diagnosis is made with ultrasound and upper GI series.
- Administer IV fluids.

Treatment

- Surgical repair: pyloromyotomy

GASTROSCHISIS

- Abdominal wall defect with protrusion of bowel/herniation
- No covering membrane
- Right of the umbilicus
- Possible matted surface
- Diagnosed prenatally on ultrasound
- Decompress stomach
- IV fluids

Treatment

- Protect the bowel: Place in bowel bag. Monitor perfusion. Apply warm saline-soaked gauze to the herniated viscera.
- Monitor for evaporative fluid loss.
- Surgical repair is necessary.

DIAGNOSTIC PROCEDURES

X-Rays

- Chest (if esophageal pathologies are suspected)
- Frontal view
- Left lateral decubitus/cross-table lateral view if perforation, ischemia, or obstruction is suspected to evaluate for free air or portal venous gas
- Prone view to evaluate for rectal gas
- Upper GI to evaluate the esophagus, stomach, and proximal small bowel; barium contrast introduced by bottle (swallow study) or via NG tube; x-rays taken while the barium is swallowed; if an upper GI with small bowel follow-through is ordered, x-rays to be taken every 30 minutes as the barium travels all the way through the small intestine

Orogastric Tube Placement

- Prior to insertion, measure the tube from the tip of the nose to the earlobe, to the midpoint between the xiphoid process and the umbilicus. Confirm placement with auscultation of air and aspiration of fluid.
- Tube is used for aspiration, suction, decompression, or gravity drainage.

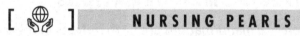

[🌐]   **NURSING PEARLS**

If respiratory support is needed, avoid nasal continuous positive airway pressure (CPAP) or high-flow oxygen (in order to prevent filling the intestine with air). Intubate with an endotracheal tube if necessary.

Ultrasound

- Hypertrophic pyloric stenosis; typically diagnosed by ultrasound
- Limited role in depicting GI pathology
- Pneumatosis intestinalis: small echogenic dots
- Volvulus: may show twisting of mesenterial vessels

COMMON PROCEDURES

Surgical

- Laparotomy: bowel resection, ostomy, and reanastomosis
- Primary percutaneous peritoneal drainage: incision in the right lower quadrant, irrigated with warm saline; performed at the bedside
- Pyloromyotomy: leaves the mucosa intact and separates the muscle fibers; treatment for hypertrophic pyloric stenosis

RESOURCES

Bielicki, I. N., Somme, S., Frongia, G., Holland-Cunz, S. G., & Vuille-Dit-Bille, R. N. (2021). Abdominal wall defects-current treatments. *Children (Basel, Switzerland)*, *8*(2), 170. https://doi.org/10.3390/children8020170

Eichenwald, E. C., Cummings, J. J., Aucott, S. W., Goldsmith, J. P., Hand, I. L., Juul, S. E., Poindexter, B. B., Puopolo, K. M., & Stewart, D. L. (2018). Diagnosis and management of gastroesophageal reflux in preterm infants. *Pediatrics, 142* (1), e20181061. https://doi.org/10.1542/peds.2018-1061

Kimura, K., & Loening-Baucke, V. (2000). Bilious vomiting in the newborn: Rapid diagnosis of intestinal obstruction. *American Family Physician. 61*(9), 2791–8. PMID: 10821158.

Ngo, A. V., Stanescu, A. L., & Phillips, G. S. (2018). "Neonatal bowel disorders: Practical imaging algorithm for trainees and general radiologists." *American Journal of Roentgenology*, *210*(5), 976–988., https://doi.org/10.2214/ajr.17.19378

Rysavy, M. A., Watkins, P. L., Colaizy, T. T. & Das, A. (2020). Is routine evaluation of gastric residuals for premature infants safe or effective? *Journal of Perinatology*, *40*(3), 540–543. https://doi.org/10.1038/s41372-019-0582-8

Sakala, M. D., Oliphant, M., & Anthony, E. Y. (2018). "Bright red rectal bleeding: The bottom line from neonates to older adults." *RadioGraphics*, *36*(5), 1600–1601. https://doi.org/10.1148/rg.2016160063.pres

Thiagarajah, J. R., Kamin, D. S., Acra, S., Goldsmith, J. D., Roland, J. T., Lencer, W. I., Muise, A. M., Goldenring, J. R., Avitzur, Y., Martín, M. G., & PediCODE Consortium (2018). Advances in evaluation of chronic diarrhea in infants. *Gastroenterology*, *154*(8), 2045–2059.e6. https://doi.org/10.1053/j.gastro.2018.03.067

Westaway, J. A., Huerlimann, R., Miller, C. M., Kandasamy, Y., Norton, R., & Rudd, D. (2021). Methods for exploring the faecal microbiome of premature infants: A review. *Maternal Health, Neonatology and Perinatology*, *7*(1). https://doi.org/10.1186/s40748-021-00131-9

Wood, R. J., & Levitt, M. A. (2018). "Anorectal malformations." *Clinics in Colon and Rectal Surgery*, *31*(02), 061–070. https://doi.org/10.1055/s-0037-1609020.

APPENDIX 7.1 MEDICATIONS FOR GASTROINTESTINAL DISORDERS

INDICATIONS	MECHANISM OF ACTION	CONTRAINDICATIONS, PRECAUTIONS, AND ADVERSE EFFECTS
Prokinetic agents (metoclopramide, domperidone, erythromycin)		
• Reduced GER symptoms	• Improved gastric emptying, reduced regurgitation, and enhanced LES tone	• These medications have not been shown to reduce GER symptoms in preterm infants. • They have the potential for higher risk of pyloric stenosis, cardiac arrhythmia, and neurologic side effects.
Sodium alginate (alginic acid)		
• Reduced GER symptoms with alginate-containing formulations combined with sodium bicarbonate • Reduced frequency of acidic GER episodes, with total esophageal acid exposure and decreased regurgitation	• Alginate formulations which precipitate into a low-density viscous gel, which acts as a physical barrier to the gastric mucosa • Combined with sodium bicarbonate, a carbon dioxide foam forms and protects the lower esophagus from acidification	• Long-term safety in preterm infants has not been evaluated.
Histamine-2 receptor blockers (ranitidine, famotidine)		
• Prescribed in infants with clinically diagnosed GER with symptoms secondary to acid reflux in the lower esophagus	• Compete with histamine for the H2 receptor in the parietal cells in the stomach, decreasing hydrochloric acid secretion and increasing intragastric pH	• Research has not assessed the efficacy of H2 blockers on the symptom profile of preterm infants with presumed reflux. • H2 receptor blockers have been linked to increased incidence of necrotizing enterocolitis, late-onset infections, and death in preterm infants.
PPIs (lansoprazole, omeprazole)		
• Prescribed in infants with clinically diagnosed GER with symptoms secondary to acid reflux in the lower esophagus	• Block the gastric proton pump, decreasing basal and stimulated parietal cell acid secretion	• PPIs in older children have been associated with a higher risk of gastric bacterial overgrowth, gastroenteritis, and community-acquired pneumonia. • PPIs are considered largely ineffective in relieving clinical signs of GER in preterm infants.

GER, gastroesophageal reflux; LES, lower esophageal sphincter; PPI, proton pump inhibitors.

8 RENAL/GENITOURINARY SYSTEM

DEVELOPMENT OF THE RENAL/GENITOURINARY SYSTEM

Overview

- The urinary system begins forming during the fourth week of gestation.
- The functioning adult kidney, the metanephros, begins to form in the sacral region in the fifth week, becomes fully functional around the 11th week, and is fully formed at 32 weeks.
- The kidneys separate and ascend between 6 and 9 weeks. The bladder begins development from weeks 4 to 7.
- By day 10, all fetuses have undifferentiated gonads.
- Gonads develop into either testes or ovaries, depending on the possession of an XX or XY chromosome.

Male

- By weeks 8 to 10, the gonads start to differentiate.
- Testosterone begins to secrete and the urogenital sinus and external genitalia form into the penis and scrotum by weeks 9 to 12.
- The mesonephric ducts differentiate into the epididymis, vas deferens, ejaculatory duct, and seminal vesicles.
- Descent of the testes occurs due to intra-abdominal pressure causing the migration through the abdominal wall via the inguinal canal at 28 weeks' gestation. The scrotum is reached by week 33.

Female

- The absence of anti-mullerian hormone (AMH) and estrogen influences the formation of fallopian tubes and the upper third of the vagina, cervix, and uterus. This process is completed by the end of week 12.
- Estrogen is also essential for the development of the clitoris, labia, and lower vagina.

PHYSIOLOGY OF THE RENAL/GENITOURINARY SYSTEM

Overview

- The renal system is also referred to as the genitourinary system. It rids waste from the body and manages the homeostasis of the body. It controls blood pressure and the fluid balance in the body.
- Components of the urinary system include the kidneys, ureters, bladder, and urethra.
- The main functions of the kidney are filtration, reabsorption, and secretion.
- The renin–angiotensin system supports blood pressure, electrolytes, and circulating blood volume.
- The loop of Henle manages the pressure difference that moves fluids and molecules (electrolytes) across a membrane.
- The bladder temporarily retains urine, which then passes through the urethra.

GLOMERULAR FILTRATION RATE

- Glomerular filtration rate (GFR) is usually low at birth. It develops rapidly and doubles in the first 2 weeks of life.
- GFR is about 20 mL/min/1.73 m² in term neonates. It is lower in premature infants and varies on gestational age.
- Estimated GFR (eGFR) = k × Ht/SCr, where k = 0.33 for preterm and k = 0.45 for term infants.
- Creatinine levels are used to calculate GFR along with race, sex, and age.

ALERT!

Neonates born small for gestational age (SGA) have a 16.2% reduction in drug clearance, observed from birth to 4 weeks old.

TUBULAR FUNCTION

- It is dependent on gestational age and postnatal age.
- It maintains fluid balance regulation.
- The kidneys regulate water and solute homeostasis through the processes of filtration, reabsorption, secretion, and excretion.
- Blood filters through the glomeruli and adjusts urine composition throughout the nephron.
- The primary segments of the tubular system include collecting ducts, distal convoluted tubule, loop of Henle, and proximal tube.

PROXIMAL TUBULAR FUNCTION

- It reabsorbs all the filtered glucose and amino acids, most of the filtered phosphates, 80% filtered bicarbonate, and two-thirds of filtered chloride.
- It is responsible for bulk reclamation of the glomerular filtrate.
- The rate of volume absorption by proximal tubular transport is dependent on the combined rate of transport of the individual solutes absorbed.

Sodium

- Normal sodium levels are 130 to 140 mEq/L.
- Sodium and water are reabsorbed at the same rate.
- Sodium exchange occurs in the distal tubule.

Potassium

- It is filtered at the glomerulus and reabsorbed in the proximal tubules.
- Normal potassium levels are 4.1 to 5.3 mmol/L.

Acid–Base Balance

- Regulation of acid–base balance improves with gestational age.
- Preterm neonates frequently present with mild to moderate normal anion gap acidosis, which is the consequence of the low renal bicarbonate threshold of the premature kidney.
- The renal system affects pH by reabsorbing bicarbonate and excreting fixed acids that are either reabsorbed or excreted.
- Imbalances may lead to metabolic acidosis, respiratory acidosis, or respiratory alkalosis.

Normal Acid–Base Values in Neonates
- pH: 7.35 to 7.45
- Bicarbonate (HCO_3): 22 to 26
- Partial pressure of carbon dioxide ($PaCO_2$): 35 to 45
- Base excess: −10 to −2

Uric Acid

- Uric acid is transported to the kidneys through blood and excreted in the urine.
- Increased uric acid may cause urate crystals to form and cause a pink, orangey red color to form in the infant's diaper, commonly called brick dust.
- This can cause concern for parents while changing the infant's diaper as it may be mistaken for blood.
- Uric acid accumulation can lead to kidney stones.
- Normal uric acid levels are 2 to 6.2 mg/dL.

ASSESSMENT OF RENAL/GENITOURINARY SYSTEM HISTORY

Overview

- Family history may lead to an underlying renal genetic disorder or congenital anomaly.
- Oligohydramnios, a decreased amount of amniotic fluid, may lead to pulmonary hypoplasia, bilateral renal agenesis, polycystic kidney disease, or urethral obstruction.
- Polyhydramnios, an excessive accumulation of amniotic fluid, may indicate fetal anemia, blood incompatibilities between the mother and the infant, infection, or possible birth defects of the infant's central nervous system (CNS) or gastrointestinal (GI) tract.
- Hypoxic ischemic encephalopathy may lead to acute kidney injury (AKI).

Physical Assessment

Clinical findings suggestive of renal/genitourinary disease include:
- Dysmorphic features: abnormal ears, hypospadias, single umbilical artery, anorectal abnormalities, and vertebral anomalies
- Abdominal mass: polycystic kidneys, hydronephrosis, and tumor
- Ascites: rupture of obstructed urinary tract
- Suprapubic mass: enlarged bladder due to urethral obstruction
- Abdominal wall defects: "prune belly"
- Failure to palpate kidney: renal agenesis, and renal malposition
- Hypertension: due to renal disease
- Anuria/oliguria
- Fluid overload
- Cardiac dysrhythmias
- Hematuria

PATHOPHYSIOLOGY: RENAL/GENITOURINARY SYSTEM DISORDERS

Overview

- Renal/genitourinary system disorders that affect the kidney(s) or urinary tract include congenital or acquired disorders.
- Congenital disorders include hydrocele, hydronephrosis, hypospadias, epispadias, neurogenic bladder, and rectourethral fistulas. ▶

Overview (*continued*)

■ Acquired disorders may develop due to congenital disorders or may be acquired after both, including AKI, end-stage renal disease, hypertension, inguinal hernia, testicular torsion, and renal vein thrombosis (RVT).

ACUTE KIDNEY INJURY

■ *AKI* is an abrupt reduction in kidney function measured by a rapid decline in GFR.
■ AKI results in impairment of nitrogenous waste product excretion, loss of water and electrolyte regulation, and loss of acid–base regulation.
■ Certain medications can be nephrotoxic, such as vancomycin, indomethacin, ibuprofen, and aminoglycosides. Trough levels, serum creatinine, and urine output should be closely monitored.
■ Anuric AKI: The kidneys stop producing urine.
■ Oliguric AKI: There is low output of urine.
■ Nonoliguric AKI: Urine is still produced but GFR begins to be affected and there is less clearance in the tubules.
■ Neonates are more susceptible due to immature renal function, limited urine concentrating ability, and increased risk of hypovolemia due to large insensible water losses.
■ Maintain fluid and electrolyte balance and treat the underlying cause.

Treatment

Supportive management includes:
■ Replacing insensible fluid loss
■ Maintaining nutrition
■ Correcting electrolyte imbalances
■ Diuretics

END-STAGE RENAL DISEASE

■ Common causes include congenital abnormalities of the kidneys and urinary tract.
■ Chronic kidney injury can lead to decreased erythropoietin production and subsequent anemia.
■ Treatment includes adequate nutrition, hemodialysis, and renal transplant.
■ Palliative care may be offered.

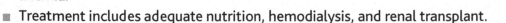

[📝]   POP QUIZ 8.1

An 8-day-old infant with acute kidney injury is experiencing acute hyperkalemia. What would the nurse anticipate administering to help with potassium excretion?

HYDROCELE

■ Collection of fluid that accumulates around the testicle. It is more likely to occur on the right testicle than on the left.
■ It is often present at birth and usually painless.
■ Physical examination reveals enlargement of the scrotum; it may transilluminate due to its cystic structure.
■ It usually resolves between 12 and 24 months of age.

HYDRONEPHROSIS

- Swelling of the kidney due to buildup of urine
- Commonly diagnosed on antenatal ultrasound; may be a benign condition or associated with congenital anomalies of the kidney
- Ultrasound postnatally with possible voiding cystourethrogram (VCUG)

Signs and Symptoms

- Fever
- Flank pain
- Increased frequency of urine
- Nausea
- May be asymptomatic

Treatment

- Antibiotic prophylaxis for prevention of urinary tract infection (UTI)
- Mild to moderate: monitoring and follow up
- Severe: antibiotics and possible surgery

HYPERTENSION

- It occurs when persistent systolic or diastolic blood pressure exceeds 95% for postconceptional age.
- It may be found in patients with renal artery stenosis and renal parenchymal disease.
- Diagnosis includes three or more elevated blood pressure (BP) measurements over a 6- to 12-hour period, assessment, laboratory testing, and ultrasound.

Risk Factors

- AKI
- Bronchopulmonary dysplasia (BPD)
- Cardiac disease
- Low birth weight
- Polycystic kidney disease
- Prematurity
- Umbilical artery catheters: thrombosis

Signs and Symptoms

- Apnea
- Failure to thrive
- Feeding difficulties
- Heart failure
- Irritability or lethargy
- Tachypnea

HYPOSPADIAS

- It is a condition where the opening of the urethra is positioned on the underside of the penis.
- It occurs most commonly within the head of the penis but may be located in the middle or the base of the penis as well. ▶

HYPOSPADIAS (*continued*)

- It may cause a downward curve of the penis (chordee).
- It may cause abnormal spraying during urination.
- Surgery restores the appearance and allows for normal urination and reproduction.

EPISPADIAS

- It is the condition when the urethra does not fully develop. Meatus is on top of the penis rather than at the tip.
- Penis may be short, wide, and curved up (dorsal chordee).
- The closer the meatus is to the base of the penis, the more likely the condition may affect the bladder sphincter and urine control.
- Surgery restores the appearance and allows for good urine control and future fertility.

INGUINAL HERNIA

- It occurs when the intestines herniate into a patent processus vaginalis.
- The incidence is higher in premature and low-birthweight infants.
- Occurrence is three to four times more likely in males than females.
- Family history of hernia, prematurity, and undescended testicle are associated with inguinal hernias.
- Infants may experience a painful bulging in the groin area especially with straining and crying.
- Surgical repair is recommended.

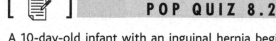

POP QUIZ 8.2

A 10-day-old infant with an inguinal hernia begins vomiting, has a high-pitched cry, and is unable to be consoled. Upon examination, the infant has redness and bruising around the bulge. What would the nurse expect has happened?

INTRINSIC RENAL PARENCHYMAL ABNORMALITIES

Overview

Renal parenchymal disease includes conditions that damage parts of the kidney, such as:

- Autoimmune diseases, like lupus nephritis or purpura
- Bacterial and viral infections
- Diabetes
- High blood pressure
- Kidney stones
- Polycystic kidneys

Signs and Symptoms

- Abdominal swelling
- Anemia
- Blood in the urine
- Edema: hands, feet, and eyes
- Fatigue
- Hypertension
- Itching
- Nausea and vomiting

Treatment

- Depends on the underlying cause

NEPHROCALCINOSIS

- *Nephrocalcinosis* refers to calcium salt deposition in the renal parenchyma.
- It is diagnosed by ultrasound, laboratory evaluation, and urinalysis.
- Infants are typically asymptomatic.

Risk Factors

- Administration of medications (loop diuretics)
- Bartter syndrome
- Hypercalcemia
- Hypercalciuria
- Neonatal primary hyperparathyroidism
- Renal tubular immaturity
- Subcutaneous fat necrosis
- Supplements that promote calcium salt deposition (calcium, vitamin D)
- Williams syndrome

NEPHROLITHIASIS

- *Nephrolithiasis* is also called "kidney stones."
- It is diagnosed by CT scan, laboratory evaluation, urine culture, and 24-hour urine.

Risks Factors

- Cystinuria
- Family history
- Hypercalciuria
- Hyperuricosuria
- Renal dysfunction

Signs and Symptoms

Although rare in neonates, symptoms may include:

- Decreased urine output
- Fever
- Pain/crying

NEUROGENIC BLADDER

- May cause neurospinal dysraphism
- Difficulty holding or releasing urine caused by nerve damage
- Occurs with spina bifida, open back lesion, and CNS tumor
- Diagnosed via ultrasound, urinalysis, and urodynamic study

Signs and Symptoms

- UTI
- Swollen kidneys
- Thickened bladder wall

Treatment

- Timed voiding catheter
- Surgery: artificial sphincter

RECTOURETHRAL FISTULAS

- A *rectourethral fistula* is an abnormal connection of the urethra to the anus or rectum.
- Diagnosis includes assessment for a patent anus and MRI.

Signs and Symptoms

- Not passing feces 1 to 2 days post birth
- Solid waste and urine empty through the urethra
- Swollen abdomen
- Repeated UTI

Treatment

- Temporary colostomy
- Surgical repair of fistula

RENAL VEIN THROMBOSIS

- RVT is characterized by reduced renal blood flow, hyperosmolality, hypercoagulability, and increased blood viscosity.
- Diagnosis includes RVT imaging, such as Doppler ultrasound, and coagulation studies.

Risk Factors

- Congenital heart disease
- Dehydration
- Inherited thrombophilia
- Perinatal asphyxia
- Prematurity
- Respiratory distress syndrome
- Sepsis
- Shock

Signs and Symptoms

- Flank mass
- Hematuria
- Hypertension/chronic kidney disease due to thrombosis
- Thrombocytopenia

Treatment

- Correction of fluid disturbances
- Heparin
- Anticoagulation therapy
- Treatment of underlying pathophysiologic abnormalities

TESTICULAR TORSION

- *Testicular torsion* occurs when a loose testicle twists around the spermatic cord cutting off blood flow to the testicle.
- There might be a medical emergency if blood supply is cut off. Testis may atrophy.
- Diagnosis includes assessment. One testis may not drop into the scrotum, may twist before birth, and shrink in size. An ultrasound or nuclear scan must be done to confirm.
- Treatment is usually futile if testicular torsion occurs prenatally. If it happens postnatally, surgery can help if it is within a few hours, or to prevent the other testicle from twisting.

Signs and Symptoms

- Firm or red testicle
- "Missing" testicle
- Tenderness

WILMS TUMOR

- Most common pediatric solid renal tumor
- Neuroblastoma
- Rare in neonates

MESOBLASTIC NEPHROMA

- Presents with a palpable abdominal mass
- Usually identified in the first 3 months of life
- Typically benign
- Treated by nephrectomy

URINARY TRACT INFECTION

- *UTI* is associated with bacteremia and congenital anomalies of the kidney and urinary tract.
- Evaluate for systemic infection or anatomic/functional abnormalities.
- Diagnosis includes urinalysis, urine culture, and radiographic evaluation.
- Treatment includes antibiotics.

Signs and Symptoms

- Apnea and bradycardia (premature infants)
- Fever
- Jaundice
- Lethargy
- Poor weight gain
- Vomiting/loose stools

DIAGNOSTIC PROCEDURES

Laboratory Data

- GFR: determines specific kidney injury or efficacy of kidney filtration
- Creatinine levels: compare serum creatinine with the amount of creatinine cleared by kidneys ▶

Laboratory Data (*continued*)

- Blood urea nitrogen (BUN): monitor kidney function
- Complete blood count: infection/inflammation or anemia
- Comprehensive metabolic panel: liver function and electrolyte balance

Urinalysis

- Bag urine
- Clean-catch urine
- Suprapubic bladder puncture
- First void of the morning is most suitable for testing. Attempt to collect at the same time of day so findings are comparable.
- Do not keep urine before testing for longer than 1 to 2 hours at room temperature or 4 hours refrigerated to prevent increase in bacterial count or pH.

URINALYSIS RESULTS

- Bilirubinuria: presence of bilirubin in urine
- Glucosuria: glucose in the urine
- Hematuria: presence of blood in the urine
- Ketonuria: presence of ketones in the urine
- Leukocytes: may indicate presence of UTI
- Nitrates: may indicate presence of UTI
- pH: measures acidity or basicity of the urine
- Proteinuria: presence of protein (albumin) in urine
- Specific gravity: estimate of urine concentration
- Urobilinogen: formed by reduction of bilirubin

Serum Creatinine Concentration

- Creatinine levels and GFR are inversely related.
- High creatinine levels are indicative of a poorly functioning kidney.
- Normal value is 0.1 to 1 mg/dL.
- Levels undergo a rapid decline from birth through the first year.

Imaging Studies

- CT scan: provides a panoramic image of the kidney and urinary tract
- MRI: useful in detecting renal artery stenosis and RVT
- Ultrasonography: provides useful images of the genitourinary structures without radiation exposure; full bladder helps provide better images
- VCUG: radiopaque liquid placed in the bladder through a catheter, with images taken before, during, and after voiding
- X-ray: monitors the position and growth of kidney stones

COMMON PROCEDURES

Hemodialysis

- Blood is filtered by a dialyzer via a cannula (usually an atrioventricular [AV] fistula).
- Central venous catheter placements are preferred.
- It may cause rapid shifts in intravascular and third space volume and can possibly result in hypovolemia and shock. ▶

Hemodialysis (*continued*)

- It may cause difficulty balancing due to circuit volume versus the infant's circulating blood volume.
- It is used in situations that require urgent correction or failure of peritoneal dialysis.

Continuous Renal Replacement Therapy

- It may achieve continuous ultrafiltration and solute clearance with fewer hemodynamic changes.
- It is useful in removing inflammatory mediators, like cytokines and chemokines.
- It is typically used after sepsis or necrotizing enterocolitis, or inborn errors of metabolism.
- Early initiation and prevention of fluid overload results in better treatment outcomes.

Peritoneal Dialysis

- Dialysate fluid flows through a catheter in the abdomen and eliminates waste products from the blood.
- It is preferred for neonates for ease of use and fewer complications, although infants may experience peritonitis, an inflammation of the peritoneum.
- It provides more gradual, steady, and predictable clearance.
- It is less efficient in removing free water and ammonia.
- The most common indication for peritoneal dialysis is oliguric AKI.

Nurses' Role in Dialysis

- Catheter care and dressing changes
- Close monitoring of volume and BP control
- Communicating with dialysis nurse and nephrologist
- Administering prescribed medications
- Obtaining vital signs (VS) and drawing any required bloodwork
- If not certified in dialysis, have basic knowledge of dialyzer, cannulating access, and signs and symptoms of adverse reactions

[🧠]   **COMPLICATIONS**

Peritoneal dialysis (PD) cannot effectively manage cases involving severe fluid overload. Complications of PD may include catheter-related leakage at insertion sites and infection of the peritoneal cavity. Terminate PD temporarily in the event of infection.

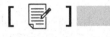

[📝]   **POP QUIZ 8.3**

An infant is receiving peritoneal dialysis. After a session, the infant has a temperature of 102.8°F (39.3°C), is irritable, and appears to be in pain. The nurse notes that the peritoneal fluid was cloudy. The nurse alerts the physician. The fluid is cultured and is gram-positive, and the white blood cell count is 120/mm. Which complication is suspected and what should the next action be?

RESOURCES

Basalely, A., Liu, D., & Kaskel, F. J. (2020). Big equation for small kidneys: A newly proposed model to estimate neonatal GFR. *Pediatric Nephrology*. 35(4), 543–546. https://doi.org/10.1007/s00467-019-04465-7

Burke, A. B. (2021). *Genitourinary Systems*. RegisteredNursing.org. Retrieved May 1, 2022, from https://www.registerednursing.org/teas/genitourinary-system

Das, C. J., Razik, A., & Sharma, S. (2020). Hemodialysis in infants: Challenges and new paradigms. *Journal of Vascular and Interventional Radiology*, 31(5), 787. https://doi.org/10.1016/j.jvir.2020.02.011

Dionne, J. M., Bremner, S. A., Baygani, S. K., Batton, B., Ergenekon, E., Bhatt-Mehta, V., Dempsey, E., Kluckow, M., Pesco Koplowitz, L., Apele-Freimane, D., Iwami, H., Klein, A., Turner, M., & Rabe, H. (2020). Method of blood pressure measurement in neonates and infants: A systematic review and analysis. *The Journal of Pediatrics*, 221. https://doi.org/10.1016/j.jpeds.2020.02.072

Gattineni, J., & Baum, M. (2015). Developmental changes in renal tubular transport—an overview. *Pediatric Nephrology*, 30, 2085–2098. https://doi.org/10.1007/s00467-013-2666-6

Knobel, R. B., & Smith, J. M. (2013). Laboratory blood tests useful in monitoring renal function in neonates. *Neonatal Network*, *33*(1), 35–40. https://doi.org/10.1891/0730-0832.33.1.35

Lowe, L. H., Isuani, B. H., Heller, R. M., Stein, S. M., Johnson, J. E., Navarro, O. M., & Hernanz-Schulman, M. (2000). Pediatric renal masses: Wilms tumor and beyond. *RadioGraphics*, *20*(6), 1585–1603. https://doi.org/10.1148/radiographics.20.6.g00nv051585

Moudgil, A. (2014). Renal venous thrombosis in neonates. *Current Pediatric Reviews, 10*(2), 101–6. https://doi.org/10.2174/157339631002140513101845. PMID: 25088263.

Muhari-Stark, E., & Burckart, G. J. (2018). Glomerular filtration rate estimation formulas for pediatric and neonatal use. *The Journal of Pediatric Pharmacology and Therapeutics : JPPT : The Official Journal of PPAG*, *23*(6), 424–431. https://doi.org/10.5863/1551-6776-23.6.424

Sajjad, Y. (2010). Development of the genital ducts and external genitalia in the early human embryo. *Journal of Obstetrics and Gynaecology Research*. *36*(5), 929–37. https://doi.org/10.1111/j.1447-0756.2010.01272.x. Epub 2010 Sep 16. PMID: 20846260.

Sulemanji, M., & Vakili, K. (2013). Neonatal renal physiology. *Seminars in Pediatric Surgery*, *22*(4), 195–8. https://doi.org/10.1053/j.sempedsurg.2013.10.008. Epub 2013 Oct 15. PMID: 24331094.

Utsch, B., & Klaus, G. (2014). Urinalysis in children and adolescents. *Deutsches Arzteblatt International*, *111*(37), 617–626. https://doi.org/10.3238/arztebl.2014.0617

Viteri, B., Calle-Toro, J. S., Furth, S., Darge, K., Hartung, E. A., & Otero, H. (2020). State-of-the-art renal imaging in children. *Pediatrics*. *145*(2), e20190829

Walker, K. A., Sims-Lucas, S., & Bates, C. M. Fibroblast growth factor receptor signaling in kidney and lower urinary tract development. *Pediatric Nephrology*. 31, 885–895 (2016). https://doi.org/10.1007/s00467-015-3151-1

APPENDIX 8.1 MEDICATIONS FOR THE RENAL/GENITOURINARY SYSTEM

INDICATIONS	MECHANISM OF ACTION	CONTRAINDICATIONS, PRECAUTIONS, AND ADVERSE EFFECTS
Loop diuretics (furosemide)		
• Volume management, kidney disease, and edema	• Inhibit sodium–potassium–chloride cotransporter in the ascending loop of Henle	• It may result in anuria and severe states of electrolyte depletion.
Adrenergic (dopamine)		
• Improves blood flow to the kidneys, improves pumping strength of the heart	• Produces positive chronotropic and inotropic effects on the myocardium, results in increased heart and cardiac contractility	• It may result in tumors of the adrenal gland and metabolic acidosis.
Erythropoiesis-stimulating agent (erythropoietin)		
• Treats anemia	• Binds to erythropoietin receptor and activates intracellular signal transduction pathway	• It may result in changes in blood pressure and probability of seizures.
Antibiotics (ampicillin, gentamicin)		
• Treat infection or prophylaxis	• Target bacterial cell wall	• Renal disease may interfere with metabolism.
Antihypertensives (angiotensin-converting enzyme inhibitors, calcium channel blockers)		
• Relax blood vessels, prevent calcium from entering the cells of vessel walls	• Inhibit angiotensin-converting enzyme vasodilation	• It may cause volume depletion; special caution with abnormal renal function.

9 NERVOUS SYSTEM

DEVELOPMENT OF THE NERVOUS SYSTEM

Overview

- *Neurulation* is the process of neural tube formation and occurs at 3 to 4 weeks' gestation.
- The embryo has three main layers: ectoderm, mesoderm, and endoderm.

FORMATION OF THE SPINAL CORD

There are four stages of development of the spinal cord:
- Neural plate: Neural plate forms from elongation of the ectoderm.
- Neural fold: Neural plate begins to bend, creating a neural groove and neural folds.
- Neural tube: Neural folds fuse together creating the neural tube.
- Spinal cord: Spinal cord arises from the neural tube.

SEGMENTATION

- *Segmentation* refers to the division of the brain into the right and left cerebral hemispheres, diencephalon, brainstem, and cerebellum.
- Disruptions during segmentation can result in holoprosencephaly, a disorder characterized by the forebrain failing to develop.

MIGRATION AND CORTICAL ORGANIZATION

- Migration and cortical organization refer to the remaining development of the brain, including cellular proliferation, myelination, gyration, and sulcation.

PHYSIOLOGY OF THE NERVOUS SYSTEM

Overview

- The nervous system consists of the central nervous system (CNS) and the peripheral nervous system (PNS).
- The CNS consists of the brain and spinal cord and acts as the integrating and command center of the nervous system.
- The PNS consists of the nerves that extend from the CNS.

BRAIN

The brain is divided into four major regions:

- Cerebral hemispheres
- Diencephalon
- Brainstem
- Cerebellum

Cerebral Hemispheres

The paired cerebral hemispheres are collectively called the cerebrum; the two hemispheres are connected by the corpus callosum. There are four lobes within the cerebrum: parietal, frontal, occipital, and temporal.

- Parietal lobe: sensory area
- Frontal lobe: motor area
- Occipital lobe: visual area
- Temporal lobe: auditory and olfactory areas

Additional Brain Anatomy

- The thalamus and hypothalamus are located within the diencephalon.
- The brainstem has three main structures: the midbrain, pons, and medulla oblongata.
- The cerebellum controls muscle activity, balance, and equilibrium.

Peripheral Nervous System

- The PNS consists of both spinal and cranial nerves (CNs).
- Spinal nerves are considered efferent or afferent.
- Efferent nerves, or motor nerves, send impulses from the CNS to the limbs and organs.
- Afferent nerves, or sensory nerves, receive information from sensory organs and carry these impulses toward the CNS.
- There are 12 pairs of cranial nerves.

ASSESSMENT OF THE NERVOUS SYSTEM

Overview

- Assessment of the nervous system includes inspection and palpation of the head and spine, measuring the head circumference, and assessment of the level of alertness, cranial nerves, motor system, reflexes, and sensory system.

HEAD

Fontanel/Suture Assessment

- Palpate the anterior and posterior fontanelles using the flat pads of the fingers. Visible pulsations in the anterior fontanelle are normal findings.
- Palpate the principal sutures of the skull, including the sagittal, coronal, lambdoid, and metopic sutures. Note whether the sutures are approximated or separated. Pressure on the neonate's head during birth may cause molding, a temporary asymmetry of the skull caused by overriding sutures.

Head Circumference

- Head circumference, or occipitofrontal circumference, is an indicator of brain growth.
- Obtain an initial head circumference at birth to establish a baseline measurement. ▶

Head Circumference (*continued*)

- Place paper measuring tape in a line just above the eyebrows to the pinna of the ears and around the widest part of the back of the head.

Skull Inspection/Palpation

- Evaluate the overall size and shape of the neonate's head and the presence of hair patterns.

SKIN/SPINE

Skin/Spine Assessment

- Gently place the neonate prone to assess the back and spinal region.
- The spine should be symmetrical, straight, and palpable along the length of the back.
- Assess for presence of a sacral dimple. This usually appears in the gluteal crease. It is a normal finding in the neonate unless it is associated with the following: base unable to be visualized, tuft of hair, and skin tags.
- Assess the skin along the spinal column and back for any lesions or discoloration. Large hemangiomas crossing the midline may be associated with spinal lesions.

NEUROLOGIC FUNCTION ASSESSMENT

Level of Alertness

Observe neonates to determine their state of alertness.

- Active sleep (REM sleep): sleeping quietly with eyes closed, regular breathing, limited movement with minimal arousal to external stimuli
- Quiet sleep (non-REM sleep): sleeping with eyes closed, but eye movement notable; shallow and irregular breathing; movements such as twitching, grimacing, or sucking
- Awake/drowsy: eyes open and close, but glazed when open; faster breathing; arm and leg movement
- Alert: eyes open, responds to stimuli, crying

Neurologic Alertness Assessment

- Prematurity is associated with more time spent in light sleep.
- The infant's ability to smoothly transition between states of alertness is known as modulation. Premature neonates are easily overwhelmed by external stimuli and may not be able to transition between states as smoothly as term newborns.
- The ideal time for neurologic assessment is when the neonate is quiet and awake. This is typically after feeding but before the neonate has fallen back to sleep.
- Altered level of alertness is associated with acute neurologic dysfunction.

Cranial Nerves

- CN I (olfactory): These are rarely tested in the neonate.
- CN II (optic): Visual response matures with gestational age. At 26 weeks' gestation, the neonate can blink to light. At 32 weeks' gestation, the neonate may fixate on objects. At 34 weeks' gestation, the neonate can track. At 37 weeks' gestation, neonates can turn their eyes toward the light.
- CN III, IV, and VI (extraocular movements): Doll's eye phenomenon can be performed as early as 25 weeks' gestation. Move the neonate's head and neck from side to side, which leads to eye deviation to the opposite side. Note any abnormal eye movements, unreactive pupils, or unilaterally dilated or constricted pupils.
- CN V (trigeminal): Note response to tactile stimuli over the face. ▶

Cranial Nerves (*continued*)

- CN VII (facial): During crying, observe facial movements for symmetry.
- CN VIII (auditory): Term infants respond to sound by the startle response or increased level of alertness. By 28 weeks' gestation, the neonate startles or blinks at a sudden loud noise.
- CN V, VII, IX, X, and XII: Sucking/swallowing assesses the function of these cranial nerves. Impairments of these nerves may present in the neonate as difficulty sucking or swallowing and a weak or absent gag reflex.
- CN XI (spinal accessories): These are rarely tested in the neonate.

Motor System

- To evaluate the motor function, assess the neonate's passive tone/posture and active muscle activity.
- Passive tone and posture are observed while the infant is at rest; normal resting tone and posture depends on gestational age (see Chapter 3, Adaptation to Extrauterine Life).
- Assess muscle tone when the neonate is active; movements should be spontaneous, symmetric, and smooth.

Primitive Reflexes

Primitive reflexes are present at 32 weeks' gestation and include:

- Moro reflex: This reflex is also known as the startle reflex. Raise the infant's head about 30° from the supine position, then drop it suddenly while supporting the head to avoid impact. This results in abduction and extension of the arms and opening of the hands, followed by flexion.
- Stepping reflex: Hold the neonate in a vertical upright position with feet in contact with a flat surface. This results in a slow, alternating stepping pattern with flexion and extension of the legs.
- Grasp reflexes (palmar and plantar/Babinski): To elicit palmar reflex, place a finger in the palm of the neonate's hand. This results in finger closure and clinging. To elicit plantar/Babinski reflex, stroke the outer part of the neonate's foot in an upward motion. This results in the toes fanning out.
- Asymmetrical tonic neck reflex: This reflex is also known as fencing posture reflex. Turn the neonate's head and neck to one side. This results in extension of the upper and lower extremities on the side to which the head and neck are facing, and flexion of the opposite upper extremity. This reflex is present at 35 weeks' gestation.
- Galant reflex: Hold the neonate in a prone suspension and stroke the paravertebral region from the thorax to the lumbar area. This results in movement of the neonate's trunk and hips toward the side of the stimulus.

NEUROLOGIC DISORDERS

Overview

- Disorders of the nervous system include birth injuries and defects and can occur due to prematurity or traumatic birth.
- Nervous system disorders may lead to a wide variety of complications, including learning disabilities, neurodevelopmental delays, and cerebral palsy.

BIRTH INJURIES

- *Birth injury* is defined as an impairment of the neonate's body function or structure caused by an adverse event that occurred during labor, delivery, or after delivery.
- Risks for birth injury include macrosomia, abnormal presentation, use of obstetrical instruments during delivery, maternal obesity, and maternal pelvic abnormalities.

Scalp

- Extracranial injuries occur during delivery and are associated with swelling or bleeding in different locations within the scalp or skull. These present at birth due to prolonged pressure on the fetal head while in the birth canal or after vacuum extraction, and often require no treatment and resolve within a few days to weeks.
- *Caput succedaneum*: This is scalp edema above the periosteum that crosses suture lines.
- *Cephalohematoma*: This is a collection of blood under the periosteum that does not cross suture lines. It presents as swelling with or without discoloration; swelling typically does not expand. Complications of cephalohematomas include jaundice, infection, and sepsis.
- *Subgaleal hemorrhage*: This is a collection of blood in the subgaleal space, not limited by sutures. It presents as a fluctuant, mobile mass and diffuse swelling from the back of the neck to the ears. It places the neonate at risk of blood loss, hypovolemic shock, and seizures. It requires continuous monitoring, serial head circumference measurements, hematocrit, and coagulation studies, and may require imaging such as head ultrasound, CT, or MRI for diagnosis. Treatment includes fluid replacement via blood transfusion and intravenous (IV) fluid administration.

Skull

- Skull fractures caused by birth trauma are associated with an increased risk of intracranial hemorrhage and cephalohematoma.
- Skull fractures are less likely to occur in unassisted vaginal or elective Cesarean deliveries but may occur if there is enough pressure on the soft fetal skull.
- Most skull fractures resolve spontaneously and only require observation.

Intracranial

- Birth injury may lead to various types of intracranial hemorrhages, including subdural, subarachnoid, epidural, and intraventricular hemorrhages (IVH; Table 9.1).

Interventions

- Monitor for signs of expansion and increased intracranial pressure.
- Monitor serial hematocrits and imaging studies.
- Most resolve spontaneously.
- Monitor for posthemorrhagic hydrocephalus.
- Provide supportive therapy for small lesions.
- Surgical intervention is necessary for large or unstable hemorrhages.

TABLE 9.1 **Classification of Intracranial Hemorrhages**

TYPE OF HEMORRHAGE	LOCATION	PRESENTATION
Subdural	• Between the dura mater and the arachnoid membrane	• May be asymptomatic • Symptoms appear within 24–48 hours • Apnea, respiratory depression, and seizures
Subarachnoid	• Below the arachnoid mater	• Symptoms appear within 24–48 hours • Apnea, respiratory depression, and seizures
Epidural	• Between the dura and the inner table of the skull	• Seizures, hypotonia, bulging fontanelle, vital sign changes, and altered LOC
Intraventricular	• Germinal matrix	• Symptoms depend on the severity of the bleed • Apnea, respiratory depression, seizures, hypotension, and acidosis

LOC, level of consciousness.

Spinal Cord

- Risk factors include instrument-assisted vaginal delivery and breech vaginal delivery.
- Injuries are most likely to occur in the upper cervical spine due to traction or rotation of this area during delivery.
- Severity of the injury determines the clinical presentation. High cervical or brainstem injuries are associated with high mortality rate. Low spinal lesions are associated with high morbidity and neurologic impairment.

Plexus Injuries

- *Brachial plexus injuries* are injuries of the brachial plexus nerves, a complex network of nerves between the neck and shoulders.
- Symptoms include the following: muscle weakness or paralysis of the arm or hand on the affected side, reduced movement in the upper extremity, and decreased or absent sensation in the upper extremity.

Types of Plexus Injuries

- Stretch: The nerve is stretched, but not torn. The injury is outside of the spinal cord. Affected nerves recover spontaneously.
- Rupture: The nerve is torn, but not at its attachment to the spine. The injury is outside of the spinal cord. It may require surgical intervention.
- Avulsion: Nerve roots tear apart from the spinal cord. The injury occurs at the spinal cord. Surgical repair requires replacement of damaged nerve tissue.

Types of Brachial Plexus Injuries

- Erb palsy: This is an upper brachial plexus injury (C5–C7) causing adduction and internal rotation of the shoulder and pronation of the forearm. It is the most common type of injury. Moro reflex is asymmetric. Treatment includes physical therapy and protective positioning.
- Horner syndrome: The injury is located in the T2 to T4 region and is usually associated with an avulsion. It presents with miosis, ptosis, and anhidrosis, and is usually the most severe injury with lasting neurosensory deficits.
- Klumpke palsy: The injury is located in the lower roots (C8, T1). Grasp reflex may be absent. It may present similar to Horner syndrome if T1 is involved. Treatment includes range of motion exercises and proper positioning.
- Total plexus involvement: This injury involves C5 to T1 and all five nerves of the brachial plexus. It results in flaccid upper extremity with little to no sensation and absent reflexes. It typically requires imaging via MRI.

Cranial and Peripheral Nerve Injuries

- Phrenic nerve injury is typically associated with brachial plexus injury and is caused by traction of the head and neck. It presents as respiratory distress and diminished breath sounds on the affected side. Treatment includes respiratory therapy such as continuous positive airway pressure (CPAP) or mechanical ventilation until the injury resolves. Surgical intervention is required if the injury persists.
- Facial nerve injury is usually caused by compression of the facial nerve during delivery. It presents with decreased movement of the face on the affected side and resolves spontaneously within 2 weeks.
- Laryngeal nerve injury may lead to vocal cord paralysis and presents as stridor, respiratory distress, a hoarse, weak or absent cry, and difficulty swallowing or aspiration. Paralysis resolves spontaneously with time.

CRANIOSYNOSTOSIS

- *Craniosynostosis* is a birth defect in which the skull bones join together too early, prior to the brain being fully formed.

Risk Factors

- Genetic syndromes
- Environmental factors
- Maternal thyroid disease
- Clomiphene citrate (fertility medication)

Signs and Symptoms

- Abnormally shaped head (plagiocephaly)
- Absent or abnormal fontanelles
- A firm raised edge where the suture closed
- Slow or no growth of the infant's head over time
- Very noticeable scalp veins
- Irritability and high-pitched cry
- Sleepiness
- Poor feeding

Treatment

- Mild craniosynostosis treatment includes helmet therapy to help reshape the infant's head.
- Moderate to severe cases will require surgical treatment to reshape the skull, allow room for brain growth, and relieve increased intracranial pressure.
- Supportive therapies such as physical, occupational, and speech therapies may be needed to support and promote normal functioning and activities.

HYDROCEPHALUS

- Hydrocephalus is a condition where there is an imbalance in the production and absorption of cerebrospinal fluid (CSF). This causes the accumulation of CSF within the cerebral ventricles and/or subarachnoid spaces. The result is either impaired absorption of CSF within the subarachnoid space, malfunction of the arachnoid villi (noncommunicating), or an obstruction to the flow of CSF in the ventricular system (communicating hydrocephalus).
- This results in ventricular dilation and often increased intracranial pressure.

Risk Factors

- Brain hemorrhage, infections, or tumor
- Birth weight less than 1500 grams
- CNS malformations
- Inherited genetic abnormalities
- Male sex
- Myelomeningocele

Signs and Symptoms

- Bulging anterior fontanel
- Cushing triad (late sign) ▶

[🧠] **COMPLICATIONS**

Complications of craniosynostosis include abnormal head shape, increased intracranial pressure, seizures, vision or eye movement disorders, developmental delays, brain damage, and breathing difficulties.

[📝] **POP QUIZ 9.1**

Neonatal brain growth is assessed most accurately by which method?

[🧠] **COMPLICATIONS**

The most common complication of a ventriculoperitoneal (VP) shunt is shunt malfunction. Shunt malfunctions are caused by either an infection or mechanical failure. If shunt malfunction or infection is suspected, refer for a neurologic assessment and neuroimaging. Keep patient NPO (nothing by mouth) for possible surgical intervention.

Signs and Symptoms (*continued*)

- Enlarged head circumference
- Hypertension
- Irritability
- Lethargy
- Papilledema
- Poor coordination and feeding
- Seizures
- Vomiting

Treatment

- First-line treatment: placement of a ventriculoperitoneal (VP) shunt, with the catheter connected to a one-way valve that opens when the pressure reaches a certain level, and with the distal end of the catheter placed in the peritoneal cavity and the proximal end placed in the ventricle
- Diuretics for short periods if the patient is too unstable for surgery
- Asymptomatic patients: watchful waiting with monthly CTs and measuring head circumference in infants if indicated
- Ventricle to atria shunt possible if VP shunt cannot be placed

[⚡] **ALERT!**

Cushing triad is a medical emergency that is a nervous system response to increased intracranial pressure and affects three vital signs (VS):

- Heart rate: bradycardia
- Respiration: irregular respirations (slow, deep respirations with periods of apnea)
- Blood pressure: sudden hypertension or a widened pulse pressure (a large difference between the systolic and diastolic blood pressure)

Nurses should anticipate contacting a provider immediately if they note Cushing triad as this is a late sign of increased intracranial pressure (ICP).

Nursing Interventions

- Assess patient for signs of VP shunt malfunction: Signs include irritability, lethargy, papilledema, and vomiting. Mechanical failure malfunction is most common in the first year after placement. Shunt mechanical failure malfunction is usually caused by obstruction of the catheter. Other causes are broken tubing, shunt migration, and excessive drainage.
- Assess patient for signs of VP shunt infection: Signs include abdominal pain and fever. Approximately 40% of shunts malfunction in the first year. Infections are most common in the first 6 months after placement. Infected shunt may be removed and an external shunt placed in the presence of infection.

Patient Education

- Learn about hydrocephalus and the signs and symptoms of shunt malfunction.
- Several shunt revisions may be needed throughout the patient's lifetime as the infant grows.

[⚡] **ALERT!**

If shunt malfunction or infection is suspected, refer for a neurologic assessment and neuroimaging. Keep patient NPO for possible surgical intervention.

HYPOTONIA

- Hypotonia, or low tone, may be an indicator of a CNS or neuromuscular disorder.

Risk Factors

- Prematurity
- Neuromuscular or CNS disorder
- Congenital infections
- Hypoglycemia or other endocrine abnormalities
- Drug toxicity (perinatal magnesium sulfate exposure)
- Genetic syndromes (Down syndrome, trisomy 18, trisomy 13, Prader–Willi syndrome)
- Inborn errors of metabolism

Signs and Symptoms

- "Floppy" or limp
- Poor head/neck control
- Extended limbs
- Difficulty sucking or swallowing
- Delayed developmental milestones

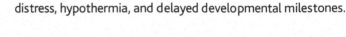

COMPLICATIONS

Complications of hypotonia include difficulty feeding, respiratory distress, hypothermia, and delayed developmental milestones.

Treatment

Once a diagnosis is made, the underlying condition is treated first, followed by supportive and symptomatic therapy such as:

- Physical/occupational therapy
- Speech therapy
- Sensory stimulation

Nursing Interventions

- Promote proper positioning and flexion of extremities.
- Ensure airway patency at all times; avoid chin-to-chest positioning.
- Insert nasogastric feeding tube if the infant is unable to orally feed.

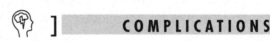

COMPLICATIONS

Complications of hypoxic ischemic encephalopathy (HIE) range from mild to severe neurologic sequelae. Mild complications include learning difficulties and attention deficit disorder. Severe complications include cerebral palsy, epilepsy, visual impairment, and severe cognitive and developmental disorders.

HYPOXIC ISCHEMIC ENCEPHALOPATHY

- *Hypoxic ischemic encephalopathy (HIE)* is a serious birth complication and brain injury affecting infants greater than 35 weeks' gestation and results from impaired cerebral blood flow during the prenatal, intrapartum, or postnatal period.
- HIE is a common cause of neonatal encephalopathy, a syndrome marked by acute neurologic dysfunction.
- HIE has three stages (Table 9.2).

Signs and Symptoms

- Low Apgar scores
- Metabolic or mixed acidosis
- Abnormal level of alertness (hyperalert, irritable, lethargic, obtunded)
- Decreased spontaneous movement
- Respiratory distress/depression
- Hypotonia
- Abnormal posturing and seizure activity
- Absent primitive reflexes

TABLE 9.2 Stages of Hypoxic Ischemic Encephalopathy			
CATEGORY	STAGE 1: MILD	STAGE 2: MODERATE	STAGE 3: SEVERE
LOC	Hyperalert	Lethargic	Stupor/coma
Spontaneous activity	Normal	Decreased	None
Tone	Normal	Mild hypotonia	Hypotonia/flaccid
Suck reflex	Weak	Weak or absent	Absent
Respirations	Normal	Periodic	Apnea
Seizures	None	Common	Uncommon
EEG	Mild depression	Moderate depression	Severe depression

LOC, level of consciousness.

Treatment

■ See Neonatal Cooling under Common Procedures section.

Nursing Interventions

■ Immediately after birth: Assist with neonatal resuscitation.

Active Cooling Phase

■ Insert and secure esophageal and/or rectal temperature probes for continuous temperature monitoring.
■ Ensure the infant's full body is in contact with the cooling blanket at all times.
■ Reposition the infant at least every 3 hours and assess the skin for areas of redness, breakdown, or fat necrosis.
■ Monitor vital signs (VS) and EEG background for abnormalities or seizures.
■ Administer IV fluids and seizure medications as ordered (Appendix 9.1).
■ Assess the infant for shivering and administer morphine to treat agitation/shivering.
■ Limit handling of the infant by both staff and family.

Rewarming Phase

■ Gradually increase the infant's core body temperature by manually increasing the cooling unit's set point.
■ Continue to monitor VS and EEG background,
■ Transport the infant to MRI once rewarming is completed and if the infant is stable.

[⚡] **ALERT!**

Infants are most at risk of seizures during the active rewarming phase. Ensure rewarming is done gradually over 12 hours or according to facility policy. Closely monitor EEG and the infant for any seizure-like activity.

[🌐] **NURSING PEARLS**

During the active cooling and rewarming phase, the nurse should expect the following changes in vital signs (VS), electrolytes, and urine output:

During cooling, expect:
• Decreased heart rate (HR)
• Increased blood pressure (BP) initially due to peripheral vasoconstriction
• Increased urine output initially due to shunting of blood to the internal organs
• Decreased calcium, magnesium, phosphorus, and potassium
• Labile glucose due to relative insulin resistance, decreased metabolic rate, and shivering

During rewarming, expect:
• Increased HR
• Decreased BP due to decreased peripheral vascular resistance
• Decreased urine output due to third spacing and shunting of blood to the periphery
• Electrolyte shifts, as renal and liver clearance rates change

INTRAVENTRICULAR HEMORRHAGE

- IVH occurs when blood vessels in the germinal matrix rupture and bleed into the ventricles of the brain, the spaces that hold CSF.
- Premature infants have underdeveloped and fragile blood vessels in the brain, which can easily rupture with alterations in blood pressure (BP) and cerebral blood flow.
- IVH typically occurs within the first 3 to 4 days of life.

Risk Factors

- Prematurity: the number one risk factor for IVH
- Prenatal: intrauterine infection, prolonged labor, lack of antenatal steroids, and premature rupture of membranes (PROM)
- Postnatal: resuscitation, sepsis, respiratory distress syndrome (RDS), patent ductus arteriosus (PDA), pulmonary hemorrhage, metabolic acidosis, pneumothorax, surfactant administration, and male sex
- Low birth weight

Grading of Intraventricular Hemorrhage

- Grade I: hemorrhage limited to the germinal matrix
- Grade II: IVH without ventricular dilation
- Grade III: IVH with ventricular dilation occupying greater than 50% of the ventricle
- Grade IV: IVH extending into the intraparenchymal area

Signs and Symptoms

- Apnea, bradycardia, and desaturations anemia
- Hypotension
- Altered neurologic examination

Treatment

The primary treatment is prevention, which includes the following:

- Administer antenatal steroids.
- Delay cord clamping.
- Grades I and II IVH will resolve on their own.
- Management of IVH includes serial head ultrasounds and monitoring of symptoms.
- A VP shunt may need to be placed if the infant develops posthemorrhagic hydrocephalus.
- Limit alterations in cerebral blood flow and BP by implementing IVH protocols after birth.

Intraventricular Hemorrhage Protocols

- Midline head positioning for 72 hours
- Slow arterial line lab draws
- Adequate respiratory support
- Limiting oral and endotracheal suctioning
- Limited handling of the infant (clustered care times, no position changes, no weighing, etc. until 72 hours of life) ▶

[🧠] **COMPLICATIONS**

Complications of intraventricular hemorrhage (IVH) include posthemorrhagic hydrocephalus, periventricular leukomalacia (PVL), cerebral palsy, seizures, and neurodevelopmental delays.

[⚙] **ALERT!**

Grades III and IV intraventricular hemorrhage (IVH) are considered severe IVH. The risk of poor neurodevelopmental outcomes significantly increases with grade III or IV IVH diagnosis.

[📝] **POP QUIZ 9.2**

A 1-day-old, 25 weeks' gestation infant requires blood gas from the umbilical arterial catheter. How can the nurse minimize the risk of intraventricular hemorrhage (IVH) during this procedure?

Intraventricular Hemorrhage Protocols (continued)
- Legs-down diaper changes
- Interventions to minimize pain

MICROCEPHALY

- *Microcephaly* is a smaller than normal head size.

Risk Factors

- Certain infections during pregnancy: cytomegalovirus (CMV), Zika, rubella, and toxoplasmosis
- Exposure to toxins in utero such as alcohol or drugs
- Lack of blood supply to the brain during pregnancy
- Genetic factors

Treatment

- There is no known treatment for microcephaly.
- Patients with mild microcephaly typically develop normally; patients with moderate to severe microcephaly will need regular follow-up appointments to monitor their growth and development, as well as physical, occupational, and speech therapies.

[🧠]   **COMPLICATIONS**

Microcephaly can lead to seizures, developmental delays, intellectual disabilities, mobility complications, difficulty feeding, hearing loss, and vision problems.

NEONATAL SEIZURES

- *Seizures* are caused by abnormal, excessive, or synchronous discharges of neurons in the cerebral cortex.
- An acute provoked seizure is the most common type of neonatal seizure and is one that is caused by an acute illness or brain injury.
- *Epilepsy* is a disorder where the infant has a predisposition to recurrent seizures. Severe neonatal epilepsy syndromes such as early infantile developmental and epileptic encephalopathy are associated with poor neurologic exam and outcomes.

Common Causes

- Preterm birth
- Neonatal encephalopathy/HIE
- Neonatal abstinence syndrome (NAS)
- CNS infection
- Acute and inherited metabolic conditions
- Genetic factors

[🧠]   **COMPLICATIONS**

Complications of seizures include:
- Aspiration of food or saliva during a seizure
- Further brain injury
- Neurologic impairment
- Developmental delay
- Postneonatal epilepsy

Classification/Types

- Neonatal seizures are defined by their electroencephalographic structure and are all considered focal, not generalized.
- Neonatal seizures have several classifications.

[⚡]   **ALERT!**

Neonatal seizures may be the first and only sign of central nervous system (CNS) disorders in the newborn. An immediate evaluation should be done to determine the cause and begin treatment.

Signs and Symptoms

- Focal clonic: slow, repetitive, rhythmic contractions of the limbs, face, or trunk that cannot be stopped with restraint; may be unifocal or multifocal, with contractions closely associated with EEG discharges ▶

Signs and Symptoms (*continued*)

- Focal tonic: sustained, but transient, asymmetrical posturing of the trunk or extremities; tonic deviation of the eyes; associated with focal EEG seizure activity
- Myoclonic: contractions of the muscle groups of well-defined regions (proximal or distal limb regions, entire limbs, trunk or diaphragm, or face); movements may be isolated or repetitive with varying speeds; may or may not be associated with EEG
- Epileptic spasms: flexion followed by extension/relaxation of the truncal muscles and limbs; on EEG, may show diffuse, high-voltage, slow-wave transient or generalized voltage attenuation
- Subclinical (electrographic only): presence of seizure on EEG without clinical manifestations; most common type of neonatal seizure
- Autonomic: abrupt changes in VS reported to be manifestations of neonatal seizures, including alterations in heart rate (HR), respirations, and BP; other autonomic changes including apnea, flushing, abrupt hypotonia, and pupil dilation or abnormal eye movement

Treatment

- Prior to initiating antiseizure medications, determine and treat the underlying cause.
- If seizures persist or are prolonged, initiate antiseizure medication therapy (Appendix 9.1).

Nursing Interventions

- Maintain seizure precautions.
- Maximize the patient's safety, when actively seizing. Do not put anything in the patient's mouth. Ensure the airway is patent and protect the patient's head.

Patient Education

- Learn the signs and symptoms of seizures.
- Make sure to administer medication as directed by the healthcare provider.

NEURAL TUBE DEFECTS

- *Neural tube defects (NTDs)* are birth defects of the brain, spinal cord, or spine that occur when the neural tube does not close properly. They develop during the first month of pregnancy.
- The two most common types of NTDs are spina bifida and anencephaly.

[ ]   **NURSING PEARLS**

Instruct the family not to put anything in the patient's mouth during a seizure. This is not necessary.

Risk Factors

- Obesity
- Diabetes
- Opioid use
- Antiseizure medications
- High body temperature early in pregnancy
- Family history of NTDs
- Genetic or chromosomal abnormalities
- Folic acid deficiency

Anencephaly

- *Anencephaly* is a type of NTD in which part of the brain or skull does not develop. It occurs when the upper part of the neural tube does not completely close. ▶

Anencephaly (continued)

- Most often, the infant is born without the forebrain and cerebellum. The remaining parts of the brain are usually uncovered.
- There is no known cure or treatment for anencephaly.

Myelomeningocele

- *Myelomeningocele* is a severe type of spina bifida in which the neural tube fails to close, causing a fluid-filled sac that protrudes from the infant's back. The sac contains part of the spinal cord, meninges, nerves, and CSF.
- Myelomeningocele usually causes moderate to severe disabilities.

Encephalocele

- Encephalocele is a rare type of NTD in which the brain and membranes surrounding it protrude from the back of the head through an opening in the skull.

Signs and Symptoms

Anencephaly

- Missing bones in the head
- Folding of the ears
- Cleft palate
- Large areas of the brain missing

Myelomeningocele

- Malformations on the back such as a bulging sac, tuft of hair, or dimple
- Lack of sensation below the defect, including paralysis of the legs or urinary/bowel elimination issues
- Hydrocephalus

Encephalocele

- Bulging sac at the back of the head
- Facial defects
- Hydrocephalus
- Arm/leg weakness
- Small head
- Seizures

[🧠]   **COMPLICATIONS**

Neural tube defects (NTDs) can lead to paralysis or mobility problems, orthopedic complications, bowel and bladder elimination impairment, hydrocephalus, trouble breathing or swallowing, infection, learning disorders, and latex allergy.

[⚙]   **ALERT!**

To prevent neural tube defect (NTDs), pregnant patients should take 400 mcg of folic acid daily and consume foods high in folate. Patients who are at high risk of having a baby with NTDs should supplement with 4,000 mcg of folic acid daily during the first 12 weeks of pregnancy.

Treatment

- Surgical intervention is needed for NTD repairs and may be done prenatally or after birth.
- In patients who develop hydrocephalus, a VP shunt may need to be placed.

Nursing Interventions

- Apply sterile dressing to the sac with sterile saline or antibiotic solution as prescribed after birth and until surgery. Change dressings when dry or as needed.
- Assess defect for redness, swelling, or purulent drainage before and after surgery.
- Assess for fever, cloudy or foul-smelling urine, irritability, and nuchal rigidity. ▶

Nursing Interventions (*continued*)

- Keep the anal area clean and apply shield between the anus and the sac.
- Assess for impaired urinary elimination.
- Provide therapeutic prone or side-lying positioning as tolerated to avoid putting pressure on the defect.
- Prevent hypothermia from large area of exposed and moist sac.

Patient Education

- Keep the sac protected. The baby should be positioned lying on their stomach or side.
- Perform diaper changes with the baby lying on their stomach or side.

DIAGNOSTIC PROCEDURES

Computed Tomography/Magnetic Resonance Imaging

- *CT* and *MRI* identify the presence and the type of brain injury.
- MRI is used more frequently as it is not associated with radiation exposure.

[📝]   **POP QUIZ 9.3**

The neonatal nurse attends the delivery of an infant with known myelomeningocele. What nursing intervention is the highest priority after initial stabilization of the infant after delivery?

Laboratory Tests

- Complete blood count (CBC): assess for infection and anemia
- Cultures: assess for sepsis
- Glucose: rules out hypo/hyperglycemia as a cause of seizures
- Electrolytes: assess for electrolyte imbalances, which may be a cause or result of nervous system disorders
- Coagulation studies: assess for coagulation factors, which may be affected during therapeutic hypothermia
- Alpha-fetaprotein (AFP) screening: a blood test done during pregnancy that measures the amount of AFP in the blood; amount higher than normal in pregnant women carrying a baby with NTD
- Genetic testing
- Metabolic testing

Electroencephalogram

- Detects and confirms the presence of seizures
- Objective method of measuring the function of the brain

Head Ultrasound

- Detects and determines the grade of IVH

Lumbar Puncture

- Detects pathogens in CSF
- Used to rule out meningitis

Prenatal Ultrasound

- May identify certain neurologic disorders such as microcephaly and NTDs

COMMON PROCEDURES

Shunt

- See Hydrocephalus section.

Neonatal Cooling

- Neonatal cooling, or therapeutic hypothermia, is the first line of treatment for neonates with presumed HIE and meet the needed criteria.

Criteria

- Gestational age greater than 36 weeks
- Less than 6 hours old
- One or more of the following: metabolic or mixed acidosis with a pH less than 7.0 or base deficit greater than 16 in a blood sample from the umbilical cord within the first hour of life; a 10-minute Apgar score of 5 or less; and resuscitation initiated at birth and continued for at least 10 minutes
- Moderate to severe encephalopathy on exam

Initiating Neonatal Cooling

- Therapeutic hypothermia preserves cerebral energy metabolism and reduces cytotoxic edema, resulting in a decreased incidence of disability and death.
- Whole-body cooling is initiated by 6 hours of life and maintained at a goal temperature of 92.3°F (33.5°C) for 72 hours; rectal temperature should be maintained at 91.4°F to 95°F (33°C to 35°C), with target temperature set to 92.3°F (33.5°C).
- Rewarming may start once goal temperature has been maintained for 72 hours. Rewarming is typically done gradually over the course of 12 hours.
- Prognosis after therapeutic hypothermia is dependent on the severity of encephalopathy. Infants with mild encephalopathy typically recover well and develop normally. Infants with moderate to severe encephalopathy are at increased risk of having neurologic deficits.

RESOURCES

Bodamer, O. (2021). Approach to the infant with hypotonia and weakness. *UpToDate*. https://www.uptodate.com/contents/approach-to-the-infant-with-hypotonia-and-weakness

Boston Children's Hospital. *Brachial plexus birth injury*. https://www.childrenshospital.org/conditions/brachial-plexus-birth-injury

Cedars Sinai. *Open Neural Tube Defects (ONTDs) in children*. https://www.cedars-sinai.org/health-library/diseases-and-conditions---pediatrics/o/open-neural-tube-defects-ontds-in-children.html

Centers for Disease Control and Prevention. (2020a). *Facts about craniocynostosis*. U.S. Department of Health and Human Services, Centers for Disease Control and Prevention. https://www.cdc.gov/ncbddd/birthdefects/craniosynostosis.html#:~:text = Craniosynostosis%20is%20a%20birth%20defect,skull%20can%20become%20more%20misshapen

Centers for Disease Control and Prevention. (2020b). *Facts about microcephaly*. U.S. Department of Health and Human Services, Centers for Disease Control and Prevention. https://www.cdc.gov/ncbddd/birthdefects/microcephaly.html#:~:text = Microcephaly%20is%20a%20condition%20where,in%20a%20smaller%20head%20size

Centers for Disease Control and Prevention. (2020c). *Facts about neural tube defects*. U.S. Department of Health and Human Services, Centers for Disease Control and Prevention. https://www.cdc.gov/ncbddd/birthdefects/facts-about-neural-tube-defects.html

Cleveland Clinic. (2022). *Neural tube defects*. https://my.clevelandclinic.org/health/diseases/22656-neural-tube-defects-ntd#prevention

Fuloria, M., & Kreiter, S. (2002). The newborn examination: Part II. Emergencies and common abnormalities involving the abdomen, pelvis, extremities, genitalia, and spine. *American Family Physician*. https://www.aafp.org/afp/2002/0115/p265.html#sec-4

Gilbert, S. (2000). *Developmental biology*. (6th ed.). Sinauer Associates. Formation of the Neural Tube. https://www
.ncbi.nlm.nih.gov/books/NBK10080

Kotagal, S. (2020). Neurologic examination of the newborn. *UpToDate*. https://www.uptodate.com/contents
/neurologic-examination-of-the-newborn

Leigh, B. (2016). Six states of alertness for newborns. *Centre for Perinatal Psychology*. https://www.centreforperinat
alpsychology.com.au/states-of-alertness

Lewis, M. (2014a). A comprehensive newborn examination: Part I. General head and neck, cardiopulmonary.
American Family Physician. https://www.aafp.org/afp/2014/0901/p289.html#sec-2

Lewis, M. L. (2014b). A comprehensive newborn exam: Part II. Skin, trunk, extremities, neurologic. *American Family
Physician*, *90*(5), 297–302. https://www.aafp.org/afp/2014/0901/p297.html#sec-1

McKee-Garrett, T. (2021). Neonatal birth injuries. *UpToDate*. https://www.uptodate.com/contents
/neonatal-birth-injuries

Medline Plus. (2021). *Intraventricular hemorrhage of the newborn*. https://medlineplus.gov/ency/article/007301.htm

Nurselabs. (2021). *Nervous system anatomy and physiology*. https://nurseslabs.com/nervous-system

Prescriber's Digital Reference. (n.d.-a). *Levetiracetam*. https://www.pdr.net/drug-summary
/Levetiracetam-Injection-levetiracetam-23988

Prescriber's Digital Reference. (n.d.-b). *Lidocaine*. https://www.pdr.net/drug-summary/Lidocaine-Hydrochloride
-Injection-lidocaine-hydrochloride-3301.2673#11

Prescriber's Digital Reference. (n.d.-c). *Phenobarbital*. https://www.pdr.net/drug-summary/Phenobarbital-Elixir
-phenobarbital-2669.3876

Prescriber's Digital Reference. (n.d.-d). *Phenytoin*. https://www.pdr.net/drug-summary/Dilantin-Infatabs
-phenytoin-1814.6158

Shellhaas, R. (2022a). Treatment of neonatal seizures. *UpToDate*. https://www.uptodate.com/contents
/treatment-of-neonatal-seizures

Shellhaas, R. (2022b). Treatment of neonatal seizures. *UpToDate*. https://www.uptodate.com/contents
/clinical-features-evaluation-and-diagnosis-of-neonatal-seizures

Wu, Y. (2021). Clinical features, diagnosis, and treatment of neonatal encephalopathy. *UpToDate*. https://www
.uptodate.com/contents/clinical-features-diagnosis-and-treatment-of-neonatal-encephalopathy

APPENDIX 9.1 NEUROLOGIC MEDICATIONS

INDICATIONS	MECHANISM OF ACTION	CONTRAINDICATIONS, PRECAUTIONS, AND ADVERSE EFFECTS
Anticonvulsants (fosphenytoin)		
• Treat myoclonic and tonic-clonic seizures • Treat epileptic spasms	• Limit the spread of seizure activity by reducing seizure propagation • Decrease seizure activity by decreasing influx of sodium ions across cell membranes in the motor cortex	• Medication is contraindicated with bradycardia and heart block. • Monitor for possible arrhythmias, hypotension, or ventricular defibrillation. • Patients with a history of blood conditions may be at higher risk. • Adverse reactions include pruritus, drowsiness, and nystagmus. • Medication is compatible with dextrose and NSS IV.

(continued)

APPENDIX 9.1 NEUROLOGIC MEDICATIONS (*continued*)

INDICATIONS	MECHANISM OF ACTION	CONTRAINDICATIONS, PRECAUTIONS, AND ADVERSE EFFECTS
Anticonvulsants (levetiracetam)		
• Seizure prophylaxis	• Mechanism of action unknown • Possibly inhibit sodium channels • Possibly facilitate GABA • Possibly decrease K+ current • Possibly bind to synaptic proteins which modulate neurotransmitter release	• Use with caution in patients with hepatic and renal disease. • Precautions include monitoring blood pressure for higher-than-normal diastolic pressure. • Adverse effects include drowsiness, headache, fatigue, increased blood pressure, dizziness, somnolence, and vomiting.
Anticonvulsants (lidocaine)		
• Seizure prophylaxis • Treat status epilepticus	• Decrease neuronal excitability	• High dosages can cause seizures. • Adverse effects include bradycardia, hypotension, neonatal depression, and cardiac arrest.
Anticonvulsants, barbiturates (phenobarbital)		
• Treat myoclonic and tonic-clonic seizures • Treat epileptic spasms • Seizure prophylaxis	• Depress sensory cortex, decrease motor activity, and alter cerebellar function • With sedative, hypnotic, and anticonvulsant properties	• Contraindications include severe hepatic impairment and dyspnea. • Precautions include CNS depression, paradoxical stimulation, respiratory depression, and asthma. • Use caution in patients with anemia, cardiac disease, hepatic impairment, hyperthyroidism, and renal impairment. • Adverse effects include nausea, rash, apnea, bradycardia, hypotension, headache, and lethargy. • Give slowly to avoid the possibility of respiratory depression, laryngospasm, hypertension, and severe hypotension.
Anticonvulsants (phenytoin)		
• Treat myoclonic and tonic-clonic seizures • Treat epileptic spasms • Seizure prophylaxis	• Limit the spread of seizure activity by reducing seizure propagation • Decrease seizure activity by decreasing influx of sodium ions across cell membranes in the motor cortex	• Contraindications include sinus bradycardia and heart block. • Patients with a history of blood conditions may be at higher risk. • Monitor for possible arrhythmias, hypotension, or ventricular fibrillation. • Monitor liver function. • Use caution in patients with hypoalbuminemia, hypothyroidism, and renal impairment. • Adverse reactions include cardiac rhythm abnormalities, CNS dysfunction, dermatitis, constipation, and nausea/vomiting. • Give slowly over a minimum of 30 minutes. • Medication is compatible only in NSS IV solution

CNS, central nervous system; GABA, gamma-aminobutyric acid; IV, intravenous; NSS, normal saline solution.

10 MUSCULOSKELETAL SYSTEM

- The musculoskeletal system is vital for movement, support and protection of the internal organs, heat generation, and blood circulation.
- Variations in the musculoskeletal assessment are expected in preterm neonates as their musculoskeletal system continues to grow and develop.

NORMAL EMBRYOLOGY

- Bone and muscle development begins at 4 weeks' gestation.
- During the embryonic period (first trimester), the musculoskeletal system differentiates. Abnormalities or interruptions (such as teratogens or genetic abnormalities) during this period produce congenital musculoskeletal malformations.
- During the fetal period (second and third trimesters), the musculoskeletal system undergoes further growth and development. Interruptions (such as teratogens or infections) during this period produce deformations or alterations in the configuration of normal musculoskeletal parts.

ASSESSMENT OF THE MUSCULOSKELETAL SYSTEM

Extremities

- Musculoskeletal assessment of the extremities should include inspection, palpation, and range of motion.
- Inspect the limbs.
- Check the hands and feet for visible deformities, correct amount of digits, asymmetry, or abnormal skinfolds.
- Palpate the joints for tenderness, swelling, or lumps.
- Perform passive and active range of motion on all extremities; assess muscle tone and strength.

Hip

- The newborn should have a hip examination within 72 hours of birth to assess for congenital dysplasia of the hips by performing the Ortolani and Barlow methods.
- The Ortolani method can identify a dislocated hip that can be reduced into the socket. The hip is abducted, and gentle pressure is applied to the thigh from behind in an attempt to relocate an already dislocated hip. A "clunk" sound is heard when the hip pops back into the joint.
- The Barlow method can identify a loose hip that can be pushed out of the socket with gentle pressure. Posterior/lateral pressure is applied to the hip. Normally, there is no motion in this direction; however, a dislocated hip will pop out of the joint. This makes a distinct "clunk" sound.

[📝] **POP QUIZ 10.1**

The nurse is performing a hip examination on a newborn and can dislocate and relocate the infant's hip. How should the nurse interpret the test results?

Spine

- Place the infant in a prone position.
- Assess the spine for asymmetry and the spinal curves (scoliosis, kyphosis).
- Palpate the height and symmetry of the shoulders and pelvis; inspect for any bruising around these areas.

PATHOPHYSIOLOGY: MUSCULOSKELETAL SYSTEM DISORDERS

Overview

- Musculoskeletal disorders of the spine, pelvis, and extremities are relatively common in neonates.
- Most disorders are pathologic; however, some may be physiologic, resulting from abnormal in-utero positioning.

CONGENITAL DYSPLASIA OF THE HIP

- Congenital dysplasia of the hip occurs because the ball and socket joint of the hip does not develop appropriately.
- The hip socket (acetabulum) is too shallow to cover the head of the femur, resulting in a loose hip joint.
- This may occur in one or both hips.

Risk Factors

- Breech presentation
- Family history of congenital dysplasia of the hip
- Female sex
- First-born children
- Tight swaddling with the legs in an extended position

Signs and Symptoms

- Hip clunk with abduction
- Restricted hip abduction
- Shorter affected leg
- Uneven gluteal folds

Diagnosis

- Barlow test
- Ortolani test
- Hip ultrasound for infants up to 6 months of age
- Hip x-ray for infants older than 6 months of age

Treatment

- Nonsurgical treatment options include observation and Pavlik harness.
- Surgical treatment options include closed and open reduction.

Nursing Interventions

- Assess the infant's hips and extremities for abnormalities.
- Educate the family about the possible need for modified car seats or securement devices. ▶

[🧠] **COMPLICATIONS**

Without early treatment, congenital dysplasia of the hip may lead to mobility issues such as a limp or trouble walking, pain, and osteoarthritis of the hip and back.

Nursing Interventions (*continued*)

- Evaluate for complications related to spica cast. Assess for signs of infection. Monitor neurovascular status and perform frequent neurovascular checks. Ensure the skin is clean and dry. Reposition frequently.
- Optimize skin integrity with Pavlik harness use. Ensure the harness does not cause skin breakdown. Keep the skin clean and dry.

Patient Education

- Avoid swaddling with legs together; allow room for flexion and extension of legs.
- Pavlik harness: Adhere to the harness schedule. It is most often worn for 23 hours per day and is only removed for bathing. Do not adjust the Pavlik harness.
- Spica cast: Do not put anything in the spica cast. Help with frequent position changes. Keep spica cast dry. Watch out for pain, swelling, or blue toes.

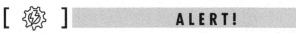

ALERT!

Do not put lotion, creams, or powder on the skin under a Pavlik harness as it will cake onto the skin and cause further breakdown.

FRACTURES AND DISLOCATIONS

- Birth injuries such as fractures and dislocations may occur during labor, delivery, or after delivery.
- Clavicular fractures are the most common type of neonatal fractures.
- Neonatal dislocations may include dislocation of the shoulder, knee, or hips (see Congenital Dysplasia of the Hip section).
- Dislocations caused by birth trauma are rare; most are due to congenital malformations and intrauterine positional deformities.

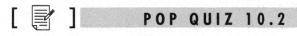

POP QUIZ 10.2

The nurse is assessing a 2-day-old infant with suspected congenital dysplasia of the hip. What assessment findings should the nurse expect to find?

Risk Factors

- Abnormal fetal presentation
- Forceps or vacuum-assisted vaginal delivery
- Macrosomia
- Maternal obesity
- Maternal pelvic anomalies
- Shoulder dystocia
- Small maternal stature

Signs and Symptoms

Clavicular Fractures

- Affected shoulder: may appear lower than the uninjured shoulder
- Bruising around the clavicular area
- Crepitus along the clavicle
- Crying with movement of the affected arm
- Decreased movement of the affected arm
- Pain with lifting the infant under the arms

Dislocations
- Crying with movement of the affected limb
- Bruising and swelling
- Decreased movement of the affected limb

Diagnosis
Clavicular Fractures
- Ultrasound
- X-ray

Dislocations
- X-ray
- MRI

Treatment
Clavicular Fractures
- Treatment is not typically needed as clavicular fractures heal spontaneously. The infant may need the affected arm strapped to the body to avoid moving the arm while it heals.

Dislocations
- Treatment depends on the severity of the dislocation and may range from observation to surgical intervention.

Nursing Interventions
- Assess neurovascular status of the affected extremity and compare it with the unaffected extremity.
- Assess pain levels and administer medications as ordered and necessary.
- Assist with position changes and perform passive range of motion as able in the fingers or toes of the affected extremities and unaffected extremities.

Patient Education
- Continue passive and active range of motion exercises.
- Follow up with orthopedics, pediatrician, and physical and occupational therapy as indicated.
- Keep affected extremity supported by a sling.

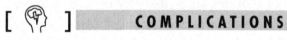

COMPLICATIONS

The most common complication of a clavicular fracture is an associated brachial plexus injury.

COMPLICATIONS

Fractures can cause a painful medical emergency called compartment syndrome. Compartment syndrome can result after a fracture when edema occurs. Pressure increases within that enclosed space and compromises circulation to the muscles, blood vessels, and nerves within that space. This can lead to decreased blood flow, ischemia, infection, and deformity. Important nursing interventions include performing frequent neurovascular assessments and monitoring the six Ps.

NURSING PEARLS

The six Ps of compartment syndrome are pain, pallor, paresthesia, pulselessness, paralysis, and pressure.

HAND AND FOOT MALFORMATIONS
- Fetal hand and arm development takes place during weeks 4 to 6 of gestation; any disruption during this time may lead to hand malformations.

Types of Hand Malformations
- Cleft hand: missing finger/fingers in the center of the hand, leaving a V-shaped space (cleft) ▶

Types of Hand Malformations (*continued*)

- Polydactyly: presence of extra digits
- Radial club hand: malformed radius, causing a short and curved forearm
- Syndactyly: fingers fused together

Types of Foot Malformations

- Metatarsus adductus: metatarsal bones that have deviated toward the middle of the body, usually caused by abnormal position in utero and improves over 6 to 12 weeks; treatment possibly needed after 3 to 4 months with possible bracing, casting, shoes, or rarely surgery
- Clubfoot: a multifactorial deformity including internal rotation of the leg, inversion and adduction of the forefoot, inversion of the heel, and limitation of extension of the ankle
- Polydactyly: presence of extra digits
- Syndactyly: toes fused together
- Overlapping toes

Risk Factors

- Genetic and environmental factors
- Family history of hand/foot malformations
- Fetal malpresentation in utero
- Most cases with no known cause

[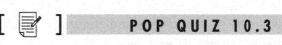]   **COMPLICATIONS**

Complications of hand/foot malformations include decreased range of motion of the affected hand/foot, mobility issues, and arthritis.

Diagnosis

Diagnostic Testing

- Most hand or foot malformations can be diagnosed on inspection of the deformity at birth; however, an x-ray may be needed to determine the extent of tissue or bone involvement.

Treatment

- Physical therapy
- Splinting/casting
- Stretching
- Surgery

[ ] **POP QUIZ 10.3**

An infant has just been casted for a clubfoot deformity and has been crying for the past hour. What interventions should the nurse perform?

LIMB MALFORMATIONS

Congenital limb malformations occur when an upper or lower limb does not form at all or does not form appropriately.

- Congenital constriction band syndrome (fibrous bands of amniotic tissue get tangled around the limbs/extremities of the fetus)
- Duplication
- Failure of differentiation of parts
- Failure of formation of parts (arrested development)
- Overgrowth (limb is larger than normal)
- Undergrowth (limb is smaller than normal)

Risk Factors

- Abnormal fetal presentation in utero
- Certain medications
- Genetic abnormalities ▶

Risk Factors (continued)

- Growth restrictions
- Maternal exposure to chemicals, smoke, or viruses while pregnant

Diagnosis

- Most limb malformations can be diagnosed on inspection of the deformity at birth; however, an x-ray may be needed to determine the extent of tissue or bone involvement.

Treatment

- Physical therapy
- Prosthetics
- Splinting/bracing
- Surgery

[🧠]   COMPLICATIONS

Complications of limb malformations include delayed mobility and developmental milestones.

SKELETAL DYSPLASIA

- *Skeletal dysplasia* is a group of conditions that affect the formation and growth of an infant's cartilage and bones.
- Most skeletal dysplasias are due to genetic abnormalities.

Types of Skeletal Dysplasia

- Achondroplasia: This is a type of short-limbed dwarfism characterized by short forearms and legs, larger head, and normal-sized torso.
- Achondrogenesis: Achondrogenesis severely affects bone formation. In addition to short limbs, infants have small, narrow chests and underdeveloped lungs, leading to pulmonary hypoplasia. These infants do not survive long after birth.
- Campomelic dysplasia: This is a fatal type of skeletal dysplasia resulting in severe bowing of the long bones. It also causes disorders of sexual development.
- Short-rib polydactyly syndrome: This is characterized by short limbs, short ribs, and polydactyly of the fingers and/or toes. Short ribs lead to pulmonary hypoplasia, which prevents survival after birth.
- Osteogenesis imperfecta: This is also known as "brittle bone" disease. Bones break easily. Signs and symptoms include small stature, curved spine, scleral blueness, breathing difficulties, and muscle weakness.

Types of Osteogenesis Imperfecta

- Type I: mildest and most common form; does not cause bone deformity
- Type II: causes multiple broken bones prior to birth; infants often do not survive
- Type III: causes multiple broken bones at birth and severe physical disabilities
- Type IV: causes mild to moderate bone deformity

[🧠]   COMPLICATIONS

Complications of osteogenesis imperfecta can include osteoporosis, hearing loss, and permanent deformities.

Diagnosis

Laboratory Testing

- Prenatal genetic testing

Diagnostic Testing
- Prenatal ultrasound
- X-ray

Treatment
- Bracing
- Physical therapy
- Growth hormone therapy
- Surgery

DIAGNOSTIC PROCEDURES

Fetal Imaging
- Fetal ultrasound: monitors growth and development and identifies birth defects and abnormalities in the anatomy

Imaging
- MRI
- Ultrasound
- X-ray

RESOURCES

Boston Children's Hospital. *Hip Dysplasia*. https://www.childrenshospital.org/conditions/developmental-dysplasia -hip#hip-dysplasia-in-babies

Children's Hospital of Philadelphia. *Congenital Limb Defects*. https://www.chop.edu/conditions-diseases /congenital-limb-defects

Children's Minnesota. *What is skeletal dysplasia?* https://www.childrensmn.org/services/care-specialties -departments/fetal-medicine/conditions-and-services/skeletal-dysplasia

Cleveland Clinic. *Congenital Hand Differences*. https://my.clevelandclinic.org/health/diseases/16890-congenital -hand-differences

Cleveland Clinical. *Osteogenesis Imperfecta (OI)*. https://my.clevelandclinic.org/health/diseases/15807-osteogenesis -imperfecta-oi

Gore, A., & Spencer, J. (2004). *American Family Physician*. The Newborn Foot. https://www.aafp.org/afp/2004 /0215/p865.html#:~:text = Common%20newborn%20foot%20abnormalities%20include,overlapping%20 toes%2C%20and%20amniotic%20bands

Liu, R., &Thompson, G. (2017). *Obgyn Key*. Musculoskeletal Disorders in Neonates. https://obgynkey.com /musculoskeletal-disorders-in-neonates

Nationwide Children's. *Newborn Clavicle Fractures*. https://www.nationwidechildrens.org/conditions /newborn-clavicle-fractures

McKee-Garrett, T. (2021). Neonatal birth injuries. *UpToDate*. https://www.uptodate.com/contents/neonatal-birth -injuries

INTEGUMENTARY SYSTEM

DEVELOPMENT OF THE INTEGUMENTARY SYSTEM

Overview

- Newborn skin serves a pivotal role in the transition from the fluid-filled intrauterine environment to extrauterine life.
- Newborn skin is vital to thermoregulation, mechanical protection, and immunosurveillance. It acts as a barrier to prevent insensible water loss.
- Skin is made up of three layers: the epidermis, dermis, and subcutaneous fat.

TERM NEWBORN VARIATIONS

- Full-term infants have a well-developed epidermis and stratum corneum.
- *Vernix*, a thick, waxy substance, protects the fetus' skin from amniotic fluid in the womb. It helps maintain skin hydration, thermoregulation, and skin acidification. Vernix has antimicrobial properties and should be rubbed into the newborn's skin after birth. Premature infants may have less vernix depending on what gestation they are born as vernix typically begins producing around 28 weeks.
- *Lanugo* is soft, fine hair covering the fetus while inside the uterus. It helps protect the fetus' skin and keep them warm. Lanugo begins to develop around 16 to 20 weeks' gestation. Premature infants typically have more lanugo when they are born as it tends to shed prior to becoming a full-term newborn. If a full-term baby is born with lanugo, it will fall out on its own over a few weeks.
- *Milia* are tiny, white, firm raised bumps on the newborn's face that will disappear on their own.
- Mild acne may appear, caused by the mother's hormones. Acne clears on its own in a few weeks.
- *Erythema toxicum* is a common harmless rash that looks like pustules on the face, trunk, legs, and arms. It disappears by 1 week of age.
- *Harlequin sign* is a phenomenon that presents as a well-demarcated color change, with half of the body displaying erythema and the other half pallor. The condition is seen in 10% of healthy newborns, is benign, and fades away in 30 seconds to 20 minutes. It may be more prone to happening if the newborn is placed on their side. Harlequin sign is most common between 2 and 5 days of life but may happen up to a few weeks.

Birthmarks

Stork Bites

- Small pink or red patches often found on a newborn's eyelids, between the eyes, the upper lip, and the back of the neck
- Caused by a concentration of immature blood vessels and may be most visible when the newborn is crying
- Fade or disappear completely over time

Congenital Dermal Melanocytosis

- Also known as Mongolian spots ▶

Congenital Dermal Melanocytosis (continued)

- Blue or purple-colored areas typically seen on the lower back or buttocks
- Usually found in darker skinned newborns
- Caused by a concentration of pigmented cells
- Usually disappear in the first 4 years of life

Hemangiomas

- Bright or dark red, raised or swollen bumpy areas that usually occur on the head but may surface on other areas of the body
- Formed by a concentration of tiny, immature blood vessels
- May not be present at birth but usually develop in the first 2 months of life
- Typically grow over several months and gradually fade by 9 years of age

Port-Wine Stain

- Flat, pink-, red-, or purple-colored birthmark usually occurring on the head or neck
- Caused by a concentration of dilated tiny capillaries
- May be small or cover large areas of the body
- Does not change color when pressed and does not disappear over time
- May become darker or thicker as a person gets older

[🌐] **NURSING PEARLS**

Due to immature skin structure and lack of vernix caseosa, preterm infants have an alkaline skin surface for a longer period of time compared with full-term infants.

PHYSIOLOGY OF THE INTEGUMENTARY SYSTEM

Stratum Corneum

- *Stratum corneum* is composed of several layers of flattened corneocytes arranged in an overlapping fashion.
- Thickness varies by body region. The thinnest are on the face, eyelids, and genitalia. The thickest are on the palms and soles.
- Term infants have a well-developed stratum corneum which contains about 10 to 20 layers.
- Preterm infants may only have two to three layers.
- Immaturity of the stratum corneum causes increased fluid and heat loss, leading to electrolyte imbalances, increased infection risk, and reduced thermoregulation ability.

Diminished Cohesion of Epidermis and Dermis

- Preterm infants have fewer and more widely spaced fibrils providing cohesion between the epidermis and the dermis. This increases the risk of skin injury.
- Skin breakdown is likely with the use of adhesives due to a stronger bond forming with the epidermis than the epidermis to the dermis.

Skin pH

- Skin pH (acidification) is vital to epidermal barrier maturation and maintaining bacterial and chemical resistance of the skin.
- pH is higher (more alkaline) at >6.0 immediately after birth and decreases (becomes more acidic) over the first few weeks of life.
- A term infant's pH is <5.0. ▶

Skin pH (*continued*)

■ A preterm infant's pH is <5.5 by 1 week and <5.1 by 1 month. This makes them more susceptible to infection during this time.

ASSESSMENT OF THE INTEGUMENTARY SYSTEM

The Neonatal Skin Condition Score

■ This is a tool used to evaluate the skin condition in neonates.

■ It evaluates erythema, breakdown, and dryness.

■ Scores range from 3 to 9, with 3 indicating a perfect score and 9 indicating the worst score.

■ High scores indicate the presence of serious skin disease.

■ Low scores indicate normal skin.

Risk Factors for Skin Injury

■ The infant's gestational age or condition at birth has a direct relation to their risk of skin injury.

■ Specific risk factors include edema, immobility, impaired tissue perfusion, ostomy, skin integrity, surgery, sepsis, and malnutrition.

THERMOREGULATION

Overview

■ *Thermoregulation* involves maintaining a neutral thermal environment to ensure the minimal metabolic activity and oxygen consumption required to conserve body temperature.

■ Effective thermoregulation requires adequate energy stores (glucose), insulation (fat deposits), hypothalamic function, and muscle tone.

NEUTRAL THERMAL ENVIRONMENT

■ Maintenance of the infant's temperature, including a stable metabolic state as well as minimal oxygen and energy expenditure

■ Best achieved when infants can maintain core temperatures between 97.7°F and 99.5°F (36.5°C and 37.5°C)

[📝] **POP QUIZ 11.1**

A 26-week infant is about to be delivered. What interventions can the nurse take to reduce evaporative heat loss?

Nursing Interventions

■ Provide environmental thermostability by preventing heat loss and applying adequate radiant warmth in infants unable to maintain a neutral thermal environment on their own. This can be achieved by utilizing incubators and radiant warmer beds.

HEAT LOSS PRINCIPLES

■ *Evaporation*: heat loss occurring during conversion of liquid to vapor (e.g., delivery or after a bath)

■ *Convection*: heat transfer from the body surface to the surrounding air (e.g., newborn is exposed to cold air)

■ *Conduction*: transfer of heat from one object to another object in direct contact with the body (e.g., when a newborn is placed naked on a cold bed or scale) ►

HEAT LOSS PRINCIPLES (*continued*)

■ *Radiation*: transfer of heat to cooler solid objects not in direct contact with the body (e.g., indirect exposure to a cold window or wall in the room)

HYPOTHERMIA CRITICAL FINDINGS

■ Occurs at core body temperatures below 97.7°F (36.5°C)
■ Cold stress: 96.8°F and 97.5°F (36°C and 36.4°C)
■ Moderate hypothermia: 89.6°F and 96.6°F (32°C and 35.9°C)
■ Severe hypothermia: <89.6°F (32°C)
■ Caused by the infant's use of chemically mediated thermogenesis in an attempt to increase core temperature
■ Nonshivering thermogenesis: This is the mechanism by which the sympathetic nervous system is triggered by cold stress. Neonates use norepinephrine-directed lipolysis of brown adipose (around the neck, scapular area, kidney regions) to create local heat reactions that are carried throughout the rest of the bloodstream to warm the body.

Signs and Symptoms

■ Palpable cold temperature
■ Acrocyanosis
■ Irritability
■ Hypotonia
■ Decreased feedings
■ Hypoglycemia

Complications

Neonates subsequently experience a rapid increase in overall metabolic rate that can lead to:.
■ Hypoxia
■ Hypoglycemia
■ Bradycardia
■ Hematologic and coagulation dysfunction
■ Gastrointestinal and renal changes
■ Metabolic acidosis
■ Organ damage
■ Intraventricular hemorrhage
■ Mortality

HYPERTHERMIA CRITICAL FINDINGS

■ Core temperature above 37.5°C
■ Usually secondary to an external source but may also be caused by sepsis, hypermetabolism, neonatal abstinence syndrome (NAS), and maternal hyperthermia

Signs and Symptoms

■ Irritability
■ Poor feeding
■ Flushing ▶

Signs and Symptoms (*continued*)

- Hypotension
- Tachypnea
- Apnea
- Lethargy
- Abnormal posturing
- Elevated peripheral or core temperature

Complications

- Seizures
- Coma
- Neurologic damage
- Death

[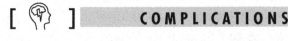] **COMPLICATIONS**

Rapid reduction in temperature is associated with the potential for cold stress shock. External heat source temperatures should only be adjusted 0.5 of a degree or less at a time. Continuous monitoring of temperature is needed.

PREVENTION OF HEAT/COLD STRESS

- Dry the infant immediately post delivery and place skin-to-skin or on a radiant warmer.
- Use incubators and radiant warmers.
- Use hats for newborns to prevent heat loss from scalp.
- Delay bathing in newborns.
- Continuously monitor temperature.
- Position probe on the abdomen in a supine infant, and on the back over the flanks in prone position to avoid hypo- or hyperthermia. Do not place the probe on areas of brown adipose tissue to avoid activating brown fat metabolism.
- Adjust incubator temperatures by 0.5 degrees or less at a time to avoid sudden changes in the infant's temperature.
- Rewarming after hypothermia should be well-controlled to avoid hyperthermia.

Incubators

- Provide a controlled, enclosed heat environment to ensure neutral thermoregulation
- Support neurodevelopmental health for preterm babies
- Reduction in noise and light
- Can be operated in servo where the temperature is regulated by a temperature probe attached to the newborn's skin or through environmental control where the infant is dressed and wrapped and the air temperature of the incubator is set
- Allow for the addition of humidification (see next section) for thermoregulation
- Not effective if frequent access to the baby is required for procedures or surgery
- Temperature stability: cannot be maintained with open portholes or sides down

Humidification

- *Humidification* reduces transepidermal water loss (TEWL) and supports temperature regulation, fluid and electrolyte management, and skin integrity.
- It is used in infants born less than 30 weeks' gestation. 80% humidity may be used for the first 7 days of life. Gradually reduce humidity by 5% each day until 2 weeks of age.

Radiant Warmers

- It is an open-care crib system that allows easy access to the infant requiring frequent intervention, continuous direct observation, and temperature support. ▶

Radiant Warmers (*continued*)

- Since it is not an enclosed system, the temperature can fluctuate depending on the surrounding environment.
- Humidification is not applicable in this setting.

Other Methods

- Plastic or polyurethane wraps reduce the incidence of hypothermia. They should be used in the delivery room for infants born less than 28 weeks' gestation. The infant should not be dried and should be placed immediately into the wrap or bag after delivery.
- Warming mattresses may be used in all premature infants after delivery, during transport to the NICU, and for up to 2 hours post delivery.
- Infants older than 28 weeks should be double-wrapped in warm blankets post delivery until placed under a heat source for assessment.
- Use kangaroo care or skin-to-skin practices (see Chapter 17, Neonatal Foundations).
- Hybrid beds such as the General Electric Giraffe bed act as incubators and can also raise the hood and function as an open-radiant warmer. They are beneficial in premature infants.

Open Crib

- Infants are typically ready to transfer into an open crib when they weigh >1700 grams, have consistent weight gain over the previous week, have stabilized apneic and bradycardic events in medically stable condition, and the incubator air temperature has been 89.6°F (32°C) or less over a 24-hour period.
- Replacement back to an incubator should be considered if the infant's temperature consistently drops below 97.7°F (36.5°C) within 4 hours, the infant fails to gain weight and is expending too many calories, or the infant has increased apnea or bradycardia episodes or increased work of breathing.

PATHOPHYSIOLOGY: INTEGUMENTARY SYSTEM DISORDERS

Overview

- Preterm infants are at an increased risk of integumentary system disorders.
- Neonates have a greater risk of infection and injury due to epidermal barrier immaturity and antimicrobial skin defenses.
- Careful assessment is needed to prevent and appropriately treat skin injury, diaper dermatitis, and extravasations.

SKIN INJURY

- Mechanical: pressure, shear/friction abrasions, skin stripping-tape removal, trauma
- Chemical: irritants, incontinence-diaper dermatitis, extravasation
- Thermal: contact with hot or cold objects
- Infectious: invasion by microorganisms
- Congenital: genetic mutations causing errors in epidermal and dermal maturation
- Vascular compromise: necrosis caused by interruption of blood supply

DIAPER DERMATITIS

- Inflammatory reaction of the skin of the perineal areas known as diaper rash
- Most common skin disorder seen in infants
- May be caused by chemical irritation or infection (*Candida*) atopic dermatitis
- Usually mild and self-limited, requiring minimal intervention

Types

- Contact diaper dermatitis: skin that is irritated from urine and stool; skin appears red and shiny; may be seen on the buttocks, thighs, abdomen, and waist; creases or folds usually not affected
- *Candida* diaper dermatitis: yeast infection of the diaper area; may also appear in the mouth (thrush); skin is a deep red color with patches outside the diaper area; folds of the thighs may be affected
- Seborrheic diaper dermatitis: skin is red with yellow, oily patches; may affect the face, scalp, or neck at the same time; affects skinfolds in the diaper

Treatment

- Skincare
- Adequate hygiene: frequent diaper changes
- Avoidance of irritants
- Topical emollients for prevention and treatment
- Corticosteroids: may be used if no improvement is seen within 2 to 3 days and rash is moderate to severe
- Topical antifungals like nystatin for *Candida* infections
- Topical antibiotics for bacterial infections

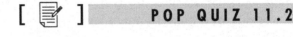

POP QUIZ 11.2

An infant has a reoccurring diaper rash that has not resolved in several days. The nurse notes tiny little raised red bumps throughout the diaper area. What would be the next course of action?

INTRAVENOUS EXTRAVASATIONS

- These are caused by intravenous (IV) fluids that escape into the surrounding tissue.
- These can occur with parenteral nutrition.
- Peripheral IVs are the most common cause.
- 70% of extravasation injuries occur in extremely premature infants.

Signs and Symptoms

- Redness
- Swelling
- Blanching
- Pain and tenderness
- Cool skin temperature around the IV site

Complications

- Pain
- Necrosis
- Tendon and nerve damage
- Compartment syndrome
- Scars
- Contractures
- Deformities leading to function restriction/amputations

COMMON PROCEDURES AND PREVENTIVE CARE

Overview

- Bathing should be delayed after birth to allow antimicrobial properties to be absorbed.
- Emollients and skin barriers can help prevent injury in a fragile newborn skin. ▶

Overview (*continued*)

- Medical adhesives should be used cautiously to prevent skin breakdown.
- Careful attention to skin integrity and prompt wound management are imperative in the premature infant.

BATHING

- Bathing in the immediate postbirth period puts the infant at risk of hypothermia, respiratory distress, hypoglycemia, and increased oxygen consumption.
- Current research supports delayed bathing to allow the antimicrobial properties of the vernix to be absorbed. Delay time varies depending on the institution; typically, it is recommended to wait at least 8 to 24 hours or longer.
- Antiseptic cleansers should be avoided. Bathe with infant appropriate soap.
- Neonates do not require frequent bathing; limit to one to three times a week as bathing can dry out skin and cause distress.

Types of Baths

- Sponge bath: Use prior to umbilical stump falling off. It is used in premature infants with breathing equipment and IV lines.
- Immersion tub bathing: Place the infant's entire body up to the head and neck into warm water to decrease evaporative heat loss.
- Swaddled bathing: Infant is swaddled in a flexed, midline position before being immersed in the water. This promotes a calm, quiet state.

EMOLLIENTS

- Mild emollients can be applied to the skin of neonates after bathing to help hydration of the skin.
- Emollients supply necessary lipids and water to the stratum corneum layer of skin to help preserve hydration, decrease TEWL, and improve structural integrity of the skin.
- The use of emollients may improve the overall barrier function of the skin.
- They may also be helpful in reducing infective dermatitis in preterm infants.

SKIN DISINFECTANTS

- Use of antiseptic disinfectants should be avoided.
- Antiseptic disinfectants may cause chemical burns in neonates.

UMBILICAL CORD CARE

- The cord should be cut using sterile scissors/blade at birth.
- The cord should be clamped, and the clamp kept on for at least 24 hours.
- The cord should be allowed to dry and fall off naturally; no antimicrobial or drying agents are necessary. The cord should be kept clean and exposed to air or loosely covered by clothing. Submerging baths should be avoided until the cord falls off.
- Educating parents on the signs and symptoms of omphalitis can decrease morbidity and mortality. Symptoms include tenderness, erythema, bleeding, and purulent drainage.

MEDICAL ADHESIVES

- Extra caution is needed when applying or removing adhesive tapes.
- Adhesives are associated with skin tears, tensions blisters, and contact dermatitis.
- Use organic, oil-based solvents or silicon-based removers for safe removal.
- Duoderm, a skin barrier, can be used under tape for nasogastric tubes, or applied to areas like the nasal bridge or septum to prevent injury from respiratory devices.

WOUND MANAGEMENT

Evaluation

Evaluate if wounds are a result of:

- Skin fragility
- Genetic disorders (epidermolysis bullosa)
- Pressure injury
- Immobility
- Sepsis
- Previous surgeries
- Chemical burns from antiseptics
- Medical devices (nasal breakdown from continuous positive airway pressure [CPAP])
- IV line extravasation injuries
- Adhesive-related

Nursing Interventions

Monitor neonates for irritant or allergic contact dermatitis. Potential causes include:

- Leakage of body fluids
- Antiseptic use
- Adhesives
- Topical ointments (consider need carefully)
- Wound dressings

Considerations

- Wound closure in infants is faster than adults due to an increased number of fibroblasts producing granulation tissue.
- The process of wound repair depends on the type of tissue that has been injured.
- Epithelium and endothelial cells have regenerative capacities for replacement of damaged tissue. If the wound is confined to the epithelium and upper layers of the dermis, scar tissue is not formed.
- Full thickness: Skin injury extends through the dermis to the hypodermis, muscle, or tendon tissues. Repair requires scar tissue formation (surgical wound, deep extravasation injury).
- Wound healing can be divided into four stages: hemostasis, inflammation, proliferation/repair, and maturation/remolding.
- Adequate tissue perfusion and oxygenation are necessary for optimal wound healing.

Treatment

- Cover dressings; provide protection by limiting exposure to microbial contamination, maintaining temperature, and additional trauma. Caution is needed when removing dressings to prevent further trauma.
- Remove necrotic tissue and slough to promote healing and decrease risk of infection. ▶

Treatment (*continued*)

- For autolytic wounds, debridement includes leaving the dressing for several days to maintain moisture and allowing for tissue breakdown.
- For sharp wounds (scalpel, forceps, scissors), debridement includes wet to dry dressings and irrigation.
- Wounds with significant depth should be packed with dressing materials to avoid abscess. The material should make contact with the wound bed but avoid excess pressure.

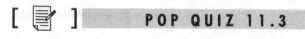

NURSING PEARLS

Two people should provide wound care so that one can focus on comforting the infant and the other can perform wound care.

POP QUIZ 11.3

Local wound infections can cause tissue death, increase wound size, and decrease oxygen to the wound, which delays wound healing. What are the classic hallmarks that indicate acute wound infection?

RESOURCES

El-Atawi, K., & Elhalik, M. (2016). Neonatal skin care. *Pediatrics and Neonatal Nursing: Open Access, 2*(2). http://doi.org/10.16966/2470-0983.e103

Fox, M. D. (n.d.). *Wound care in the neonatal intensive care unit*. Neonatal network: NN. Retrieved May 9, 2022, from https://pubmed.ncbi.nlm.nih.gov/21846624

Johns Hopkins Medicine. (2021). *Diaper dermatitis*. Retrieved May 30, 2022, from https://www.hopkinsmedicine.org/health/conditions-and-diseases/diaper-dermatitis

Hackenberg, R. K., Kabir, K., Müller, A., Heydweiller, A., Burger, C., & Welle, K. (2021). Extravasation injuries of the limbs in neonates and children—development of a treatment algorithm. *Deutsches Arzteblatt International, 118*(33–34), 547–554. https://doi.org/10.3238/arztebl.m2021.0220

Kuller, J. M. M. (2015). *Update on newborn bathing*. Medscape. Retrieved May 9, 2022, from https://www.medscape.com/viewarticle/838253_3

Lara-Corrales, I., Sibbald, C. J., Ayello, E. A., & Sibbald, G. R. (n.d.). *Focus on skin and wounds in neonates and children*. Advances in skin & wound care. Retrieved May 9, 2022, from https://pubmed.ncbi.nlm.nih.gov/32427782

Royal Children's hospital. (n.d.). *Key differences in infant skin*. Retrieved May 7, 2022, from https://www.rch.org.au/uploadedFiles/Main/Content/rchcpg/hospital_clinical_guideline_index/Key%20Differences%20in%20Infant%20Skin.pdf

Stewart, D., Benitz, W., Committee on fetus and newborn. (2016). Umbilical cord care in the newborn infant. *Pediatrics, 138* (3), e20162149. https://doi.org/10.1542/peds.2016-2149

APPENDIX 11.1 MEDICATIONS FOR THE INTEGUMENTARY SYSTEM

INDICATIONS	MECHANISM OF ACTION	CONTRAINDICATIONS, PRECAUTIONS, AND ADVERSE EFFECTS
Topical aminoglycosides (bacitracin/neomycin/polymyxin B)		
• Neomycin and polymyxin B: effective against gram-negative aerobic bacteria • Bacitracin: effective against gram-positive bacteria • Used for wound management, skin abrasions, and minor burns	• Bacitracin: inhibits bacterial cell wall synthesis • Neomycin: prevents formation of functional proteins and inhibits DNA polymerase • Polymyxin B: binds to phospholipids on cell membranes of gram-negative bacteria	• Adverse reactions include hypersensitivity reactions, diarrhea, hearing loss, and pruritus. • Medication is contraindicated for use against viral or fungal infections. • Take precaution for systemic exposure, especially in children with renal failure.

(continued)

APPENDIX 11.1 MEDICATIONS FOR THE INTEGUMENTARY SYSTEM (*continued*)

INDICATIONS	MECHANISM OF ACTION	CONTRAINDICATIONS, PRECAUTIONS, AND ADVERSE EFFECTS
Glycopeptide antibiotics (vancomycin)		
• Treat bacterial infections • Treat gram-positive osteomyelitis bacterial infections • Treat bloodstream infections, pneumonia, meningitis, and skin and soft tissue infections	• Bind to bacterial cell wall, inhibiting synthesis	• Adverse effects include vancomycin flushing syndrome, chest pain, chills, and dizziness; medication can have ototoxic effects. • Adverse effects may include pruritus, Stevens–Johnson syndrome, leukopenia, thrombocytopenia, myalgia, vertigo, malaise, dyspnea, wheezing, and fever. • Adverse effects include ototoxicity, renal toxicity, extravasation, and phlebitis. • Administer over at least 60 minutes and monitor for adverse effects including redness in the face, neck, torso, and upper extremities (vancomycin flushing syndrome, formerly known as red man/neck syndrome), and hypotension.
Antibacterials: topical (mupirocin)		
• Treat skin infections	• Inhibit bacterial protein and RNA synthesis	• Adverse effects include headache, localized burning, and rash. • Medication is contraindicated for use in infants less than 3 months old and also contraindicated for use on burns. • Use caution with prolonged use due to overgrowth of resistant organisms.
Antifungals: topical (nystatin)		
• Treat candidiasis (cutaneous candidiasis and candidal diaper dermatitis)	• Bind to sterols in the cell membrane of fungal cells	• Adverse reactions include Stevens–Johnson syndrome, eczema, bronchospasm, and angioedema. • Use caution in patients with paraben hypersensitivity and diabetes mellitus.
Zinc oxides: diaper cream (Desitin, Boudreaux's Butt Paste, Balmex)		
• Mineral used to treat diaper rash and minor skin irritations	• Provide physical barrier to prevent irritation and help heal damaged skin	• Stop using if worsening of diaper rash occurs.

12 HEAD, EYES, EARS, NOSE, AND THROAT

ASSESSMENT OF THE HEAD, EYES, EARS, NOSE, AND THROAT

Overview

- HEENT assessment is important in detecting abnormalities in the head, eyes, ears, nose, and throat.

HEAD

- Assess molding, fontanelles, swelling, and symmetry.
- Measure head circumference.

EYES

- Inspect the eyes, eyelids, sclerae, irises, pupils, and conjunctiva.
- Eyelids should open and close completely.
- Sclera should be white in appearance.
- Iris should be round with the appropriate color (permanent color at 6 to 12 months of age).
- Pupils should be equal, round, and assessed for reactivity to light and accommodation.
- Conjunctiva should be pink.
- Red reflex should be present in infants.

EARS

External Structures

- Inspect the pinna on each side of the head.
- Assess ear alignment by visualizing a horizontal line from the outer orbit of the eye. The pinna should reach the horizontal line.
- Measure the angle of the ear by visualizing a perpendicular vertical line across that horizontal line. The pinna should be within 10° of the vertical line.
- Palpate the pinna for tenderness.

Internal Structures

- Assess the internal structures with an otoscope.
- Inspect the tympanic membrane.
- The tympanic membrane should be a light pearly pink or gray color.
- Light reflex is a cone-shaped reflection and will be seen at 5 o'clock position in the right ear or 7 o'clock position in the left ear.

NOSE

- Internal mucosa and turbinates should be pink and free of swelling.
- Nostrils should be present and patent.
- Septum should be midline and intact.
- The nose should be midline and skin color consistent throughout the head and face.
- Abnormal findings include discharge, redness, or septum deviation.

THROAT

- Inspect the cheeks, tongue, gums, teeth, hard and soft palate, and uvula.

ABNORMAL FINDINGS OF THE HEAD AND FACE

Overview

- Abnormal findings of the head and face may include congenital abnormalities or trauma from birth.

CLEFT ABNORMALITIES

- *Cleft lip* and *cleft palate* are birth defects where the lip and/or palate do not close properly.
- Cleft lip may be a small notch in the lip, or there can be a separation from the upper lip toward the nose.
- Cleft palate is an opening in the roof of the mouth connecting the mouth and nasal cavity.
- Infants may have one condition or both.
- The cause is unknown but thought to be genetic and/or the baby's environment in utero.

Risk Factors

- Maternal smoking
- Gestational diabetes
- Maternal exposure to certain medications while pregnant

Nursing Interventions

- The infant will need a specialized nipple for feeding.
- The infant's respiratory rate and effort should be monitored continuously throughout feedings.

Treatment

- Cleft lip: Surgery should be performed within the first year of life, usually around 3 months old.
- Cleft palate: Surgery should be performed before 18 months, usually at 10 to 12 months. A bone marrow is grafted to the palate, usually from the hip.
- Additional surgeries are as needed.

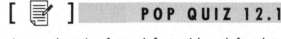

[📝] POP QUIZ 12.1

A nurse is caring for an infant with a cleft palate who is due to eat. Which approach will the nurse take while feeding the infant?

TRAUMA: CEPHALOHEMATOMA AND CAPUT SUCCEDANEUM

- See Chapter 9, Nervous System.

HAIR WHORLS

- *Hair whorls* are patches of hair growing in a circular direction around a visible center.
- One main hair whorl is typically seen over the vertex of the head.
- When there are multiple hair whorls, or they are in unusual locations, abnormal brain growth may be present.

MICROGNATHIA

- Condition in which the lower jaw is undersized; sometimes called mandibular hypoplasia
- Fairly common in infants and may correct itself as the child grows
- Can cause abnormal tooth alignment

Signs and Symptoms

- Apnea
- Feeding difficulties
- Noisy breathing
- Poor sleeping

Treatment

Nonsurgical Therapy

- Continuous positive airway pressure (CPAP) or bilevel positive airway pressure (BiPAP)
- Nasopharyngeal airways
- Prone positioning

Surgical Treatment

- Mandibular distraction osteogenesis, where the lower jaw is made larger by lengthening the lower jawbone and relieving airway obstruction
- Tongue-lip adhesion
- Tracheostomy

ABNORMAL FINDINGS OF THE EYES

Overview

- Abnormal findings in the eyes that may cause issues with vision and may possibly require surgical intervention include retinopathy of prematurity (ROP), cataracts, and glaucoma.
- Ophthalmia neonatorum refers to any conjunctivitis occurring within the first 28 days of life. It is often caused by a blocked lacrimal duct but may also be caused by a bacterial or viral infection.

RETINOPATHY OF PREMATURITY

- *ROP* is a developmental vascular proliferative disorder which occurs in the retina of premature infants with incomplete retinal vascularization.
- Initial injury may be caused by hypotension, hypoxia, or hyperoxia.
- Free radical formation may injure newly developing blood vessels.
- ROP advances irregularly until 40 to 45 weeks' postmenstrual age and resolves spontaneously in most infants.
- Screening consists of a comprehensive eye exam by an ophthalmologist.
- The pupil must be dilated to visualize the vitreous and retina.
- Laser photocoagulation may be needed in infants who progress further in disease.

International Classification

- Zone: disease location on the retinal surface in relation to the disc—central zone (I) to the outer crescent (zone III)
- Stage: severity from mild disease (flat white line of demarcation; stage 1) to most severe (total retinal detachment; stage 5)
- Extent: divides the retinal surface into 12 sections, similar to the hours of a clock
- Presence or absence of plus disease

CATARACTS AND GLAUCOMA

Cataracts

- *Cataracts* are opacity of the lens of the eye causing partial or total visual loss.
- Early detection and intervention is critical for good visual outcome.
- Asymmetry of the red reflex is a common finding.
- Infants with 20/50 vision or better, small opacities (less than 3 mm), or extra-axial opacities can be managed conservatively with glasses or contact lens correction.
- Otherwise, surgical correction is necessary.

Glaucoma

- Characterized by progressive optic neuropathy, cupping of the optic disc, and increased intraocular pressure
- May lead to optic nerve damage and visual loss
- Often asymptomatic
- Acetazolamide: may be given to reduce intraocular pressure in glaucoma (Appendix 12.1)
- Surgical intervention necessary

[📝]   **POP QUIZ 12.2**

Which postoperative education should the nurse provide to parents following cataract surgery of an infant?

INFECTIONS

- Infections of the eye may be viral or bacterial.

Bacterial

Examples of infections caused by bacteria include:

- *Chlamydia trachomatis*
- *Escherichia coli*
- Group A and B streptococci
- *Haemophilus influenzae*
- *Neisseria gonorrhoeae*
- *Pseudomonas*
- *Staphylococcus aureus*
- *Streptococcus pneumonia*

Treatment

- May require antibiotic eye ointment or drops depending on culture results

Viral

Examples of infections caused by viruses include:

- Adenovirus
- Herpes simplex

Treatment
- Regularly cleansing and warm soaks are typically sufficient treatment.

CONJUNCTIVITIS

- Conjunctivitis is inflammation of the conjunctiva. It is also known as pink eye.
- Causes include infections from birth such as bacteria, chlamydia, gonorrhea, and herpes simplex virus (HSV).

Signs and Symptoms
- Crusting of the eyelids
- Purulent drainage
- Swollen eyelids
- Watery drainage

Treatment
- Antibiotic drops or ointment for bacterial infections
- Erythromycin drops or ointment in newborns' eyes immediately after birth for neonatal conjunctivitis prevention
- Warm compress

[🧠]   **COMPLICATIONS**

If untreated, neonatal conjunctivitis can lead to severe illness, pneumonia, and permanent visual impairment.

CHORIORETINITIS

- Characterized by inflammation of the uvea (middle portion of the eye), the anterior portion of the uvea that includes the iris and ciliary body, and the posterior portion of the uvea or choroid
- Also known as uveitis

Subsets
- Infections
- Masquerade syndromes, such as lymphoma, leukemia, or retinal degeneration
- Systemic immune-mediated disease
- Syndromes confined to the eye

Signs and Symptoms
- Cells in the anterior chamber
- Floaters
- Red eye

Treatment
- Treatment varies depending on the etiology.

ABNORMAL FINDINGS OF THE EARS

Overview
- The location of the defect of the ear characterizes the hearing impairment.
- Abnormal findings in the alignment and formation of the ears may indicate certain conditions or hearing impairments.

HEARING IMPAIRMENT

- *Conductive* hearing loss originates in the middle ear and can result from recurrent otitis media. It affects the loudness of sounds.
- *Sensorineural* hearing loss is related to an inner ear or auditory nerve (cranial nerve [CN] VIII) problem. It is a result of congenital disabilities, ototoxic drugs, and exposure to excessive noise.
- The severity of hearing impairment is classified from slight to profound based on the hearing level in decibels.

ALIGNMENT

- Ears are considered low-set if the superior rim of the auricle is below a line drawn posteriorly from the superior orbital rim.
- Low-set ears are associated with trisomy 18 and 21, Treacher Collins syndrome, and Potter sequence.
- If the external ear is displaced anteriorly and outward, the infant may have mastoiditis, external otitis, or cellulitis.

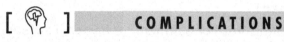

COMPLICATIONS

Commonly used ototoxic drugs include aminoglycosides, such as gentamicin, and high-dose loop diuretics, such as furosemide. These can cause acquired sensorineural hearing loss.

FORMATION

- Preauricular skin tags may be occasionally associated with hearing loss.
- Ear pits involving the auricle and preauricular skin pits are unlikely to be associated with hearing loss.
- A pit located in front of the tragus may infrequently extend into a subcutaneous cyst and become infected.

ABNORMAL FINDINGS OF THE NOSE AND THROAT

Overview

- Abnormal findings of the nose and throat are usually congenital. They may be mild and not found until later in childhood, or they may be more severe and require surgical intervention.

CHOANAL ATRESIA

- *Choanal atresia* is a congenital condition resulting in nasal tissue blocking the nasal airway.
- It may affect one or both sides of the nose.
- It may be made completely out of bone or a combination of bone and soft tissue.
- Infants may have difficulty breathing with bilateral choanal atresia unless they are crying. Bilateral choanal atresia requires intubation.
- Unilateral symptoms may include unilateral nasal drainage or obstruction. Symptoms may be mild and go unrecognized until the child is older.
- It is diagnosed by CT scan and a nasal endoscopy.
- Surgical treatment is necessary.

TRANSESOPHAGEAL FISTULA

- It is a congenital anomaly resulting in an abnormal connection between the esophagus and the trachea.
- Not being able to pass a nasogastric tube is usually the first cause of concern for transesophageal fistula.

Signs and Symptoms

- Respiratory distress
- Feeding difficulties
- Choking
- Risk for aspiration
- Full abdomen

Treatment

- Surgical treatment is necessary.

TRACHEOMALACIA

- Cartilage of the trachea is soft, weak, or floppy.
- It may cause the tracheal wall to collapse and block the airway.
- Diagnosis involves chest x-ray, physical exam, and possible bronchoscopy.

Signs and Symptoms

- Difficulty breathing
- High-pitched or rattling, noisy breaths
- Noisy breathing that may improve during sleep
- Recurrent pulmonary infections
- Severe coughing
- Wheezing

Treatment

Treatment depends on the cause.

- Antibiotics for infection
- Physical therapy and stretching exercises

TRACHEAL STENOSIS

- *Tracheal stenosis* is narrowing of the trachea.
- Congenital: The cartilage that supports the structure of the trachea can cause narrowing of the airway. It may include tracheal cartilaginous sleeves prone to obstruction and crusting. It may also include complete tracheal rings, consisting of several complete rings of cartilage with a narrowed diameter.
- Acquired: This may be caused by repeated irritation or injury, such as from an endotracheal tube.
- Diagnosis includes CT scan, MRI, or bronchoscopy.

Signs and Symptoms

- Apnea
- Chest congestion
- Cyanosis
- Stridor
- Wheezing

[📝]   **POP QUIZ 12.3**

The nurse notes that the newborn has a round, full belly. The nurse is unable to pass a nasogastric tube despite several attempts. Which condition would the nurse suspect?

DIAGNOSTIC PROCEDURES

Imaging

- CT scan
- MRI
- X-ray
- *Bronchoscopy*: This is a procedure that allows direct visualization of the throat, larynx, trachea, and lungs via a bronchoscope.
- *Endoscopy*: This is a procedure that is used to diagnose and sometimes treat conditions that affect the upper part of the digestive system, including the esophagus, stomach, and duodenum via an endoscope.
- *Laryngoscopy*: This is a procedure that allows direct visualization of the throat and larynx.
- Nursing responsibilities for all procedures include administering any anesthetics as ordered, monitoring respiratory status and vital signs (VS) during and after the procedure, and assisting with the procedure including handling the specimens taken.

Laboratory Tests

- Complete blood count
- C-reactive protein (CRP)
- Surface cultures of the ear and eye

COMMON PROCEDURES

Surgery

- See individual diagnoses.

Therapy

- Chest physiotherapy
- Physical therapy
- Speech therapy

RESOURCES

Akangire, G., & Carter, B. (2016). Birth injuries in neonates. *Pediatrics in Review, 37*(11), 451–462. https://doi.org/10.1542/pir.2015-0125

Centers for Disease Control and Prevention. (2020). *Common eye disorders and diseases*. U.S. Department of Health and Human Services, Centers for Disease Control and Prevention. https://www.cdc.gov/visionhealth/basics/ced/index.html

Centers for Disease Control and Prevention. (2019). *Conjunctivitis*. U.S. Department of Health and Human Services, Centers for Disease Control and Prevention. https://www.cdc.gov/conjunctivitis/index.html

Green, G. E., & Ohye, R. G. (2021). Diagnosis and management of tracheal anomalies and tracheal stenosis. *Cummings Pediatric Otolaryngology*, 441–455. https://doi.org/10.1016/b978-0-323-69618-0.00030-5

Johnson, S. M., Wallace, D. K., & Meyers, T. M. (2005). *Ophthalmic medications in pediatric patients*. Medscape. Retrieved May 27, 2022, from https://www.medscape.com/viewarticle/504199_5

MedCrave Publishing. (2016). *Airway in the newborn patient. Journal of Anesthesia & Critical Care: Open Access*. Retrieved June 1, 2022, from https://www.medcraveonline.com/JACCOA/airway-in-the-newborn-patient.html

NHS. (n.d.). *Eye infections in the neonate: Ophthalmia Neonatorum and the management of systemic Gonococcal and Chlamydial infections*. NHS choices. Retrieved May 16, 2022, from https://www.clinicalguidelines.scot.nhs.uk/nhsggc-guidelines/nhsggc-guidelines/neonatology/eye-infections-in-the-neonate-ophthalmia-neonatorum-and-the-management-of-systemic-gonococcal-and-chlamydial-infections

O'Brien, J., Rinehart, T., Orzechowski, K. M., & Terrone, D. A. (2009). The normal neonate: Assessment of early physical findings. *The Global Library of Women's Medicine's Welfare of Women Global Health Programme*, (ISSN: 1756-2228). https://doi.org/10.3843/GLOWM.10147

Coats, D. K. (n.d.). Retinopathy of prematurity: Pathogenesis, epidemiology, classification, and screening. *UpToDate*. Retrieved May 16, 2022, from https://www.uptodate.com/contents/retinopathy-of-prematurity-pathogenesis-epidemiology-classification-and-screening#!

Smith, R. J. H., & Gooi, A. (2021). Hearing loss in children. *UpToDate*. https://www.uptodate.com/contents/hearing-loss-in-children-etiology?search=ototoxic%20drugs&source=search_result&selectedTitle=4~150&usage_type=default&display_rank=4#H29

Drutz, J. E. (n.d.). The pediatric physical examination: HEENT. *UpToDate*. Retrieved May 17, 2022, from https://www.uptodate.com/contents/the-pediatric-physical-examination-heent#!

APPENDIX 12.1 MEDICATIONS FOR HEAD, EYES, EARS, NOSE, AND THROAT

INDICATIONS	MECHANISM OF ACTION	CONTRAINDICATIONS, PRECAUTIONS, AND ADVERSE EFFECTS
Ophthalmologic anti-infectives (erythromycin)		
• Prevention of conjunctivitis in the newborn • Treatment of superficial eye infections	• Inhibit bacterial protein synthesis	• Adverse effects include eye irritation. • There are no contraindications.
Carbonic anhydrase inhibitors (acetazolamide)		
• Reduce intraocular pressure in glaucoma	• Reversible carbonic anhydrase inhibitor	• Medication is contraindicated in angle closure glaucoma.
Corticosteroids (prednisolone acetate)		
• Treat inflammatory conditions affecting the eye	• Penetrating and binding to cytoplasmic receptor proteins	• Medication can cause blurred vision. • Medication can cause watery eyes.
Antimicrobials (ampicillin, gentamicin, vancomycin, cefotaxime)		
• Infection • Sepsis	• Bind to penicillin-binding proteins to inhibit bacterial cell wall synthesis	• Monitor renal and hepatic function. • Use caution not to infuse rapidly with vancomycin as "red person/red neck" syndrome may occur.

13 ENDOCRINE/METABOLIC SYSTEM

PATHOPHYSIOLOGY: COMMON ENDOCRINE SYSTEM DISORDERS

Overview

- The *endocrine system* is responsible for regulating many bodily functions through the release of hormones.
- Disorders of the endocrine system place the newborn at risk of developing long-term complications. Early diagnosis and treatment is important.

DISORDERS OF THE PITUITARY GLAND

- The *pituitary gland* is responsible for regulating growth, metabolism, reproduction, and homeostasis.
- It produces eight hormones: human growth hormone, follicle-stimulating hormone (FSH), luteinizing hormone (LH), adrenocorticotropic hormone (ACTH), thyroid-stimulating hormone (TSH), prolactin, oxytocin, and antidiuretic hormone (ADH; vasopressin).
- Hyperpituitarism is rare in infancy.
- Congenital hypothyroidism (CH) is defined as a deficiency of one or more hormones produced by the pituitary gland.
- Hypopituitarism has both congenital and perinatal causes. Congenital causes include congenital infections, developmental defects of the pituitary gland, and genetic mutations. Perinatal causes include birth trauma/asphyxia and sepsis.

Signs and Symptoms

- Cholestasis
- Hypoglycemia
- Jitteriness
- Lethargy
- Midline defects (cleft lip, cleft palate)
- Polyuria
- Poor feeding and weight gain
- Prolonged hyperbilirubinemia
- Respiratory distress
- Temperature instability
- Undescended testes and micropenis
- Growth issues and short stature

DISORDERS OF SEXUAL DIFFERENTIATION

- *Disorders of sexual differentiation* (DSD) is defined as a discrepancy between the external genitalia, gonads, and chromosomal sex. ▶

DISORDERS OF SEXUAL DIFFERENTIATION (*continued*)

- Neonates with DSD can present with partial sets of both male and female reproductive organs, atypical appearances in their genitalia, or atypical sex chromosomes.
- DSDs are congenital and are caused by genetic, hormonal, or environmental factors during pregnancy.
- Congenital adrenal hyperplasia (CAH), the most common etiology, is an inherited disorder of the adrenal cortex resulting in hormone deficiencies.

Most Common Types of Disorders of Sexual Differentiation

- 46,XX DSD: female chromosomes, male or ambiguous genitalia
- 46,XY DSD: male chromosomes, female or ambiguous genitalia
- 46,XX ovotesticular: female chromosomes, tissue from both ovaries and testicles, genitals may be female, male, or ambiguous
- Sex chromosome DSD: atypical arrangement of chromosomes (XO or XXY), female or male genitalia
- Rokitansky syndrome: females who have XX chromosomes but are missing female reproductive organs such as the cervix, uterus, and ovaries

Signs and Symptoms

- Symptoms vary but most often present as ambiguous or mixed external genitalia.
- DSD may present with typical external genitals with abnormal or mixed internal reproductive organs.

Diagnostic Imaging

- MRI
- Ultrasound

Treatment

- Medications such as hormone replacement therapy may correct hormonal imbalances.
- Surgery may be done to correct the appearance of the genitals and improve fertility.

[ ]   **COMPLICATIONS**

The most severe complication can result from life-threatening salt wasting in CAH. If untreated, it can lead to shock and brain damage.

[ ]   **COMPLICATIONS**

Prolonged, severe hypothyroidism can cause myxedema coma, which is an endocrine emergency.

[⚡]   **ALERT!**

Congenital hypothyroidism is one of the most preventable causes of intellectual disability. However, most newborns with congenital hypothyroidism do not present with clinical manifestations, making an early diagnosis difficult. For this reason, this disease is included in the newborn screening program to detect cases as early as possible.

HYPOTHYROIDISM

Two kinds of hypothyroidism affect children:

- Acquired: most often caused by autoimmune thyroiditis (Hashimoto thyroiditis); can also be caused by thyroid disease and hypothalamus–pituitary disease
- Congenital: most often caused by an embryologic defect in the thyroid gland during development; can also be caused by iodine deficiency

Signs and Symptoms

- Constipation
- Facial/periorbital edema ▶

Signs and Symptoms (*continued*)

- Feeding difficulties
- Hoarse cry
- Hyperbilirubinemia
- Hypothermia
- Large fontanels
- Large, thick tongue
- Lethargy and hypotonia
- Pallor/mottling

Diagnosis

Labs

- Elevated T3 and TSH
- Low free T4
- Newborn screening

Diagnostic Testing

- Thyroid radionuclide uptake and scan
- Thyroid ultrasound

Treatment

- Levothyroxine (Appendix 13.1); ideal dose determined by normal TSH levels and improved symptoms

Nursing Interventions

- Palpate the thyroid to determine if firm or tender; assess for nodules or goiter.
- Assess the thyroid from the front and side.
- Monitor for irritability or restlessness.
- Monitor temperature and protect against temperature extremes.

Patient Education

- Adhere to frequent follow-up visits.
- Avoid soy formulas as they may decrease the effectiveness of levothyroxine.
- Take levothyroxine at the same time every day on an empty stomach. It may be crushed and mixed with milk, formula, or water to administer.

HYPERTHYROIDISM

- *Hyperthyroidism* is a hormonal imbalance caused by overproduction of thyroid hormone that affects growth and puberty.
- An insidious onset is characteristic of hyperthyroidism.
- Graves disease is the primary cause of hyperthyroidism. Autoantibodies bind to the thyrotropin receptor, stimulating the growth of the thyroid gland and the overproduction of thyroid hormone.

[✍] **POP QUIZ 13.1**

What medication education should the nurse teach the parents of a newborn being discharged on levothyroxine?

[ ] **COMPLICATIONS**

Thyroid storm is an acute, life-threatening event that presents with exaggerated hyperthyroidism symptoms: tachycardia, atrial fibrillation, agitation, fever, jaundice, nausea/vomiting, and restlessness. It can be caused by untreated hyperthyroidism, thyroid surgery, trauma, infection, or iodine overload. Labs show a low TSH and high T4/T3.

Signs and Symptoms

- Goiter
- Hepatosplenomegaly
- Hyperbilirubinemia
- Hyperthermia, flushing, and sweating
- Irritability and restlessness
- Jitteriness
- Petechiae
- Poor weight gain
- Tachycardia

Diagnosis

Labs

- Elevated total T4
- Low TSH 1
- Serum thyroid antibody test

Diagnostic Testing

- Radionuclide uptake and scan

Treatment

- Beta blockers to treat symptoms until a definitive solution
- Medications: antithyroid medications (Appendix 13.1)

Nursing Interventions

- Identify and manage symptoms.
- Provide a quiet, nonstimulating environment.

Patient Education

- Recognize signs of thyroid storm and notify the provider.

INBORN ERRORS OF METABOLISM

- Inborn errors of metabolism are rare genetic disorders that block the metabolism of nutrients and energy production.
- These disorders may affect either the breakdown or the storage of fats, proteins, or carbohydrates.

Signs and Symptoms

- Metabolic acidosis
- Unexplained hypoglycemia
- Lethargy and hypotonia
- Poor feeding
- Vomiting
- Abnormal breathing
- Seizures
- Liver dysfunction

[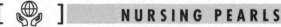] **NURSING PEARLS**

On physical exam, patients with hyperthyroidism may stare and have lid lag when closing their eyes.

[📝] **POP QUIZ 13.2**

A term newborn is noted to have a large goiter. What interventions should the nurse prioritize?

[🧠] **COMPLICATIONS**

If undiagnosed or untreated, inborn errors of metabolism may lead to neurologic abnormalities such as developmental delay, poor tone, and seizures; they also often cause gastrointestinal disturbances such as food intolerance, vomiting, diarrhea, and dehydration.

[⚡] **ALERT!**

Signs and symptoms of inborn errors of metabolism are often indistinguishable from sepsis. If a newborn being treated for suspected sepsis is not responding to antibiotics, an inborn error of metabolism disorder should be considered in the differential diagnosis.

■ Encephalopathy

Treatment

■ Initial treatment should focus on ceasing the buildup of toxic metabolites by placing the newborn on nothing by mouth (NPO). Administer a continuous infusion of 10% dextrose at a one-and-a-half maintenance rate.

■ Long-term treatment includes dietary restrictions and enzyme replacement therapies.

DISORDERS OF CALCIUM HOMEOSTASIS

■ Calcium is the most abundant mineral in the body and is important for muscle contraction, neural transmission, and blood coagulation.

■ Calcium levels are regulated by parathyroid hormone (PTH), vitamin D_3, and calcitonin.

HYPOCALCEMIA

■ *Hypocalcemia* is classified into serum calcium less than 7.0 mg/dL or ionized calcium less than 1 mmoL/L in preterm newborns, and serum calcium less than 8.0 mg/dL or ionized calcium less than 1.10 mmoL/L in term newborns.

■ At birth, there is an abrupt cessation of maternal calcium supply, resulting in a decreased serum calcium in the newborn. This triggers the mobilization of calcium from the bones and an increase in PTH.

■ Early-onset hypocalcemia occurs during the first 1 to 2 days of life and is self-limiting. It usually occurs due to decreased dietary intake during the first few days of life and improves with increased dietary intake, increased renal phosphorus excretion, and improved parathyroid function.

■ Late-onset hypocalcemia occurs after the third day of life and is rare.

Causes

■ Cow's milk-based formulas
■ Hypomagnesemia
■ Hypoparathyroidism
■ Low birth weight
■ Maternal anticonvulsants
■ Maternal diabetes
■ Perinatal asphyxia
■ Phototherapy
■ Prematurity
■ Viral gastroenteritis

Signs and Symptoms

■ Irritability
■ Jitteriness or tremors
■ Lethargy
■ Muscle twitching or seizures
■ Poor feeding

[🌐]   **NURSING PEARLS**

Extremely low birth weight (ELBW) and asphyxiated neonates have a decreased PTH response and are more likely to become hypocalcemic in the first few days of life.

Treatment

■ Calcium gluconate (bolus or continuous infusion; Appendix 13.1); can give PO after the initial correction
■ Calcitriol or additional calcium to formula

Nursing Interventions

- Monitor vital signs (VS) and EKG for arrhythmias.
- Collect labs and monitor electrolytes.
- Administer intravenous (IV) calcium as ordered. Give slowly over at least 30 minutes and stop immediately for bradycardia. If possible, administer through a central line rather than a peripheral intravenous line (PIV). Monitor the site for signs of infiltration and extravasation.

HYPERCALCEMIA

- *Hypercalcemia* is defined as serum calcium greater than 12 mg/dL or ionized calcium greater than 6 mg/dL.

Causes

The most common causes is iatrogenic. Other cause include:

- Congenital hyperparathyroidism
- Idiopathic infantile hypercalcemia
- Low phosphorus
- Rickets of prematurity
- Subcutaneous fat necrosis

COMPLICATIONS

If prolonged, hypercalcemia may lead to metastatic calcifications, particularly nephrocalcinosis, which can cause acute or chronic kidney injury.

Signs and Symptoms

- Bradycardia
- Constipation
- Dehydration
- Hypotonia
- Lethargy
- Polyuria

Treatment

- Discontinuation of calcium and vitamin D supplements
- IV fluids and furosemide to promote calcium excretion (Appendix 13.1)
- Glucocorticoids (decreased intestinal absorption of calcium)

Nursing Interventions

- Monitor urine output, electrolytes, VS, and EKG for arrhythmias.
- Collect labs and administer IV fluids as ordered.

GLUCOSE MANAGEMENT

Overview

- Growth and development of the neonate's brain are significantly impacted by blood glucose levels.
- In the early newborn period, glucose homeostasis is regulated by gluconeogenesis and glycogenolysis.
- Hypoglycemia is defined as less than 30 mg/dL in the first 24 hours of life and less than 45 mg/dL thereafter.
- Hyperglycemia is defined as greater than 150 mg/dL.

HYPOGLYCEMIA

Etiology

- Newborns experience an expected drop in blood glucose levels immediately after birth as part of the normal transition to extrauterine life.
- Prolonged hypoglycemia may occur in newborns with low glucose supply due to low glycogen or fat stores or poor glucose production, increased glucose utilization due to excessive insulin production or increased metabolic demand, and pituitary or adrenal failure.

Risk Factors

- Congenital heart defect (CHD)
- Congenital hyperinsulinemia
- Congenital syndromes (Beckwith–Wiedemann syndrome, Soto syndrome, Costello syndrome)
- Endocrine disorders
- Hypothermia
- Infants of diabetic mothers
- Inborn errors of metabolism
- Insulin administration
- Ischemia
- Large for gestational age (LGA), small for gestational age (SGA), intrauterine growth restriction (IUGR), or very low birth weight (VLBW)
- Maternal medications (beta-adrenergic tocolytics, valproic acid, propranolol, anesthetics)
- Prematurity
- Sepsis

Clinical Signs

- Apnea, grunting, and tachypnea
- Cyanosis
- Feeding difficulties and poor suck
- High-pitched cry
- Hypothermia
- Irritability
- Jitteriness/tremors
- Lethargy or hypotonia

Treatment

- In asymptomatic at-risk newborns, treatment recommendations include early initiation of frequent feedings within the first hour of life and dextrose gel 200 mg/kg massaged into the buccal mucosa.
- In symptomatic newborns with a serum glucose less than 40 mg/dL, treatment recommendations are IV dextrose 10% bolus 2 mL/kg followed by continuous infusion of dextrose 10% at 80 to 100 mL/kg/d (Appendix 13.1).

[🌐]   **NURSING PEARLS**

If hypoglycemia persists despite dextrose 10% administration, the dextrose concentration may be increased. However, if the dextrose concentration exceeds 12.5%, a peripheral IV may not be used, as concentrations this high are caustic to the veins. A central line is needed for any infusion containing a dextrose concentration greater than 12.5%.

Nursing Interventions

■ Check blood glucose levels according to unit protocol, ideally 1 hour after feeding asymptomatic at-risk newborns and 30 minutes to 1 hour after administration of glucose gel or IV dextrose.

■ Monitor IV site for signs of infiltration and phlebitis.

Complications

■ Cerebral palsy

■ Death

■ Long-term neurodevelopmental disabilities

■ Seizures

HYPERGLYCEMIA

Etiology

■ Although less common than hypoglycemia, hyperglycemia is associated with morbidity and mortality and must be addressed promptly. Neonatal hyperglycemia is often iatrogenic due to excessive glucose infusion rates or a physiologic response to stress.

■ Inadequate insulin production, insulin resistance, or inability to suppress glucose production may contribute to hyperglycemia in premature or IUGR neonates.

Risk Factors

■ IUGR or SGA

■ Maternal medications (diazoxide, antenatal steroids)

■ Neonatal medications (dopamine, dobutamine, epinephrine, caffeine, phenytoin, corticosteroids)

■ Physiologic stress (hypoxia, sepsis, respiratory distress syndrome [RDS], pain)

■ Prematurity

Clinical Signs

■ Dehydration

■ Feeding difficulties

■ Fever

■ Increased urine output

■ Weight loss

Treatment

■ Initial evaluation of hyperglycemia includes assessing the glucose infusion rate (GIR) and decreasing it to as low as 4 mg/kg/min. Evaluation should also include ruling out underlying causes such as sepsis, stress, or medications (Table 13.1).

■ If hyperglycemia persists despite a low GIR, it may indicate insulin resistance or deficiency. Insulin may be added to maintenance fluids or run as a separate continuous infusion (Appendix 13.1). Insulin dosage should start at 0.01 to 0.05 U/kg/hr.

Complications

■ Dehydration and electrolyte imbalances

■ Intracranial hemorrhage, necrotizing enterocolitis (NEC), and retinopathy of prematurity (ROP)

■ Poor neurodevelopmental outcomes

[📝] **POP QUIZ 13.3**

A 24-hour-old, 33-week gestation newborn is NPO and receiving IV fluids of dextrose 10% (D10W). The serum glucose is 30 mg/dL via heel stick. The newborn is jittery and has a high-pitched cry. What action should the nurse anticipate taking?

TABLE 13.1 Symptomatic Treatment for Endocrine Disorders

DISORDER	SYMPTOMATIC TREATMENT
ACTH deficiency	Hydrocortisone
TSH deficiency	Levothyroxine
Gonadotropin deficiency	Testosterone injections or gel (males)
Disorders of sexual differentiation	Hormone replacement therapy
Hypothyroidism	Levothyroxine
Hyperthyroidism	PTU, methimazole
Hypocalcemia	Calcium gluconate
Hypercalcemia	IV fluids, furosemide
Hypoglycemia	IV dextrose
Hyperglycemia	Insulin

ACTH, adrenocorticotropic hormone; IV, intravenous; PTU, propylthiouracil; TSH, thyroid-stimulating hormone.

Nursing Interventions

While the newborn is receiving insulin:

- Monitor frequent serum glucose levels per hospital policy.
- Titrate insulin according to orders.
- Monitor electrolytes for hypokalemia and watch for signs such as EKG changes.

DIAGNOSTIC PROCEDURES

Laboratory Tests

Pituitary Disorders

- ACTH deficiency: ACTH stimulation test
- Gonadotropin deficiency: LH and testosterone (males), FSH (females)
- Prolactin deficiency: prolactin TSH deficiency: T4, TSH

Disorders of Sexual Differentiation

- Chromosome test
- Hormone level tests

Thyroid Disorders

- T4
- TSH

Inborn Errors of Metabolism

- Ammonia
- Creatine kinase
- Coagulation studies
- Creatinine
- Electrolytes
- Lactate
- Urine organic acids

Calcium Disorders
- Ionized calcium
- Serum calcium

Glucose Disorders
- Point-of-care testing
- Serum glucose (more accurate than point-of-care testing)

Newborn Screening

- Newborn screening is a vital screening program that tests all newborns for congenital disorders that are not apparent at birth. It allows for early diagnosis and treatment.
- Disorders may be genetic-, metabolic-, blood, or hormone-related.
- All states screen newborns for at least 29 diseases.

Common Newborn Screenings
- Phenylketonuria (PKU)
- Congenital hypothyroidism
- Galactosemia
- Sickle cell disease
- Maple syrup urine disease
- Biotinidase deficiency
- Congenital adrenal hyperplasia
- Cystic fibrosis
- Severe combined immunodeficiency

Nursing Interventions

Require proper collection to ensure accuracy:
- Prick the newborn's heel. Allow a large drop of blood to form and touch the first circle on the newborn screening card to the drop of blood, allowing blood to soak and fill the circle. Fill the remaining circles in the same way.
- Do not press the card directly against the newborn's skin.
- Apply blood to only one side of the card.
- Do not milk or excessively squeeze incision site; this may cause hemolysis and interfere with the results.
- Allow specimen to dry on a flat surface for at least 3 hours before sending to appropriate lab.

RESOURCES

American Thyroid Association. *Congenital Hypothyroidism*. https://www.thyroid.org/congenital-hypothyroidism

Bosch I Ara, L., Katugampola, H., & Dattani, M. T. (2021). Congenital Hypopituitarism During the Neonatal Period: Epidemiology, Pathogenesis, Therapeutic Options, and Outcome. *Frontiers in pediatrics*, 8, 600962. https://doi.org/10.3389/fped.2020.600962

Centers for Disease Control and Prevention. (2021). *Newborn Screening Portal*. U.S. Department of Health and Human Services, Centers for Disease Control and Prevention. https://www.cdc.gov/newbornscreening/index.html

Cleveland Clinic. *Disorders of Sexual Differentiation*. https://my.clevelandclinic.org/health/diseases/16324-disorders-of-sex-differentiation#:~:text=What%20are%20disorders%20of%20sex,atypical%20appearances%20to%20their%20genitals.

Dysart, K. (2021). Neonatal Hypocalcemia. In *Merck Manual Professional Version*. Merck & Co., Inc. Retrieved May 19, 2022 from https://www.merckmanuals.com/professional/pediatrics/metabolic,-electrolyte,-and-toxic-disorders-in-neonates/neonatal-hypocalcemia

Dysart, K. (2021). Neonatal Hypercalcemia. In *Merck Manual Professional Version*. Merck & Co., Inc. Retrieved May 19, 2022 from https://www.merckmanuals.com/professional/pediatrics/metabolic,-electrolyte,-and -toxic-disorders-in-neonates/neonatal-hypercalcemia.

Kruszka, P., & Regier, D. (2019). Inborn Errors of Metabolism: From Conception to Adulthood. *American Family Physician*. https://www.aafp.org/afp/2019/0101/p25.html#:~:text = Inborn%20errors%20of%20 metabolism%20(IEM)%20are%20genetic%20conditions%20that%20block,findings%20affecting%20 multiple%20organ%20systems

Minnesota Department of Health. *Newborn Screening Information for Providers: Blood Spot Collection*. https://www .health.state.mn.us/people/newbornscreening/providers/collection.html#:~:text = Touch%20the%20 first%20circle%20on,be%20filled%20and%20saturated%20through

Rozance, P. (2022). Management and outcome of neonatal hypoglycemia. *UpToDate*. Retrieved May 18, 2022 from https://www.uptodate.com/contents/management-and-outcome-of-neonatal-hypoglycemia/print

Segni, M. (2019). Neonatal Hyperthyroidism. *Endotext*. Available from: https://www.ncbi.nlm.nih.gov/books /NBK279019

Stark, A., & Simmons, R. (2022). Neonatal hyperglycemia. *UpToDate*. Retrieved May 18, 2022 from https://www .uptodate.com/contents/neonatal-hyperglycemia

APPENDIX 13.1 MEDICATIONS FOR THE ENDOCRINE/METABOLIC SYSTEM

INDICATIONS	MECHANISM OF ACTION	CONTRAINDICATIONS, PRECAUTIONS, AND ADVERSE EFFECTS
Antithyroid medications (methimazole, propylthiouracil)		
• Treatment of hyperthyroidism	• Directly interfere with thyroid hormone biosynthesis in the thyroid gland by inhibiting the incorporation of iodine into the thyroid hormone precursors • Inhibit conversion of thyroxine	• Use with caution in newborns with hepatic disease. • Adverse effects include lethargy, leukopenia, rash, and hepatotoxicity.
Calcium gluconates		
• Treatment of hypocalcemia	• Calcium replacement	• Medication is contraindicated in hypercalcemia or in newborns receiving ceftriaxone. • Give slowly; do not push. • Adverse effects include tissue necrosis, hypotension, bradycardia, cardiac arrhythmias, and cardiac arrest.
Corticosteroids (hydrocortisone)		
• Treatment of adrenocortical insufficiency	• Corticosteroid effect believed to be due to enzyme modifications	• Do not abruptly discontinue medication. • Use with caution in immunosuppressed patients. • Adverse effects include hyperglycemia, fluid retention, and immunosuppression.

(continued)

APPENDIX 13.1 MEDICATIONS FOR THE ENDOCRINE/METABOLIC SYSTEM (*continued*)

INDICATIONS	MECHANISM OF ACTION	CONTRAINDICATIONS, PRECAUTIONS, AND ADVERSE EFFECTS
Dextrose 10% (D10W)		
• Parenteral (IV) treatment for hypoglycemia	• Glucose replacement and supplementation	• Adverse effects include hyperglycemia. • Monitor IV site for infiltration.
Diuretics (furosemide)		
• Treatment of hypercalcemia by removing excess water and phosphorus from the body	• Secretion of electrolytes and water by preventing resorption and increasing urine output	• Medication is contraindicated in cross sensitivity with sulfonamides (thiazide diuretics). • Use caution in hypokalemia, digoxin therapy, cardiac disease, and arrhythmia.
Insulin		
• Persistent hyperglycemia	• Lowers glucose concentration by facilitating glucose uptake in the muscle and adipose tissue	• Monitor potassium levels as hypokalemia can result. • Use caution in patients with renal and hepatic impairment. • Adverse effects include hypoglycemia, hypokalemia, peripheral edema, injection site pruritus, swelling of extremities, and visual disturbance.
Thyroid hormones (levothyroxine)		
• Treat hypothyroidism	• Act as endogenous thyroid hormone	• Contraindications include adrenal insufficiency. • Adverse effects include gastrointestinal upset, goiter, weight loss, alopecia, diaphoresis, cardiac arrhythmia, flushing, tachycardia, hypertension, increased liver enzymes, anxiety, fatigue, and dyspnea. • Take on an empty stomach; may be crushed and mixed with water, breast milk, or formula. • Do not take within 4 hours of calcium- or iron-containing products.

IV, intravenous.

14 HEMATOLOGIC SYSTEM

■ The *hematologic system* is responsible for delivering oxygen and nutrients to all tissues in the body.

■ It transports blood cells, antibodies, and hormones throughout the body.

■ The hematologic system is also responsible for removing waste.

■ Neonates are at increased risk for hematologic disorders because birth causes dramatic changes in circulation and oxygenation, which affect hematopoiesis.

ANEMIA

■ *Anemia* indicates a reduction in the number or volume of red blood cells (RBCs) or a reduction in hemoglobin and hematocrit throughout the body.

■ All newborns experience a transient reduction in hemoglobin, known as physiologic anemia of the newborn; however, due to physiologic and pathologic factors, preterm neonates experience a greater degree of anemia, known as anemia of prematurity.

■ Compared with the life span of adult erythrocytes (120 days), term newborn erythrocytes have a shorter life span (60–90 days). Preterm newborns' erythrocytes have an even shorter life span (35–50 days).

■ The three etiologies of anemia are blood loss, decreased RBC production, and increased RBC destruction.

[ ]   **COMPLICATIONS**

The major physiologic impact of anemia is impaired oxygen delivery to the tissues. Complications include poor growth, limited cardiovascular reserve, and decreased movement.

Causes of Blood Loss in the Neonate

■ Obstetrical causes: placental abruption, placenta previa, and trauma to the placenta or umbilical cord during delivery

■ Feto-maternal transfusion

■ Feto-placental transfusion

■ Twin-to-twin transfusion

■ Internal hemorrhage

■ Iatrogenic blood loss secondary to blood sampling for laboratory tests (the most common cause of anemia and blood transfusions in neonates)

Causes of Decreased Red Blood Cell Production

■ Congenital disorders of erythrocyte production: Diamond–Blackfan anemia

■ Bone marrow suppression from infection: cytomegalovirus, parvovirus B-19, rubella, syphilis, and toxoplasmosis

■ Nutritional deficiencies: copper, folate, iron, and vitamins A, B_{12}, C, and E

Causes of Increased Red Blood Cell Destruction

■ Hereditary RBC disorders: RBC membrane or enzyme defects, and hemoglobinopathies (alpha and beta thalassemia) ▶

Causes of Increased Red Blood Cell Destruction (*continued*)

- Immune hemolysis: ABO or Rh incompatibility
- Acquired hemolysis: drugs and infection

Signs and Symptoms

- Pallor
- Tachycardia
- Increased oxygen requirements
- Tachypnea or apnea
- Hypotension
- Lethargy
- Jaundice
- Metabolic acidosis

Treatment

- Limit blood sampling for laboratory tests.
- Administer iron supplements or recombinant human erythropoietin (Appendix 14.1).
- Transfuse with packed RBCs.

Nursing Interventions

- Assess for signs of hemorrhage, infection, respiratory distress syndrome (RDS), or hypoperfusion.
- Administer oxygen, medications (Appendix 14.1), intravenous (IV) fluids, and blood products (Box 14.1) as ordered.
- Promote rest by clustering care and limiting handling of the neonate from the staff and the family.
- Monitor electrolytes and blood levels following transfusion of blood products.

POLYCYTHEMIA

- *Polycythemia* is defined as increased hematocrit or hemoglobin.
- At birth, newborns have higher hematocrit and hemoglobin compared with children and adults.
- A newborn is considered to have polycythemia if hematocrit is >65% and hemoglobin is >22 g/dL.
- Active polycythemia is due to excess production of RBCs in response to hypoxia.
- Passive polycythemia is due to excess RBC transfusion to the fetus.

Causes of Active Polycythemia

Maternal Factors

- Diabetes
- Increased age
- Oligohydramnios ▶

[📝] **POP QUIZ 14.1**

A 50-day-old neonate with a corrected gestational age of 36 weeks is requiring 100% oxygen at 1 L/min via a nasal cannula. The neonate is pale and lethargic and has had multiple apneic episodes in the past 24 hours. Complete blood count reveals hematocrit of 22%, hemoglobin of 7.0 g/dL, and reticulocytes of 1.8%. Based on the clinical findings, the nurse should anticipate what interventions?

[🧠] **COMPLICATIONS**

Polycythemia increases blood viscosity, which slows perfusion to organs and tissues and may lead to multisystem organ dysfunction.

> **[BOX 14.1] GENERAL INDICATIONS
> FOR BLOOD PRODUCT TRANSFUSION**
>
> - Decreased hemoglobin or hematocrit
> - Decreased platelets
> - Plasma coagulation factors deficient
> - Reversal of anticoagulation
> - Diagnosis of disseminated intravascular coagulation
> - Factor VIII replacement
> - Fibrinogen levels less than 100 mg/dL
> - Packed red blood cells
> - Platelets
> - Fresh frozen plasma
> - Cryoprecipitate

Maternal Factors (continued)

- Pregnancy-induced hypertension (PIH)
- Renal or heart disease
- Smoking

Placental Factors

- Placental dysfunction resulting in intrauterine growth restriction (IUGR)/ small for gestational age (SGA) neonates
- Placental infarction
- Placenta previa
- Postmaturity
- Viral infections (toxoplasmosis, other agents, rubella, cytomegalovirus, herpes simplex [TORCH])

Fetal Syndromes

- Beckwith–Wiedemann syndrome
- Trisomy 13, 18, and 21

Causes of Passive Polycythemia

- Delayed cord clamping
- Maternal–fetal transfusion
- Twin-to-twin transfusion

Signs and Symptoms

- Apnea
- RDS
- Pulmonary edema
- Cyanosis
- Plethora
- Lethargy
- Hypotonia
- Tremors

Treatment

- Normal saline infusion bolus (10 mL/kg)
- PET

COAGULOPATHIES AND BLEEDING

- *Coagulopathy* is any alteration in baseline hematologic function, which results in impaired clot formation.
- Coagulopathies can be acquired or genetic (inherited).

Acquired Coagulopathies

- Disseminated intravascular coagulation (DIC)
- Liver failure
- Thrombocytopenia
- Thrombosis
- Vitamin K deficiency

Genetic Coagulopathies

- Hemophilia A (factor VIII deficiency)
- Hemophilia B (factor IX deficiency)
- von Willebrand disease

Thrombocytopenia

- *Thrombocytopenia* occurs when platelets are lower than 150,000/mm³.
- Normal platelet range in newborns is 150,000 to 450,000/mm³.
- Mild thrombocytopenia is 100,000 to 150,000/mm³.
- Moderate thrombocytopenia is 50,000 to 90,000/mm³.
- Severe thrombocytopenia is <50,000/mm³.
- Platelets are essential to help the body clot and facilitate wound healing.

Causes

Maternal Factors

- Eclampsia or hypertension
- Drug ingestion
- Placental insufficiency or infarction
- Immune-mediated maternal platelet antibodies

Neonatal Factors

- Cold injury
- DIC
- Exchange transfusion
- Hyperbilirubinemia and phototherapy
- Necrotizing enterocolitis
- Perinatal asphyxia
- Polycythemia
- Sepsis
- SGA

[ ] **ALERT!**

Exchange transfusions increase the risk of gastrointestinal symptoms such as bleeding, feeding intolerance, and necrotizing enterocolitis. Feedings should not be resumed until 2 to 4 hours following completion of the exchange transfusion.

[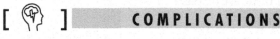] **COMPLICATIONS**

Complications of thrombocytopenia include severe internal bleeding. The most critical is cerebral bleeding, which can result in hemorrhagic stroke and death.

Signs and Symptoms

- Ecchymosis
- Petechiae
- Mucosal bleeding
- Pink or blood-tinged secretions
- Cephalohematoma
- Oozing from umbilical cord or puncture sites

Treatment

In most cases, thrombocytopenia resolves spontaneously without intervention; however, if treatment is needed, it should be focused on the underlying condition, as well as:

- Platelet transfusion
- IVIG (Appendix 14.1) for immune-mediated thrombocytopenia

Vitamin K Deficiency

- Vitamin K is a fat-soluble vitamin and is an essential cofactor for the synthesis and activation of coagulation factors.
- Vitamin K deficiency can lead to vitamin K deficiency bleeding (VKDB), which can be life-threatening.
- Newborns are born with decreased vitamin K levels and can easily develop vitamin K deficiency due to poor placental transfer of vitamin K, low vitamin K content in breast milk, and poor intestinal absorption due to immature gut flora and malabsorption.
- Preterm newborns are at higher risk for VKDB due to hepatic immaturity, delayed gut colonization, and other factors.
- Administration of intramuscular vitamin K (Appendix 14.1) shortly after birth can prevent VKDB.

Risk Factors

- Maternal use of medications such as warfarin and anticonvulsants
- Not receiving vitamin K prophylaxis after birth
- Neonatal liver disease
- Newborns with gastrointestinal disorders

Signs and Symptoms

In most cases of VKDB, there are no warning signs; however, signs and symptoms to watch for include:

- Ecchymosis (especially around the face and head)
- Mucosal bleeding
- Oozing from umbilical site
- Pallor
- Scleral jaundice
- Hematochezia or hematemesis
- Signs of intracranial hemorrhage

Treatment

- Newborns with nonlife-threatening bleeding should be given vitamin K via slow IV injection.
- For newborns with severe bleeding, treatment includes administration of fresh frozen plasma (FFP) and IV vitamin K while awaiting blood products.

[⚙]   **ALERT!**

Do not administer intramuscular vitamin K in the presence of severe bleeding or existing coagulopathy. If venous access cannot be obtained for intravenous vitamin K, it may be given subcutaneously.

Congenital Bleeding Disorders

- Congenital bleeding disorders occur due to the absence or deficiency of specific clotting proteins.
- The three most common causes are hemophilia A, hemophilia B, and von Willebrand disease.
- Hemophilia is an X-linked recessive disorder caused by factor VIII deficiency.
- von Willebrand disease is the most common bleeding disorder and is caused by a deficiency in von Willebrand factor, a blood clotting protein.

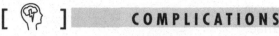

COMPLICATIONS

Congenital bleeding disorders may lead to internal bleeding, such as intracranial, gastrointestinal, or urinary hemorrhage. These are life-threatening events.

Signs and Symptoms

- Prolonged bleeding after procedures
- Ecchymosis
- Petechiae
- Hematuria
- Hematochezia
- Cephalohematoma
- Internal hemorrhage

ALERT!

Newborns with congenital bleeding disorders should wear a medical bracelet identifying the type of bleeding disorder so that they can receive proper medical attention in the event of an emergency.

Treatment

- Treatment depends on the type and severity of the bleeding disorder and includes blood product (Box 14.1) and factor replacement therapy (Appendix 14.1).

Liver Failure

- *Liver failure* is the partial or complete loss of liver function usually accompanied by encephalopathy. It may be acute or chronic.
- The main finding for diagnosis of acute liver failure is the presence of coagulopathy with either a partial thromboplastin time (PTT) >20 sec after vitamin K administration or international normalized ratio (INR) greater than or equal to 3.

Causes

- Gestational alloimmune liver disease
- Viral infections
- Metabolic disorders
- Hemophagocytic lymphohistiocytosis
- Hypoxia
- Toxic substances/drugs

Signs and Symptoms

- Lethargy
- Vomiting
- Dark urine
- Jaundice
- Ecchymosis
- Prolonged bleeding
- Abdominal ascites

Thrombosis

- *Thrombosis* occurs when a blood clot forms inside a vessel (vein or artery).
- Neonates are the most at-risk pediatric population for thrombosis due to their developing and vulnerable hemostatic system.

Causes

- Central venous or arterial catheters
- Congenital heart disease
- Dehydration
- Mechanical ventilation
- Perinatal asphyxia
- Sepsis

Signs and Symptoms

Clinical presentation depends on the type and location of the thrombosis.

Venous Thromboembolism

- Abdominal mass
- Central venous line dysfunction
- Edema
- Limb discoloration

Renal Vein Thrombosis

- Abdominal mass
- Hematuria
- Thrombocytopenia

Cerebral Sinus Venous Thrombosis

- Apnea
- Agitation
- Decreased alertness
- Seizures
- Signs of infection

Nonspecific Signs

- Apnea
- Bradycardia
- Persistent bacteremia
- RDS
- Thrombocytopenia

[🌐]   **NURSING PEARLS**

Nursing assessment of a neonate with a central catheter should include monitoring the area distal to the catheter (fingers, toes, groin) for signs of thrombosis.

Disseminated Intravascular Coagulation

- *DIC* is an acquired syndrome characterized by excessive systemic activation of coagulation, resulting in both hemorrhage and thrombosis.
- Neonates are born with slightly altered hemostasis, putting them at higher risk for DIC.

Risk Factors

- Placental abruption
- PIH
- Sepsis
- Asphyxia/RDS ▶

Risk Factors (*continued*)

- Hypotension
- IVH
- Brain injury

Signs and Symptoms

- Ecchymosis
- Petechiae
- Blood clots
- Prolonged bleeding
- Hematuria
- Change in neurologic status
- Respiratory distress

[ ] **COMPLICATIONS**

Disseminated intravascular coagulation causes microvascular thrombosis, which may lead to endothelial tissue and multi-organ damage.

WHITE BLOOD CELLS

- No established norm for normal white blood cell (WBC) count in neonates
- Preterm newborns: 6,000 to 19,000 mm^3
- Term newborns: 10,000 to 26,000 mm^3
- In neonates, very low WBC counts may be more concerning than high WBC counts.

NEUTROPENIA

- Neutropenia is defined as decreased absolute neutrophil count (ANC).
- Neutrophils are a type of WBC and are the primary defense against bacteria, often seen during acute infection.
- Generally, an ANC less than 1,500 is suggestive of infection.
- Neutropenia may be secondary to decreased production of neutrophils or increased neutrophil destruction.

Risk Factors

- PIH or preeclampsia
- Fetal growth restriction
- Prolonged rupture of membranes or chorioamnionitis
- Twin-to-twin transfusion syndrome
- Infection during pregnancy
- Alloimmunization
- Hemolytic disease

Signs and Symptoms

- Hypo- or hyperthermia
- RDS
- Increased secretions or congestion
- Loose stools

HYPERBILIRUBINEMIA

- Neonatal hyperbilirubinemia, or jaundice, is defined as elevated total serum bilirubin.
- There are two forms of bilirubin: unconjugated (indirect, lipid-soluble) and conjugated (direct, water-soluble).
- In utero, unconjugated bilirubin is transported across the placenta and excreted by maternal circulation.
- After birth, the newborn liver is responsible for metabolizing bilirubin.
- Bilirubin binds with albumin and is carried to the liver, where it is conjugated and then excreted in the bile.

[🧠]   **COMPLICATIONS**

Damage to the brain may occur if unconjugated bilirubin crosses the blood–brain barrier. Although it may be reversible, the irreversible form leads to encephalopathy.

Symptoms may include:

- Apnea
- Fever
- Hypertonia
- Opisthotonos
- Seizures

Complications caused by this encephalopathy include cerebral palsy, hearing loss, paralysis, and intellectual disability.

- Newborns produce bilirubin at a higher rate than adults due to the higher turnover and shorter life span of RBCs.
- If the bilirubin production rate exceeds the ability of the liver to conjugate and excrete it, unconjugated bilirubin will increase and jaundice will develop.
- Physiologic jaundice is due to the normal breakdown of RBCs and the newborn's immature liver. It peaks at 3 to 4 days of life, then declines over the first week after birth.
- Pathologic jaundice occurs in the first 24 hours of life and includes a rapidly rising total serum bilirubin of more than 5 mg/dL/d. Jaundice is prolonged (7–10 days). Causes include sepsis, infection, hemorrhage, and erythroblastosis fetalis.

Risk Factors

Maternal Factors

- ABO or Rh incompatibility
- Asian or Native American ethnicity
- Breastfeeding
- Certain drugs (diazepam, oxytocin)
- Gestational diabetes

Neonatal Factors

- Birth trauma (cephalohematoma, bruising, instrument-assisted delivery)
- Delayed meconium passage
- Excessive weight loss after birth
- Infections
- Infrequent feedings
- Male sex
- Prematurity
- Previous sibling with hyperbilirubinemia
- Polycythemia

Signs and Symptoms

- Yellowing of the skin and eyes
- Lethargy ▶

Signs and Symptoms (*continued*)
- Hypotonia
- High-pitched cry

Nursing Interventions
- The best prevention of hyperbilirubinemia is adequate hydration.
- Ensure breastfed newborns have 8 to 12 feedings per day in the first week of life. Formula-fed newborns should eat 1 to 2 oz. every 2 to 3 hours for the first week of life.

Treatment
- See Phototherapy and Exchange Transfusion under Common Procedures.

DIAGNOSTIC PROCEDURES

Laboratory Testing

Pertinent laboratory tests and findings for hematologic disorders include the following:

Polycythemia
- Increased hematocrit and hemoglobin
- Decreased platelets
- Elevated reticulocytes
- Hypocalcemia
- Hypoglycemia
- Hyperbilirubinemia

Thrombocytopenia
- Decreased platelets
- Abnormal coagulation studies

Vitamin K deficiency
- Prolonged PTT and PT
- Increased levels of proteins induced by vitamin K absence or antagonists (PIVKAs)

Hemophilia
- Prolonged PTT
- PT, thrombin time, and platelets usually normal

von Willebrand
- Decreased or absent von Willebrand factor antigen
- Decreased factor VIII

Disseminated intravascular coagulation
- Decreased platelets
- Prolonged PTT and PT
- Decreased fibrinogen

Neutropenia
- Elevated immature to total neutrophil (I:T) ratio
- Decreased ANC
- Increased C-reactive protein

[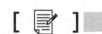]   **POP QUIZ 14.2**

A newborn male is experiencing a significant amount of bleeding after a circumcision. Coagulation studies reveal that the PTT is elevated, but the PT and platelet count are normal. The newborn's mother states that her brother experienced the same problem. Based on these findings, what is the most likely diagnosis?

Transcutaneous Bilirubin Measurement

- *Transcutaneous bilirubin (TcB) measurement* is a noninvasive method for monitoring bilirubin level.
- The measurement is taken by gently pressing the meter against the skin on the sternum or forehead.
- It provides an immediate result.
- Accuracy may be affected by gestational age, body weight, and skin color.

COMMON PROCEDURES

Phototherapy

- Phototherapy uses blue wavelengths of light to convert unconjugated bilirubin into water-soluble isomers that can bypass the liver to be excreted in the bile and urine.
- Treatment with phototherapy is implemented to avoid the neurotoxic effects of elevated unconjugated bilirubin and reduces the need for exchange transfusion.

Nursing Interventions

- Ensure the neonate has as much skin exposed as possible.
- Cover the neonate's eyes with the appropriate eye shield; only remove during care and feeding times for routine eye care.
- Monitor temperature and adjust isolette settings as needed.
- Collect and monitor serial bilirubin blood levels.
- Ensure phototherapy lights are turned off during blood sampling.
- Educate family members that the neonate is required to remain under phototherapy light at all times besides feedings; in the case of neonates nearing exchange transfusion level, all feedings should be given while under phototherapy via bottle or nasogastric tube.
- Monitor hydration status and administer IV fluids as ordered.

Exchange Transfusion

- *Exchange transfusion* is a procedure that requires removal of the neonate's blood and replacement with donor blood to remove abnormal blood components and toxins, while simultaneously maintaining adequate circulating blood volume. ▶

[🧠] **COMPLICATIONS**

Complications from phototherapy may include:
- Diarrhea
- Insensible water loss
- Overheating
- Rash
- Retinal damage

[⚡] **ALERT!**

During phototherapy treatment, ensure that petroleum-based products are not applied to areas of the neonate's skin that are exposed to the light. Phototherapy can cause burns on areas of petroleum-covered skin.

[📝] **POP QUIZ 14.3**

A 5-day-old newborn is readmitted to the NICU for intensive phototherapy due to hyperbilirubinemia. The parents question why the newborn needs intravenous fluids during phototherapy treatment. How should the nurse respond?

[🧠] **COMPLICATIONS**

Complications of exchange transfusions include:
- Arrhythmias
- Bradycardia
- Neutropenia
- Dilutional coagulopathy
- Feeding intolerance
- Necrotizing enterocolitis
- Sepsis
- Hypocalcemia, hyperkalemia, hypo/hyperglycemia, and acidosis
- Air emboli and thrombosis
- Hypo/hyperthermia

Exchange Transfusion (*continued*)

■ Indications include hemolytic disease of the newborn, hyperbilirubinemia, severe anemia, and polycythemia.

Nursing Interventions

■ Parental consent is necessary prior to initiation.

■ At least one provider and one registered nurse should be exclusively involved throughout the entire procedure.

[⚙]   **ALERT!**

To avoid major fluctuations in blood pressure, perform procedure slowly over approximately 2 hours.

■ Confirm the neonate is nothing by mouth (NPO) and stomach contents have been aspirated.

■ Remove patient blood from arterial line while infusing donor blood through venous line at the same rate.

■ Obtain and monitor labs and vital signs (VS) per hospital policy.

RESOURCES

Araki, S., & Shirahata, A. (2020). Vitamin K deficiency bleeding in infancy. *Nutrients*, *12*(3), 780. https://doi.org/10 .3390/nu12030780

Chien, M., & Glader, B. (2022). Disseminated intravascular coagulation in infants and children. *UpToDate*. Retrieved May 31, 2022 from https://www.uptodate.com/contents/disseminated-intravascular-coagulation-in -infants-and-children

Doherty, T., & Kelley, A. (2022). Bleeding disorders. *StatPearls*. https://www.ncbi.nlm.nih.gov/books/NBK541050

Fernandes, C. (2022). Neonatal thrombocytopenia: Clinical manifestations, evaluation and management. *UpToDate*. Retrieved May 23, 2022 from https://www.uptodate.com/contents/neonatal-thrombocytopenia -clinical-manifestations-evaluation-and-management/print

Haley, K. (2017). Neonatal venous thromboembolism. *Frontiers in Pediatric,* 136(5). https://doi.org/10.3389/fped .2017.00136

Karadağ, N., Okbay Güneş, A., & Karatekin, G. (2021). Acute liver failure in newborns. *Turkish Archives of Pediatrics*, *56*(2), 108–114. https://doi.org/10.5152/TurkArchPediatr.2021.190205

Porter, M., & Dennis, B. (2002). Hyperbilirubinemia in the term newborn. *American Family Physician*. https://www .aafp.org/afp/2002/0215/p599.html

Starship. (2018). *Exchange Transfusion in the Neonate*. https://starship.org.nz/guidelines/exchange-transfusion -in-the-neonate

The Royal Children's Hospital Melbourne. (2018). *Phototherapy for neonatal jaundice*. https://www.rch.org.au /rchcpg/hospital_clinical_guideline_index/Phototherapy_for_neonatal_jaundice

Walter, A. (2020). Perinatal Anemia. *Merck Manual*. https://www.merckmanuals.com/professional/pediatrics /perinatal-hematologic-disorders/perinatal-anemia

APPENDIX 14.1 MEDICATIONS FOR THE HEMATOLOGIC SYSTEM

INDICATIONS	MECHANISM OF ACTION	CONTRAINDICATIONS, PRECAUTIONS, AND ADVERSE EFFECTS
Coagulation factors (coagulation factor VIIa recombinant)		
• Coagulopathies responsive to coagulation factor administration • von Willebrand disease	• Affect tissue factor dependent and independent pathways to reduce PT and PTT	• Use caution in patients with DIC, hepatic disease, trauma, and thromboembolism due to risk of further thromboembolism.

(*continued*)

APPENDIX 14.1 MEDICATIONS FOR THE HEMATOLOGIC SYSTEM (*continued*)

INDICATIONS	MECHANISM OF ACTION	CONTRAINDICATIONS, PRECAUTIONS, AND ADVERSE EFFECTS
Erythropoietin agents (epoetin alfa)		
• Anemia	• Stimulate bone marrow to make more RBCs	• Erythropoietin agents are contraindicated in albumin or mammalian cell-derived product hypersensitivity and uncontrolled hypertension. • Use caution with history of seizures. • Adverse effects include seizures, CHF, and hypertension.
Immunoglobulins (IV immunoglobulin)		
• Immune-mediated thrombocytopenia	• Provide antibodies that activate humoral and cell-mediated immunity	• Monitor for signs of thromboembolism. • Use caution in patients at risk of thromboembolism.
Iron supplements (ferrous sulfate)		
• Low hemoglobin • Inadequate iron reserves	• Increase hemoglobin production • Allow for transportation of oxygen via hemoglobin	• Give on empty stomach between meals if possible; may mix with milk/formula to enhance taste. • Adverse effects include constipation, black tarry stools, and vomiting. • Administer iron 2 hours prior or 4 hours after calcium or antacids for optimal iron absorption. • Iron may decrease concentration of levothyroxine. • Administer iron 4 hours after levothyroxine.
Vitamin K products (phytonadione)		
• Prophylaxis or treatment of vitamin K deficiency	• With identical action to vitamin K, facilitate binding of proteins to help blood coagulate	• Adverse effects include pain and redness at the injection site, rash, hypersensitivity reactions, and hyperbilirubinemia.

CHF, congestive heart failure; DIC, disseminated intravascular coagulation; IV, intravenous; PT, prothrombin time; PTT, partial thromboplastin time; RBC, red blood cells.

15 IMMUNE SYSTEM AND INFECTIOUS DISEASES

INNATE IMMUNITY DEFICIENCIES

■ The *innate immune system* comprises cells that respond as a nonspecific response to infection without additional specialization or training. It is made up of neutrophils, monocytes, natural killer cells (NK), basophils, mast cells, and complement proteins.

■ Increased susceptibility to more frequent infections than normal is common. Examples include recurrent sinus infections, ear infections, colds, pneumonia, and yeast infections.

Causes

■ Congenital
■ Genetic mutations
■ Associations with other medical conditions

Signs and Symptoms

■ Symptoms vary widely depending on the deficiency.

ADAPTIVE IMMUNITY DEFICIENCIES

■ *Adaptive* or *acquired immune system*: the specific response to infection with cells that adapt and tailor their response to specific intruders over time (T-cells and B-cells)

■ Acquired after birth (secondary)

Causes

■ Viral infections
■ Malnutrition
■ Metabolic disorders (kidney disease)
■ Diabetes
■ Drugs
■ Cancer treatments or other medications
■ May also occur following surgery or loss of proteins from the body (bowel abnormalities)

INFECTION CONTROL PRACTICES

Handwashing

■ Handwashing is one of the most important means of preventing and controlling the spread of healthcare-associated infections in the NICU.

■ Perform hand hygiene routinely and thoroughly before entering the NICU and before and after contact with the neonate or the neonate's environment. ▶

Handwashing (*continued*)

- Current best practice includes cleaning the hands before and after patient contact, after touching patient equipment or environmental surfaces, before performing invasive procedures, and after removing gloves.
- Alcohol-based hand hygiene products are appropriate for use when hands are not visibly soiled; soap and water must be used when hands are visibly soiled or contaminated with blood or other body fluids, when exposed to potential spore-forming pathogens, and after using the restroom.
- Hands should be washed for at least 20 seconds.
- Facilities commonly require initial handwashing and scrubbing before entering the NICU. Hands and arms should be thoroughly washed with antiseptic soap to a point above the elbow. Recommendations vary regarding the length of time necessary for performing the procedure (typically 1 to 2 minutes).
- Glove use does not eliminate the need for hand hygiene.

Patient Placement

- Infants may be isolated because they are known or suspected to be colonized or infected with a pathogen based on clinical diagnosis, microbiologic confirmation, or epidemiology, or because they are particularly at risk of acquiring a hospital-acquired infection (HAI).
- Isolation or cohorts may be effective in controlling nosocomial infections by preventing horizontal spread from patient to patient.
- Guidelines from the American Academy of Pediatrics (AAP) state that it may be unnecessary to isolate a neonate (except in the case of neonatal varicella zoster or an epidemic of bacterial infection) if the following conditions are met: There is sufficient nursing staff on duty, sufficient space between stations, and two or more sinks for handwashing available in each area, and continuing instruction is provided regarding the way infections spread.
- Cohorting is the physical segregation of infants with similar exposures, colonization, or infections in separate areas where they are cared for by designated staff assigned exclusively to those infants. They are created based on clinical diagnoses, epidemiology, and mode of transmission of the infectious agent. Cohorting may be more feasible than single-room isolation during times of outbreak in the NICU.

Proper Specimen Collection

- The choice of site and procedure (venous site or heel prick) depends on the volume of blood needed for the procedure and the type of laboratory test to be done. Venipuncture is the preferred method of blood sampling for term neonates requiring more than 1 mL of blood. Heel puncture should be done on the most medial or lateral portions of the plantar surface of the heel.
- Lumbar puncture (LP) is used for ruling out sepsis in the neonate: Hold the patient in lateral decubitis position. Palpate the spinous process so that it is even with the iliac crests. Locate one interspace above (L3–L4) or one space below (L4–L5) as the site. When collecting for diagnostic purposes, spinal fluid should be collected in the following order: tube 1: culture and stat Gram stain; tube 2: glucose and protein; and tube 3: cell count.
- Urine specimens are obtained by bag urine collection or suprapubic aspiration if urinary tract infection (UTI) is suspected and antibiotics will be required. For suprapubic aspiration (SPA), place the infant supine in frog-leg position, with the insertion site 1 cm above the symphysis pubis, strictly in midline, and advance the syringe while applying minimal negative pressure. UTI should never be diagnosed or treated on the basis of a bag urine specimen alone.
- Respiratory specimen collection is done via nasal culture using a nasal swab in the nare until resistance is met or to the posterior nasopharynx (at the base of the throat), depending on which test is needed.

Employee Health and Attire

- NICU nurses should wear clean scrubs (uniforms vary depending on the hospital).
- Nails should be kept short, clean, and free of nail polish. NICU nurses should not wear artificial nails.
- Jewelry should not be worn on hands or arms.
- Nurses should not report to work if they are febrile, or have gastroenteritis, respiratory infection, or suspected communicable disease. Masks should be worn with cold sores or when a nurse has a general feeling of being unwell. See hospital infection control policies for specific units.

Skin and Cord Care

See Chapter 11, Integumentary System.

ANTIMICROBIAL THERAPY

Antibacterial

- If a neonate shows symptoms of infection, collect complete blood count (CBC) with differential, C-reactive protein (CRP), and blood culture; however, there should be a low threshold for starting broad-spectrum antibiotics (ampicillin/gentamicin).
- Isolate the organism. Choose the appropriate antibiotic.
- The decision to stop antibiotics is based on clinical response and CRP.
- Practice antibiotic stewardship to avoid antibiotic resistance.
- Common antibacterial therapies include ampicillin, gentamicin, cefotaxime, and vancomycin.

Antiviral

- Antivirals are used in the treatment and prophylaxis of viral diseases.
- They are most effective within 2 days of symptoms and may reduce serious complications.
- They are used to treat viruses such as influenza, herpes simplex virus (HSV), and cytomegalovirus (CMV).
- Common antiviral therapies include acyclovir and valganciclovir.

Antifungal

- Antifungals are used to treat fungal infections, especially candidiasis.
- Common antifungal therapies include nystatin, fluconazole, or amphotericin B.

TRANSMISSION OF INFECTION

Overview

- Almost all fetal and neonatal infections are vertically transmitted (acquired from the mother).
- Transmission may be transplacental in utero, perinatal during birth, or postnatal, including breastfeeding.
- Neonates can also acquire infections horizontally, such as nosocomial infections.

TRANSPLACENTAL (INTRAUTERINE) COMMON PATHOGENS

- Transplacental infections occur when microorganisms present in the blood of the mother transfer through the placenta to infect the fetus.
- Common pathogens include syphilis, *Toxoplasma*, CMV, hepatitis B virus (HBV), HIV, HSV, varicella, and rubella.

Human Immunodeficiency Virus

- The rate of transmission of HIV to neonates has been reduced to less than 1% with comprehensive serologic screening and treatment of HIV-infected pregnant mothers. Antiretroviral therapy (ART) can be prescribed during pregnancy, antepartum during vaginal or elective Cesarean delivery, postnatally to the neonate, and during breastfeeding to reduce vertical transmission.
- The probability of vertical transmission is about 25% without the use of appropriate ART therapy during pregnancy.
- Risk factors for transmission include elevated maternal plasma viral RNA concentrations, maternal breast milk viral load, acute maternal seroconversion, advanced maternal disease, and decreased CD4+ T-cell count of the mother. Intrapartum transmission is known to be the greatest risk for vertical infection.
- Neonates may not display any symptoms for the initial few months of life and may remain asymptomatic until 3 to 5 years of age. The most common exhibited signs of HIV infection, if left untreated, include recurrent bacteremia, increased opportunistic infections, frequent diarrhea, cardiomyopathy, hepatitis, lymphadenopathy, splenomegaly, hepatomegaly, oral candidiasis, growth delay, delayed cognition, low IQ, and global developmental delay.
- Neonates with any level of risk of exposure to HIV should be started on the appropriate ART within 6 hours of birth. Antiretroviral regimens should include two nucleoside reverse transcriptase inhibitors (NRTIs) and an additional drug from another class, either an integrase strand transfer inhibitor (INSTI), a protease inhibitor (PI) with a booster, or an non-nucleoside reverse transcriptase inhibitor (NNRTI). Zidovudine (ZDV) plus lamivudine (3TC) or emtricitabine (FTC) is the preferred dual NRTI regimen in neonates and infants <3 months. For infants ≥3 months, the preferred regimen is abacavir (ABC) plus 3TC or FTC.

Cytomegalovirus

- Primary CMV infection in pregnancy is associated with the highest risk of transplacental transmission.
- The virus is present in the saliva, blood, urine, breast milk, and genital secretions.
- The most common signs of congenital CMV in the neonate are jaundice, petechiae, hepatosplenomegaly, seizures, and microcephaly. Hearing loss, the most common issue with a congenital cytomegalovirus (cCMV), may be present at birth or later in life. Other complications include developmental delay.
- Neonates must be tested within 3 weeks of delivery via saliva, urine polymerase chain reaction (PCR), or culture.
- Symptomatic neonates should receive oral valganciclovir for 6 months, which has been shown to preserve normal hearing or prevent the progression of hearing loss. Valganciclovir administration also correlates with improved long-term neurodevelopmental outcomes.

Rubella

- It is a congenital infection occurring during pregnancy or the peripartum period. Severity of neonatal illness varies on the timing of infection.
- Congenital rubella syndrome may include eye disorders, sensorineural deafness, pulmonary stenosis, intrauterine growth restriction (IUGR), microcephaly, thrombocytopenia, hepatosplenomegaly, and hemopoietic disorders.
- It is diagnosed via immunoglobulin M (IgM) or isolation of the rubella virus (eye, throat, nasopharyngeal airway [NPA], cerebrospinal fluid [CSF], stool, urine).
- There is no specific treatment besides supportive management.

Syphilis

- *Syphilis* is a sexually transmitted infection that can be transplacental or transmitted at birth.
- Congenital infection can cause perinatal death, prematurity, low birth weight, anomalies, active congenital syphilis, rash, hepatosplenomegaly, jaundice, anemia, deafness, or neurologic impairment.
- Treat with penicillin G.
- All infants with a reactive test should receive follow-up tests until negative as well as an HIV test.

Toxoplasmosis

- *Toxoplasmosis* occurs through transplacental transmission via cats, raw meat, and unpasteurized milk.
- It may cause spontaneous abortion or intrauterine fetal demise later in pregnancy.
- Most infants will be asymptomatic; if left untreated, it can lead to severe visual and central nervous system (CNS) deficits.
- Treat with pyrimethamine, sulfadiazine, and folinic acid for up to 1 year.

Zika Virus

- Perinatal transmission, congenital defects observed in early versus late pregnancy
- May cause microcephaly, issues with hearing and vision, joints with limited range of motion, seizures, hypertonia, and developmental delays
- Supportive management only; monitor for delays and perform hearing and vision screenings

Perinatal Common Pathogens

- *Perinatal transmission* or *mucous membrane transmission* is the transmission of infections from the cervix or vagina to the neonate while the neonate goes through the birth canal.
- Common pathogens include *Neisseria gonorrhoeae*, *Chlamydia trachomatis*, HBV, and HSV.

Chlamydia Trachomatis Infection

- *C. trachomatis* is the most common sexually transmitted infection (STI) in the United States. Infants born vaginally to infected mothers are at risk.
- It usually presents as conjunctivitis or pneumonia in the neonate.
- Testing includes swabbing the conjunctiva or nasopharynx. A nucleic acid amplification test (NAAT) is considered the gold standard for diagnosis.
- Treatment depends on the infection site. Oral azithromycin is the preferred treatment for both conjunctivitis and pneumonia.

Enterovirus Infections

- These infections are typically acquired from a symptomatic mother in the perinatal period. They may be acquired via nosocomial transmission in the NICU.
- These are found in the upper respiratory or gastrointestinal (GI) tract.
- Early clinical manifestations are mild and may include transient respiratory distress.
- Clinical presentations associated with high mortality include meningoencephalitis, myocarditis, and sepsis.
- Treatment includes supportive measures.

Group B *Streptococcus*

- It is acquired in utero or via the birth canal. ▶

[📝]   **POP QUIZ 15.1**

A 6-day-old infant born precipitously to a mother without prenatal care is brought to the clinic exhibiting conjunctivitis in both eyes, with marked swelling, yellow exudate, and blood-stained eye discharge. Which infection would be suspected in the infant?

Group B *Streptococcus* (*continued*)

■ It is diagnosed through rectovaginal culture of the mother at 35 to 37 weeks. Treat positive mothers with penicillin or ampicillin.

■ There are standard algorithms for evaluation of infants based on risk factors, duration of rupture of membranes, and the mother's intrapartum temperature.

■ Asymptomatic infants should have a CBC with differential and blood culture and receive antibiotics if there is evidence of maternal infection.

■ Symptomatic infants should have a CBC with differential, LP, CSF, blood culture, and x-ray and receive antibiotics (ampicillin).

■ Early-onset Group B *Streptococcus* (GBS) infection presents at or within 24 hours of birth up to day 6 after birth. Symptoms include sepsis, pneumonia, and meningitis.

■ Late-onset GBS occurs at 4 to 5 weeks of age (range 7–89 days). Symptoms include bacteremia, meningitis, bone/joint infection, and cellulitis-adenitis.

■ Late, late-onset GBS occurs in infants older than 3 months of age. It is most common in infants born before 28 weeks' gestation or in infants with a history of immunodeficiency. Symptoms may include bacteremia, CNS infection, and bone/joint infection.

Hepatitis B

■ Maternal transmission is thought to be from contact with the mother's blood at delivery.

■ Symptoms include malaise, nausea, vomiting, abdominal pain, and jaundice.

■ Infants born to positive mothers should receive hepatitis B immune globulin (HBIG).

Hepatitis C

■ Intrauterine transmission and infection at the time of delivery are both possible. The majority of hepatitis C virus (HCV)-infected infants are infected perinatally.

■ Neonates with HCV infection are usually asymptomatic or may have slightly elevated alanine transaminase (ALT) levels.

■ HCV RNA should be tested for diagnosis. Anti-HCV antibodies should be tested at 18 months of age for all perinatally exposed infants.

■ Treatment includes supportive management. Prescription treatment for HCV infection is not yet approved for children under 3 years of age.

Varicella

■ Varicella occurs through transplacental transmission. If contracted later in pregnancy, there is a higher risk of infant mortality.

■ Congenital varicella symptoms include skin lesions, ocular defects, limb abnormality, CNS abnormalities, IUGR, and death.

■ Acyclovir is given for perinatal transmission.

Herpes Simplex Types 1 and 2

■ Elective Cesarean section should be considered with active infection.

■ Infants should be swabbed in the conjunctivae, nasopharynx, and anus for culture/PCR exposure in addition to blood.

■ Skin, eye, and mouth (SEM) infection symptoms include vesicles that affect the skin, eye, or mucocutaneous membranes. This may result in cataracts, chorioretinitis, retinopathy, or neurologic impairment. ▶

Herpes Simplex Types 1 and 2 (*continued*)

- CNS infection symptoms include temperature instability, lethargy, seizures, or encephalitis. There is a high risk of mortality if left untreated. Long-term sequelae include microcephaly, blindness, spasticity, deafness, or learning disabilities.
- Disseminated infection, the most severe, includes pneumonitis, hepatitis, encephalitis, shock, seizures, respiratory distress, or disseminated intravascular coagulation (DIC). Half of infants infected are at risk of mortality or long-term morbidity.
- Intravenous (IV) acyclovir is used for treatment for 14 to 21 days depending on the classification of the HSV disease.

Neisseria Gonorrhoeae Infection

- This is typically acquired during delivery. Perinatal transmission can occur with maternal cervical infection. Intrauterine infection can occur after rupture of membranes.
- Infection causes purulent conjunctivitis with profuse exudate and swelling of the eyelids. It can lead to blindness without treatment.
- Ophthalmia neonatorum is confirmed by positive culture of the exudate.
- It is treated with ceftriaxone or cefotaxime in infants with significant hyperbilirubinemia.

Early-Onset Bacterial Disease

- This is an infection in the first 72 hours after birth (typically present within first 24 hours).
- Causative organisms are predominantly those which are colonized in the vagina or lower GI tract of the mother, such as GBS, gram-negative bacteria, staphylococci, and *Listeria*.
- It is typically treated with antibiotics.

[⚙] **ALERT!**

Daily suppressive antiviral therapy for women with a history of genital herpes can aid in the reduction of recurrent episodes and viral shedding. It has been recommended for all pregnant women with recurrent genital herpes starting at 36 weeks' gestation However, treatment does not always prevent asymptomatic shedding so there is still a risk of transmission from the mother to the infant. According to the American College of Obstetricians and Gynecologists, women presenting with prodromal symptoms (burning or tingling) or active genital lesions at the time of delivery should have a Cesarean delivery prior to rupture of membranes to lessen the risk of perinatal transmission

[⚙] **ALERT!**

Ceftriaxone should be used with caution in infants with clinically significant hyperbilirubinemia (it displaces bilirubin from albumin and may increase the risk of encephalopathy). It should also be avoided in neonates receiving calcium-containing intravenous fluids, including parenteral nutrition (due to risk of precipitation).

[📝] **POP QUIZ 15.2**

Which prophylactic measure has significantly reduced the risk of contracting gonococcal conjunctivitis in the newborn?

POSTNATAL ACQUISITION: HOSPITAL-ACQUIRED INFECTIONS

- Hospital-acquired or nosocomial infections are infections acquired in the NICU rather than in utero or intrapartum.
- Premature infants or term infants requiring prolonged hospitalization are primarily affected. The incidence increases as birth weight decreases.
- The most common nosocomial infections are central line-associated bloodstream infections or skin infections such as with *Staphylococcus aureus*.
- Prevention includes meticulous hand hygiene, infection surveillance, and adhering to strict protocols for maintaining catheters, lines, and devices.

Late-Onset Bacterial Disease

- Late-onset sepsis (LOS) occurs over 72 hours after birth.
- Coagulase-negative staphylococci are the predominant pathogens in LOS. Other organisms include *Escherichia coli, Klebsiella, Enterobacter, Pseudomonas,* and *Candida.*
- Blood culture is the definitive diagnostic tool.
- Treatment consists of empirical antibiotic therapy until organism is isolated.

Necrotizing Enterocolitis

- See Chapter 7, Gastrointestinal System.

Neonatal Pneumonia

- See Chapter 5, Respiratory System.

Central Line–Associated Bloodstream Infections

- Central line–associated bloodstream infections (CLABSI) are the most common healthcare-acquired infections in the NICU.
- Risk factors include poor skin integrity and prolonged IV use.
- Reductions in CLABSI are possible with implementation of bundled interventions focused on central line insertion and maintenance.

Urinary Tract Infection

- See Chapter 8, Renal/Genitourinary System.

IMMUNE DEFICIENCIES

PRIMARY IMMUNE DEFICIENCIES

- Many types of primary immune deficiencies (PIDs) appear in the neonatal period. Recognizing and managing PIDs in newborns are challenging because the primitive neonatal immune system masks immune deficits and/or results in complicated analysis of clinical findings and laboratory assays. Preterm newborns have fragile skin, moderate to severe hypogammaglobulinemia, lower lymphocyte counts, plasma complement, and antimicrobial peptide levels. These defects might make preterm and/or term neonates more susceptible to infections, making it hard to differentiate a premature infant with PID from an infant who is just premature.
- The most common PIDs include antibody deficiencies, cellular/combined immunodeficiencies (with syndromic appearance or dysmorphic facial features), phagocyte defects, immunoregulatory disorders, autoinflammatory disorders, complement deficiencies, and autoinflammatory disorders.

Risk Factors

- Family history of immunodeficiency, confirmed or suspected, leading to early death or reoccurrence, or chronic illness in one or more family members
- Male sex
- Certain ethnic groups with founder mutations (ataxia telangiectasia in Amish and Bloom syndrome in Ashkenazi Jews) or nations/populations where there is a high incidence of consanguinity (Amish, Arab countries)

Signs and Symptoms

- Syndromic look (abnormal facies)
- Infection at any location, infection after live vaccines
- Failure to thrive
- Chronic diarrhea
- Abdominal distention
- Lymphadenopathy and/or hepatosplenomegaly
- Lung or cardiac problems
- Mucosal diseases (thrush, mouth sores)
- Skin rashes
- Pigmentary disorders or alopecia
- Bleeding
- Petechiae
- Melena
- Late separation of the umbilical cord

SEVERE COMBINED IMMUNODEFICIENCY

- *Severe combined immunodeficiency (SCID)* is caused by defects in genes involved in the development and function of infection-fighting T- and B-cells.
- Infants with SCID appear healthy at birth but are highly susceptible to infections.
- If left untreated, SCID is fatal, usually within the first year of life.
- Development of a newborn screening test has made it possible to detect SCID before symptoms appear.
- Hematopoietic (blood-forming) stem cell transplantation is the standard treatment for infants with SCID.

INFECTIOUS DISEASES

MENINGITIS

- Evaluation includes CBC with differential, blood culture, urine culture, and LP. Examination of the CSF is necessary to diagnose bacterial meningitis.

Signs and Symptoms

- Seizure activity
- Apnea
- Tense or bulging fontanelle
- Respiratory distress
- Rash

Treatment

- Broad-spectrum antibiotics should be administered until organisms is confirmed on CSF. Ampicillin, gentamicin, and cefotaxime are typically given.

Nursing Interventions

- Infants should undergo a repeat LP 48 to 72 hours prior to discontinuing antimicrobial therapy as well as an MRI.

CONJUNCTIVITIS

- See Chapter 12, Head, Eyes, Ears, Nose, and Throat.

STREPTOCOCCAL DISEASE

- See Group B Streptococcus section.
- It may result in sepsis, meningitis, and pneumonia.
- Intrapartum prophylaxis and postpartum neonatal prophylaxis significantly reduce early-onset disease.

COVID-19

- There is not enough evidence to support vertical transmission.
- COVID-19-positive mothers may still breastfeed their infant; mask and proper hand hygiene are required.
- Clinical presentation in neonates is nonspecific.

Signs and Symptoms

- Temperature instability
- Respiratory distress
- Poor feeding
- Lethargy
- Diarrhea
- Vomiting

Nursing Interventions

- Perform testing and supportive management.
- Monitor vitals, and respiratory and GI symptoms.

NEONATAL SEPSIS

Etiology

- Early-onset sepsis (EOS) is caused by the transmission of pathogens from the female genitourinary system to the newborn or the fetus. Pathogens may involve the vagina, the cervix, and the uterus, or the amniotic fluid. Neonates can also become infected in utero or during delivery as during passage from the vaginal canal. Typical bacterial pathogens for EOS include GBS, *E. coli*, coagulase-negative *Staphylococcus*, *Haemophilus influenzae*, and *Listeria*. Maternal factors that may increase the risk of neonatal sepsis include chorioamnionitis, GBS colonization, delivery prior to 37 weeks, and prolonged rupture of membranes greater than 18 hours.
- LOS sepsis occurs via the transmission of pathogens from the surrounding environment after delivery, such as contact from healthcare workers or caregivers. LOS may also be caused by late manifestation of vertically transmitted infection. Neonates requiring intravascular catheter insertion or other invasive procedures are at increased risk of developing late-onset sepsis.

Signs and Symptoms

- Respiratory distress
- Irritability
- Lethargy ▶

Signs and Symptoms (*continued*)

- Temperature instability
- Persistent pulmonary hypertension
- Hypotension
- Poor perfusion

Laboratory Findings

- Laboratory testing results may be abnormal but are not necessarily diagnostic. Diagnosis is made by clinical symptoms of sepsis in addition to positive blood culture, CSF, or urine cultures.
- Laboratory findings with sepsis may include positive blood cultures, elevated CRP, elevated absolute neutrophil count (ANC) levels, leukocytosis, leukopenia, decreased platelet count, and possible positive urine culture.
- CSF analysis may reveal elevated protein level, elevated white blood cells (WBC), positive cultures, decreased glucose concentration, and positive PCR.
- Laboratory findings vary depending on the organism and the neonate's inflammatory response.

Complications

- DIC
- Respiratory failure (acute respiratory distress syndrome [ARDS])
- Septic shock
- Meningitis
- Symptomatic hypoglycemia

DIAGNOSTIC PROCEDURES

Laboratory Procedures

- Neonates with clinical signs of sepsis should have a CBC, differential with smear, blood culture, urine culture, and LP.

Lumbar Puncture

- LP checks for CSF, glucose and protein concentration, Gram stain, and culture.

[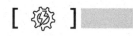]   **ALERT!**

Perform lumbar puncture prior to administering antibiotics if clinically stable.

- Hold the patient in lateral decubitis position. Palpate the spinous process that is even with the iliac crest. Locate one interspace above (L3–L4) or one space below (L4–L5) as the site.
- When collecting for diagnostic purposes, spinal fluid should be collected in the following order: tube 1: culture and stat Gram stain; tube 2: glucose and protein; and tube 3: cell count.

Imaging

- Neonates with respiratory symptoms require chest x-ray.
- MRI is done in cases of meningitis.

Kaiser Newborn Sepsis Calculator

- It is a tool used to assess the risk of EOS in infants born >34 weeks.
- It produces the probability of EOS per 1,000 babies by entering values for specified maternal risk factors and the infants' clinical presentation.
- Predictor includes incidence of EOS, gestational age, highest maternal antepartum temperature, hours of rupture of membranes (ROM), maternal GBS status, and type of intrapartum antibiotics.

COMMON PROCEDURES

Immunizations

- Infants born in the NICU follow the same schedule recommended by the Centers for Disease Control and Prevention (CDC) and the AAP. Monitor vital signs (VS) and for apnea/bradycardia postimmunization.
- Hepatitis B vaccine may be delayed in preterm infants due to low birth weight or instability.
- Palivizumab can be given in preterm infants with chronic lung disease (CLD) 1 month apart for the respiratory syncytial virus (RSV) season up to five doses.
- Deferral of rotavirus should be made until the time of discharge and should not be given in infants >15 weeks.

RESOURCES

Abbas, M., Bakhtyar, A., & Bazzi, R. Neonatal HIV. [Updated 2022 Sep 20]. In: StatPearls [Internet]. Treasure Island (FL): StatPearls Publishing; 2022 Jan-. Available from: https://www.ncbi.nlm.nih.gov/books/NBK565879

Akron Children's Hospital. (n.d.). *Specimen collection procedure - respiratory specimen collection.* Retrieved November 27, 2022, from https://www.akronchildrens.org/lab_test_specimen_procedures/Respiratory _Specimen_Collection.html

Centers for Disease Control and Prevention. (2021). Hand hygiene in healthcare settings: Healthcare providers—clean hands count for healthcare providers. Retrieved July 2021 from https://www.cdc.gov/handhygiene/providers /index.html

Centers for Disease Control and Prevention. (2022). *ACIP Vaccine Information Sources*

Centers for Disease Control and Prevention. *Guidelines for Immunization.* Retrieved December 2, 2022, from https:// www.cdc.gov/vaccines/hcp/acip-recs/general-recs/special-situations.html

IT-Development, D. O. R. (n.d.). *Infection probability calculator - neonatal sepsis calculator.* Infection Probability Calculator - Neonatal Sepsis Calculator. Retrieved December 2, 2022, from https://neonatalsepsiscalculator .kaiserpermanente.org

Kuti, B. P., Ogunlesi, T. A., Oduwole, O., Oringanje, C., Udoh, E. E., & Meremikwu, M. M. (2021). Hand hygiene for the prevention of infections in neonates. *Cochrane Database of Systematic Reviews, 1,* Article CD013326. Retrieved July 2021 from https://www.cochranelibrary.com/cdsr/doi/10.1002/14651858.CD013326.pub2/ full

Melikoki, V., Kourlaba, G., Kanavaki, I., Fessatou, S., & Papaevangelou, V. (2021). Seroprevalence of Hepatitis C in Children Without Identifiable Risk-Factors: A Systematic Review and Meta-Analysis. *Journal of Pediatric Gastroenterology and Nutrition. 72*(6), e140.

Messacar, K., Modlin, J. F., & Abzug, M. J. (2017). Enteroviruses and Parechoviruses. In: S. Long S, C. Prober, & M. Fischer (Eds.), *Principles and Practice of Pediatric Infectious Diseases.* Elsevier Saunders, Philadelphia.

Ozdemir, O. (2021). Primary immunodeficiency diseases in the newborn. *Northern Clinics of İstanbul, 8*(4), 405–413. https://doi.org/10.14744/nci.2020.43420

Pammi, M., Davis, R. J., Gordon, A., & Starke, J. (2016). Infant isolation and cohorting for preventing or reducing transmission of healthcare-associated infections in neonatal units. *Cochrane Database of Systematic Reviews. 2016*(12), CD012458. https://doi.org/10.1002/14651858.CD012458. PMCID: PMC6472529.

Rawlinson, W. D., Boppana, S. B., Fowler, K. B., Kimberlin, D. W., Lazzarotto, T., Alain, S., Daly, K., Doutré, S., Gibson, L., Giles, M. L., Greenlee, J., Hamilton, S. T., Harrison, G. J., Hui, L., Jones, C. A., Palasanthiran, P., Schleiss, M. R., Shand, A. W., & van Zuylen, W. J. (2017). Congenital cytomegalovirus infection in pregnancy and the neonate: Consensus recommendations for prevention, diagnosis, and therapy. *Lancet Infectious Diseases. 17*(6), e177–e188.

Samies, N. L., & James, S. H. (2020). Prevention and treatment of neonatal herpes simplex virus infection. *Antiviral Research. 176,* 104721. https://doi.org/10.1016/j.antiviral.2020.104721. Epub 2020 Feb 7. PMID: 32044154; PMCID: PMC8713303.

Singh, M., Alsaleem, M., & Gray, C. P. Neonatal Sepsis. [Updated 2022 Sep 29]. In: StatPearls [Internet]. Treasure Island (FL): StatPearls Publishing; 2022 Jan-. Available from: https://www.ncbi.nlm.nih.gov/books/NBK531478

University of South Florida (USF Health). "How Zika virus is transmitted from mother to fetus during pregnancy." ScienceDaily. ScienceDaily, 3 February 2021. <www.sciencedaily.com/releases/2021/02/210203101315.htm>.

Yu, J. C., Khodadadi, H., Malik, A., Davidson, B., Salles, É. D. S. L., Bhatia, J., Hale, V. L., & Baban, B. (2018). Innate immunity of neonates and infants. *Frontiers in Immunology*. 9, 1759.https://doi.org/10.3389/fimmu.2018.01759. PMID: 30105028; PMCID: PMC6077196.

APPENDIX 15.1 MEDICATIONS FOR INFECTIOUS DISEASES

INDICATIONS	MECHANISM OF ACTION	CONTRAINDICATIONS, PRECAUTIONS, AND ADVERSE EFFECTS
Antiretroviral (zidovudine)		
• Used in the management and treatment of HIV	• Functions as an antiviral agent by being incorporated into newly made viral DNA and acting as a viral DNA chain terminator • Inhibits the ability of HIV-1 reverse transcriptase to make viral DNA from the RNA template, which interferes with the HIV life cycle	• Medication may induce leukopenia, anemia, and macrocytosis.
Antiviral (acyclovir)		
• Treats neonatal herpes or varicella infections	• Taken up by infected cells and phosphorylated to the active compound acyclovir triphosphate • Acts as an inhibitor of herpes specified DNA polymerase • Prevents further viral DNA synthesis without affecting normal cellular processes	• Monitor renal function as it may increase urea and creatinine. • Medication may cause venous irritation.
Antiviral (valganciclovir)		
• Used to prevent disease in cytomegalovirus	• Valganciclovir: rapidly converted to ganciclovir in the body • Ganciclovir: inhibits binding of deoxyguanosine triphosphate to DNA polymerase, resulting in inhibition of viral DNA synthesis	• Valganciclovir should be avoided if the absolute neutrophil count is less than 500 cells/µL, platelet count is less than 25,000/µL, or hemoglobin is less than 8 g/dL.
Antifungal (fluconazole)		
• Treats candidiasis in infants	• Inhibition of the demethylase enzyme involved in the synthesis of ergosterol	• Medication may increase liver enzymes.
Antimicrobial (ampicillin, gentamicin, vancomycin)		
• Infection • Sepsis	• Binds to penicillin-binding proteins to inhibit bacterial cell wall synthesis	• Monitor renal and hepatic function. • Use caution not to infuse rapidly with vancomycin; "red person/red neck" syndrome may occur.

16 GENETIC DISORDERS

GENETICS

Genes

- A *gene* is a specific sequence of DNA and the functional unit of inheritance. Genes may contain information needed to make a protein or molecules that carry out all of a cell's vital activities.
- Humans have approximately 20,000 protein-coding genes.

Chromosomes

- The human genome consists of 23 pairs of *chromosomes* (thread-like packages of genes) and other DNA that carry genomic information from cell to cell. Chromosomes reside in the nucleus of cells.
- Each parent contributes one chromosome to each pair.

Genetic Disorders and Malformations

- Genes as well as environmental factors are believed to control the complex processes necessary for fetal development. When one or more of the processes becomes askew, they can result in genetic alterations that result in disease.
- There are four types of inherited genetic disorders: single-gene inheritance, multifactorial inheritance, chromosome abnormalities, and mitochondrial inheritance.

COMMON CHROMOSOMAL DISORDERS

Overview

- There are 46 chromosomes that present as 23 pairs. Chromosomal disorders are caused by structural changes in chromosomes.
- *Aneuploidy* is the loss or gain of a chromosome, such as in trisomy or monosomy. Common chromosomal disorders due to aneuploidy include Down syndrome, trisomy 13, trisomy 18, XXY syndrome, Turner syndrome, triple X syndrome, and XYY syndrome.
- *Deletion* is when a portion of a chromosome is lost during cell division.

Down Syndrome

- Down syndrome or trisomy 21 is the most common chromosomal disorder affecting about 1 in every 700 babies born each year.
- The prevalence of Down syndrome increases as the mother's age increases.
- Characteristic physical traits of Down syndrome include low muscle tone, a single deep crease across the palm of the hand, slightly flattened facial profile, short neck, protruding tongue, low-set ears, and an upward slant of the eyes. Mild to moderate cognitive impairment is common in people with Down syndrome.

Trisomy 18

- Trisomy 18, also known as Edward syndrome, occurs at a rate of 1 in 2,000 to 6,000 live births. 95% of babies do not survive beyond the first year.
- Characteristics include prominent back of the head; small eyes, mouth, and ears; clenched fists with overlapping fingers and thumbs; small fingernails; clubbed or rocker bottom soles of the feet; a short sternum; and extra skinfolds at the back of the neck.
- Over 90% of infants with trisomy 18 have a congenital heart defect, most commonly ventricular septal defect (VSD), atrial septal defect (ASD), or patent ductus arteriosus (PDA).

Trisomy 13

- Trisomy 13, also called Patau syndrome, occurs in about 1 out of every 10,000 newborns.
- It has a 90% mortality rate within the first year of life.
- Characteristics may include cleft lip or palate, clenched hands, close set eyes, decreased muscle tone, polydactyly, hernias, coloboma, low-set ears, seizures, single palmar crease, and intellectual disability.

Turner Syndrome

- Turner syndrome is a condition that only affects females.
- It results when one of the X chromosomes is missing.
- If Turner syndrome is apparent at birth, characteristics may include a web-like neck, low-set ears, high palate, fingernails that are turned upward, swelling of hands and feet, slowed growth, cardiac defects, low hairline at the back of the head, and a receding or small lower jaw.
- Mild cases may not be diagnosed until girls become teenagers. Young teens may have short stature and ovarian insufficiency due to ovarian failure. They will have slowed growth, slowed or stalled puberty, and early end to menstrual cycles.

SINGLE-GENE OR MENDELIAN DISORDERS

Overview

- *Single-gene* or *Mendelian disorders* are genes that can be pinpointed as a cause of a disease.
- Single-gene mutations are grouped according to whether the trait is sex-specific (X-linked) or not (autosomal).
- Mendelian disorders or single-gene disorders are relatively uncommon.

Autosomal Dominant Disorders

- Autosomal dominant disorders occur in infants who contain a single mutant copy of the disease-associated gene.
- Affected individuals are heterozygous. Inheritance of only one copied from either an affected mother or an affected father is sufficient enough to cause disease.
- Autosomal dominant diseases may include Marfan syndrome, neurofibromatosis, retinoblastoma, and polydactyly.

Autosomal Recessive Disorders

- Two copies of the mutated gene are needed in order to have an autosomal recessive disorder. One allele is inherited from the mother and one from the father.
- The risk of experiencing the effect of the disorder is 25%. 75% of affected babies will be unaffected but will be carriers of the gene.
- Phenylketonuria (PKU) is a prominent autosomal recessive disorder. Other disorders include cystic fibrosis, sickle cell anemia, and Tay-Sachs disease.

X-LINKED DISORDERS

- X-linked dominant inheritance follows a similar pattern to autosomal dominant inheritance; however, more females are affected than males. These disorders are very rare.
- X-linked recessive disorders usually only occur in males, a second X chromosome in females will be normal, while males who inherit the recessive gene on their sole X chromosome will be affected.
- X-linked disorders include hemophilia A, Duchenne muscular dystrophy, and glucose-6-phosphate dehydrogenase (G6PD).

COMPLEX OR MULTIFACTORIAL DISORDERS

Overview

- Complex or multifactorial disorders result from contributions of multiple genomic variants and genes in conjunction with significant physical and environmental influences.
- Common complex disorders include heart disease, diabetes, and cancer.

Nontraditional Inheritance

- Inheritance patterns that do not fall into single-gene or multifactorial categories are known as nontraditional.
- *Uniparental disomy* is when two copies of a chromosome come from the same parent. Examples include Angelman syndrome and Prader–Willi syndrome.
- Trinucleotide repeats occur when there are more than the usual copies that should be in a gene. This may cause the gene to no longer function. An example is fragile X syndrome.
- Mitochondrial genes are inherited from the mother only. If there is a mutation in a mitochondrial gene, it will pass from the mother to all of the children. Sons will not pass the gene; however, daughters will pass it to all of their children. An example of a mitochondrial inheritance gene is Leber hereditary optic neuropathy (LHON).

INHERITED METABOLIC DISORDERS

- Inherited metabolic disorders, also known as inborn errors of metabolism, are heritable or genetic disorders. They occur when an infant inherits two defective copies of a gene, one from each parent.
- Examples include galactosemia, maple syrup urine disease, Krabbe disease, glycogen storage disease, cystinuria, and PKU.
- Infants with inherited metabolic disorders may exhibit apnea, lethargy, poor feeding, tachypnea, jaundice, seizures, failure to thrive, vomiting, or abnormal odor of urine, breath, sweat, or saliva.
- Infants experiencing persistent hypoglycemia or jaundice may warrant further testing for inborn errors of metabolism.
- Symptoms may appear within a few weeks of birth or may take several years to develop. Routine standard newborn screening has helped to identify many inherited metabolic disorders.

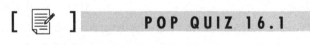

[📝]   POP QUIZ 16.1

When changing the diaper of a 2-day-old infant, the nurse notices a strong odor of maple syrup in the urine. What disorder would the nurse suspect and what steps should be taken next?

Environmental Exposure Abnormalities

- *Teratogens* are environmental agents or substances that can be physical, chemical, or biological, which harm a developing fetus. They may include drugs, alcohol, tobacco, infection, radiation, hyperthermia, and environmental toxins such as mercury, lead, pesticides, pollutants, and polychlorinated and polybrominated biphenyls (PCBs).
- The risk of teratogens to a developing fetus is usually early in the first trimester and sometimes prior to implantation.
- Living near hazardous waste has been associated with possible birth defects including spina bifida, cleft lip/palate, gastroschisis, hypospadias, Down syndrome, and heart defects.
- Teratogens may cause complications such as preterm labor, spontaneous abortions, or miscarriages.
- In addition to physical malformations such as neural tube defects, microcephaly, abdominal wall defects, and limb reduction defects, teratogens may cause behavioral or emotional development issues in a child.

[📝] 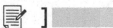 **POP QUIZ 16.2**

Hyperthermia has been recognized as teratogenic to the fetus. What measures should pregnant women avoid in their pregnancy in order to decrease the risk of hyperthermia?

DIAGNOSTIC PROCEDURES

Physical Examination

- A complete physical examination of every newborn should be performed within 24 hours of birth to detect any genetic conditions or acute condition requiring urgent diagnosis.
- Basic measurements of length, weight, and head circumference should be done, as well as assessment of gestational age.
- The cardiorespiratory system should be evaluated to rule out any obvious cardiac or respiratory defects.
- Head and neck should be inspected to rule out any craniofacial abnormalities.
- The abdomen and pelvis should be assessed to rule out hernias, masses, or genital abnormalities.
- The musculoskeletal system should be examined to rule out deformities in the extremities, missing limbs, contractures, or maldevelopment.
- The spine should be inspected for issues with the spinal cord as well as the hips for dysplasia.
- The infant's neurologic systems should be assessed for reflexes, tone, and level of alertness.
- The skin should be assessed for any abnormalities.
- Major malformations may be more apparent on physical examination than minor malformations, which may present over time.

Newborn Screening

- Newborns are routinely screened for genetic, endocrine, and metabolic disorders at birth using a simple blood test called a newborn screen.
- Newborn screening tests may include testing for PKU, congenital hypothyroidism, galactosemia, sickle cell disease, maple syrup urine disease, homocystinuria, biotinidase deficiency, congenital adrenal hyperplasia, and medium-chain acyl-coenzyme A dehydrogenase (MCAD).
- Most screenings are performed after 24 hours within 48 hours to allow the infant to have at least 24 hours of breast milk or formula. The infant may need a repeat testing if they are premature or if there is suspected disease.
- Routine hearing screens are done for all newborns as well to rule out hearing loss.

[⚡] 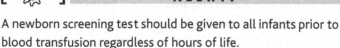 **ALERT!**

A newborn screening test should be given to all infants prior to blood transfusion regardless of hours of life.

Laboratory Data

- There is no single genetic test to detect all genetic conditions. Tests are individualized based on family and medical history and suspected genetic condition.
- Single-gene tests look for changes in one gene. This is done for conditions such as Duchenne muscular dystrophy or sickle cell disease. It can be used when there is a known genetic mutation in the family.
- Panel testing looks for changes in many genes usually grouped in categories based on different medical concerns. Examples of genetic panel tests include low muscle tone, epilepsy, and short stature.
- Large-scale genetic tests include exome sequencing, which looks at all of the genes in the DNA (whole exome) or can look at just the genes related to medical conditions (clinical exome). Genome sequencing is the largest genetic test and looks at all of a person's DNA.
- Chromosomal testing can be done as well to look for chromosomes rather than gene changes, such as karyotypes or microarrays.
- Gene expression tests compare levels between normal cells and diseased cells.

Imaging

- X-rays, CT scans, or MRI may be used to see structures within the body in order to assist in diagnosing a genetic disease. This is especially helpful in diagnosing neuromuscular, musculoskeletal, or central nervous system (CNS) disease.

RESOURCES

ACOG. (n.d.). *Cell-free DNA to screen for single-gene disorders*. Retrieved December 5, 2022, from https://www.acog.org/clinical/clinical-guidance/practice-advisory/articles/2019/02/cell-free-dna-to-screen-for-single-gene-disorders

Blencowe, H., Moorthie, S., Petrou, M., Hamamy, H., Povey, S., Bittles, A., Gibbons, S., Darlison, M., & Modell, B. (2018). Rare single gene disorders: Estimating baseline prevalence and outcomes worldwide. *Journal of Community Genetics*, 9(4), 397–406. https://doi.org/10.1007/s12687-018-0376-2

Centers for Disease Control and Prevention. (2014). *Racking network: Birth defects and the environment*. Centers for Disease Control and Prevention. Retrieved December 5, 2022, from https://www.cdc.gov/nceh/features/trackingnetwork/save/copy-1-of-index.html#:~:text = Environmental%20Exposures%20and%20Birth%20Defects&text = Living%20near%20a%20hazardous%20waste,heart%20and%20blood%20vessel%20defects

Centers for Disease Control and Prevention. (2020). *Data and statistics on down syndrome*. Centers for Disease Control and Prevention. Retrieved December 5, 2022, from https://www.cdc.gov/ncbddd/birthdefects/downsyndrome/data.html#:~:text = Down%20syndrome%20continues%20to%20be,in%20every%20700%20babies%20born

Dima, V. (n.d.). *Actualities in neonatal endocrine and metabolic screening*. Acta endocrinologica (Bucharest, Romania). Retrieved December 5, 2022, from https://pubmed.ncbi.nlm.nih.gov/35342476

Han, L. (2021). Genetic screening techniques and diseases for neonatal genetic diseases. *Journal of Zhejiang University (Medical Science)*, 50(4), 429–435. https://doi.org/10.3724/zdxbyxb-2021-0288. PMID: 34704410; PMCID: PMC8714486.

Humana Press. (n.d.). *Principles of Molecular Medicine*. SpringerLink. Retrieved December 5, 2022, from https://link.springer.com/book/10.1007/978-1-59259-963-9

National Human Genome Research Institute. (n.d.-a). *Complex disease*. Retrieved December 5, 2022, from https://www.genome.gov/genetics-glossary/Complex-Disease

National Human Genome Research Institute. (n.d.-b). *Gene*. Retrieved December 4, 2022, from https://www.genome.gov/genetics-glossary/Gene

Surveillance guidelines for children with trisomy 13. (n.d.). Retrieved December 5, 2022, from https://onlinelibrary.wiley.com/doi/10.1002/ajmg.a.62133

U.S. Department of Health and Human Services. (n.d.). *Trisomy 18 - about the disease*. Genetic and Rare Diseases Information Center. Retrieved December 5, 2022, from https://rarediseases.info.nih.gov/diseases/6321/trisomy-18

17 NEONATAL FOUNDATIONS

NUTRITION AND FEEDING MANAGEMENT

Overview

- Nutrition and feeding management in the NICU can be complex. Many infants will receive intravenous (IV) fluids and parenteral nutrition when they are premature or critically ill. Fluids need to be delicately balanced and carefully assessed for optimal nutrition and hydration.
- Infants may receive trophic feeds in the beginning of their NICU stay and progress to full feeds via orogastric tubes until they are ready for breastfeeding or bottle feeding.
- Each infant has unique requirements that are constantly assessed to ensure optimal nutrition and fluid balance.

ENTERAL NUTRITION REQUIREMENTS AND COMPOSITION

- Term infants require about 100 kcal/kg/d. Preterm caloric requirements are about 110 to 135 kcal/kg/d. Nutrition is focused on providing optimal caloric content and protein, as well as macronutrients (protein, carbohydrates, and lipids), micronutrients, and electrolytes.
- Enteral feeds are introduced as soon as possible; trophic feeds are ideally given within 4 hours of life and advanced gradually until full feeds can be attained/kg/d.
- Feeds are gradually advanced by 10 to 30 mL/kg/d to full feeds usually over 7 to 14 days. When the infant is receiving 75 to 80 mL/kg/d, breast milk may be fortified up to 24 cal/oz.

Formulas

- Formula is modeled after breast milk and usually contains 20 kcal/oz.
- The carbohydrate source is lactose and standard formula usually contains cow's milk protein unless specialty formula is required for certain feeding intolerances.
- There is formula to cater to different feeding intolerances such as lactase deficiency, enzyme deficiency, or allergy to cow's milk. There is also formula available for many specific needs such as antireflux, lactose allergy, hypoallergenic, and colic.
- Preterm infants have higher protein and caloric requirements. They require more calcium, magnesium, and phosphorus. Formulas geared toward premature infants are designed to meet the special requirements of this population. Preterm formulas contain 24 kcal/oz. Enriched formulas may also contain 22 kcal/oz. for infants not requiring 24 kcal.

Breast Milk

- The composition of breast milk (also known as human milk) varies depending on gestational age, maternal diet, and environmental factors.
- Breast milk is generally about 87% to 88% water and 124 g/L solid components as macronutrients, including 7% carbohydrates, 1% protein, and 3.8% fat. ▶

Breast Milk (*continued*)

■ Breast milk also contains live immune-boosting white blood cells, stem cells, amino acids, oligosaccharides, enzymes, growth factors, hormones, vitamins, minerals, microRNAs, long-chain fatty acids, and antibodies. All of these components boost the neonate's immune system, aid in digestion and brain development, regulate the infant's appetite, and support healthy growth and organ function.

Colostrum Feeding

■ *Colostrum* is the first type of milk the body makes. It is a thick yellowish fluid and is produced for a few days after birth.

■ It is very high in protein, minerals, and fat-soluble vitamins, and is catered to the baby's needs in the first few days after birth. Colostrum contains antibodies needed to fight off viral and bacterial infections.

■ Colostrum can be breast-, spoon-, cup-, bottle, or gavage-fed.

■ In cases where smaller amounts are produced, colostrum can be collected on swabs or in syringes, and parents or providers can provide oral care to the neonate by placing colostrum to the buccal mucosa. Early administration of colostrum via oral care may provide immunologic benefits.

Donor Breast Milk

■ Donor breast milk is available for mothers who are unable to produce enough milk or cannot breastfeed due to personal or medical reasons.

■ Donated milk is safe as long as it comes from an accredited milk bank. Milk donors undergo medical and physical screenings. The milk is pasteurized (sterilized) and tested for bacterial growth, recreational and prescription drugs, various infectious, and other substances.

■ Donor milk can help strengthen the infant's immune system and fight off infection. Human milk is easier to digest than most formulas; therefore, donor milk is a great option for infants in the NICU who are at risk of developing necrotizing enterocolitis.

■ Some nutrients may be lost in pasteurization, but pasteurized donor milk is still more beneficial for the infant than formula. While the rules for donating breast milk to a donor bank are more stringent than blood donation, there is still a chance that undetected viruses remain in the milk and this could place the infant at risk.

■ The risks versus benefits need to be considered when using human donor milk.

FEEDING TECHNIQUES

■ Feeding techniques in the NICU vary depending on gestational age and the infant's well-being and ability to feed.

■ Breastfeeding and bottle feeding are two methods of feeding. Infants who are born very prematurely or who are not ready to feed orally may be fed by gavage feeding or syringe feeding.

■ At some point in the infant's stay, they may utilize gavage or syringe, breastfeeding, and bottle feeding throughout the day until they are strong enough to exclusively breastfeed or bottle-feed.

Oral Feeding

■ Infants are typically ready for oral feeding when they are able to coordinate a suck–swallow–breathe pattern without cardiorespiratory compromise.

■ Infants are scored based on readiness and may begin to orally feed as early as 33 to 34 weeks' gestation depending on respiratory status and overall well-being. Other infants may not be ready until the 35- to 38-week mark. Each infant is evaluated on their ability to orally feed safely.

■ Oral feeds can be via bottle feeding or breastfeeding.

Infant-Driven Feeding

- Infant-driven feeding provides consistent assessment tools and feeding techniques to support the infant's feeding needs, promote positive oral feeding experiences, and decrease the length of hospital stay. It is individualized and developmentally focused rather than focusing on having the infant drink a specific volume.
- The infant-driven feeding method is composed of three behavioral assessments: feeding readiness, quality of feeding, and caregiver support.
- Infants are given a score from 1 to 5 to assess feeding readiness. Scores of 1 to 2 allow for nipple feeding, while scores of 3 to 5 determine that the infant should be gavage-fed.

Gavage Feeding

- Preterm infants born less than 32 to 33 weeks' gestation and critically ill infants require an orogastric or nasogastric tube.
- Bolus feedings are given via gravity or timed on a feeding pump. Feedings of breast milk or formula may be given via gavage.

Breastfeeding

- The same considerations will be taken for breastfeeding as for bottle feeding. Infants will be evaluated for readiness to feed.
- Nurses and lactation consultants will assist parents in breastfeeding the infant.
- Infants will typically be offered the breast one to two times a day until the infant is able to tolerate breastfeeding well.

Neonatal Intensive Care Unit Considerations

- Nonnutritive sucking can be provided prior to full breastfeeding initiation to get the infant familiar with the breast.
- Premature infants tire easily, so breastfeeding sessions may be brief and the remainder gavage-fed.
- Premature infants may require a nipple shield to breastfeed until they gain the strength to create the suction necessary to breastfeed.
- Infants will need to be carefully monitored for cardiorespiratory compromise while breastfeeding.

Contraindications to Breast Milk

- Breastfeeding may be contraindicated in infants with galactosemia and in infants whose mothers are diagnosed with HIV or T-cell lymphotropic virus. Breastfeeding may also be contraindicated if the mother is using illicit drugs, including phencyclidine (PCP) or cocaine.
- Narcotic-dependent mothers enrolled in a supervised methadone program and are free of other illicit drugs can still breastfeed because it is beneficial to the infant.
- Mothers should also temporarily not breastfeed if they are taking certain medications that are contraindicated in breastfeeding, if they are undergoing diagnostic imaging with radiopharmaceuticals, when they have brucellosis, or when they have active herpes simplex virus (HSV) lesions present on their breast.
- Infants can be fed expressed breast milk if the mother has active tuberculosis or active varicella.
- Other needs for feeding expressed breast milk include the mother not being physically present in the NICU or if the mother is not able to physically breastfeed or the infant has a difficult time latching.

NEUROPROTECTIVE/NEURODEVELOPMENTAL CARE

Overview

- Neuroprotective care is vital in the NICU to protect infants from intraventricular hemorrhage. Minimal handling of extremely premature infants is crucial especially in the first 72 hours after birth. Interventions such as midline positioning, minimal handling, maintaining normothermia, avoiding IV boluses, and maintaining normal carbon dioxide (CO_2) levels help decrease the risk of intraventricular hemorrhage. Optimal nutrition is also necessary for the developing brain.
- Neurodevelopmental care involves minimizing stress for the infant by decreasing overstimulation in the NICU by lowering noise levels, dimming lighting, providing cluster care, and encouraging kangaroo care.

TOUCH

- Touching can be stressful, uncomfortable, and overstimulating for premature infants if not done in an intentional and therapeutic manner.
- Therapeutic touch in medically stable infants is reported to improve weight gain, result in less apnea and bradycardia, and decrease length of hospital stay.
- Therapeutic touch involves containment holding, putting hands on the head and feet of the infant, and applying gentle and steady pressure on their body.
- Avoid stroking premature infants in the NICU as it can be overstimulating to their developing nervous system. Use a firm touch instead. As the infant matures, they may later enjoy stroking or patting.

Massage

- Infant massage in the NICU includes using positive mindful touch with gentle but firm pressure. Massage involves slowly kneading each part of the baby's body while extending and flexing their arms and legs.
- To ensure proper neuroprotective/neurodevelopmental care, infant massage should only be given by providers or parents who have had education and/or certification on infant massage techniques.
- Benefits of infant massage include shorter length of stay, reduced pain, feeding tolerance, and improved weight gain.

KANGAROO CARE

- Kangaroo care is the act of holding an infant skin-to-skin on a bare chest with the infant wearing only a diaper.
- To increase stimulation, it is most beneficial for the infant to be held for at least an hour, if tolerated.
- Kangaroo care can improve blood oxygen levels, improve weight gain, and maintain stable body temperature, heart rate, and respirations. It can help infants sleep better, encourage breastfeeding, and decrease the length of hospital stay.
- Holding an infant skin-to-skin encourages bonding and helps physical and emotional development.

SWADDLING AND BODY CONTAINMENT

- Swaddling in the NICU can help the infant feel secure, prevent the startle reflex from waking up the infant, promote sleeping, and help preterm infants maintain their temperature.
- It is important when swaddling to keep the swaddle loose on the infant's hips to prevent hip dysplasia. The infant should be able to move and flex their hips upward. The infant's hands should be placed midline under their chin. ▶

SWADDLING AND BODY CONTAINMENT (*continued*)

- Containment is a way of placing hands on the infant's head and body to make them feel secure. Tucking the infant's arms and legs in toward their body soothes them and helps them calm. Containment holding allows providers or parents to comfort infants without picking them up. This can be done to soothe a restless infant or during a painful procedure such as suctioning or a heel stick.
- Containment holding has been shown to reduce pain and promote a faster recovery.

POSITIONING

- Therapeutic positioning maintains the fetal midline position of flexion to support the infant and promotes comfort and self-regulation.
- Positioning may involve the time-limited use of positioning devices, including blanket rolls and commercially available developmentally supportive products such as a "snuggle up" or "bendy bumper," to help create boundaries for the infant and mimic the womb.
- Without support from these devices, the preterm infant lies flat and asymmetric with the hips and joints abducted with abnormal rotation. This may lead to musculoskeletal and neurodevelopmental abnormalities such as upper extremity hyperabduction, flexion, and generalized muscular rigidity.

Safe Sleep

- Certain medical needs in the NICU often benefit from nonsupine positioning of the infant and positioning devices. All NICU patients are on monitors and can be watched closely while in prone position. Once the infant is medically stable, they should be transitioned to a safe sleep environment like they would use at home.
- The American Academy of Pediatrics (AAP) recommends that the infant be placed on their back to sleep, with the use of a firm, flat sleep surface, free of loose bedding or soft objects like stuffed toys, a neutral thermal environment, room sharing without bed sharing, and a smoke-free environment.

[] **ALERT!**

Infants in acute respiratory distress, regardless of gestational age, may be placed in nonsupine positioning as clinically indicated to stabilize/improve respiratory function.

[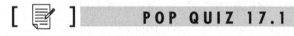] **POP QUIZ 17.1**

Which intervention is beneficial to an infant with Pierre Robin syndrome who has a moderate case of gravity-dependent, tongue-based obstruction?

ENVIRONMENTAL CARE

- The NICU environment can affect the infant's neurosensory and neurobehavioral development. Measures should be taken in the NICU to decrease stimulation and promote a calm, soothing environment.
- Environmental care includes decreasing noise below 50 decibels, dimming lights to promote sleep/wake cycles (covers can be placed over isolettes to achieve this), and promoting cluster care to avoid disturbing the infant unless necessary.

Auditory

- Auditory stimulation interventions in the NICU include music therapy, music (classical, calming music, lullabies), singing (parental or from music therapist), and implementing recordings of maternal heartbeat or voice.

Visual

- Visual stimulation in the NICU includes eye contact (eye-to-eye), eye engagement, visual contact, and visual engagement (such as a mobile, light and cycled lighting or light reduction).
- Visual stimulus can be in the form of developmentally appropriate toys or patterns.

Taste and Smell

- Oral stimulation in the NICU includes oropharyngeal colostrum, oral immune therapy, oral sucrose, flavor agents, and oral/buccal hygiene.
- Smell stimulation includes breast milk and the mother's scent.

NEURODEVELOPMENTAL DISABILITIES

- About 17% of children are born with developmental disabilities that begin during the developmental period and may be recognized at any point between birth and childhood.
- Developmental disabilities are conditions due to an impairment in physical, learning, language, or behavior areas.

Risk Factors

- Prenatal risk factors for neurodevelopmental disabilities include chronic maternal illness, certain maternal infections (cytomegalovirus [CMV], toxoplasmosis), toxin exposures, and nutritional deficiencies.
- Risk factors in the perinatal period may include pregnancy-related complications, prematurity, low birth weight, and infection exposure during pregnancy or during the birthing process.
- Lack of access to quality care during pregnancy, delivery, and soon after birth can significantly contribute to developmental disabilities and adversely affect outcomes for both the mother and the infant.

Neurodevelopmental Impairments

- Common neurodevelopmental impairments seen in former NICU patients include attention deficit hyperactivity disorder (ADHD), autism spectrum disorder, cerebral palsy, visual or hearing impairment, intellectual disability, learning disability, and other developmental delays.

PAIN ASSESSMENT AND MANAGEMENT/PALLIATIVE CARE

Overview

- Neonates may experience long-term effects to pain, including negative effects on neurologic and behavioral development, because the experience of pain occurs during a critical time of neurologic maturation.
- Assessing pain in a neonate is difficult because they are nonverbal, although multiple validated pain scoring systems exist; there is no standardized or universal approach to assessing neonatal pain. There is a lack of understanding of how neonates perceive pain and the results that occur when pain remains untreated.

PAIN RESPONSE OF THE NEONATE

- Neonates experience acute and measurable physiologic, behavioral, metabolic, and hormonal responses to pain.

Physiologic

- Increased heart rate and blood pressure
- Decreased oxygen saturation

Behavioral

- Changes in facial expression (grimacing)
- Motion activity of the body and extremities
- Sleep disturbances
- Crying

Hormonal

Major hormonal responses to pain as indicated by changes in plasma include:

- Adrenaline
- Noradrenaline
- Glucagon
- Aldosterone
- Corticosterone
- Blood glucose
- Lactate
- Pyruvate

COMMON CAUSES OF NEONATAL PAIN

- Routine patient care (gastric tube insertion, bladder catheterization, or physical examination)
- Moderately invasive procedures (suctioning, venipuncture, or heel stick)
- More invasive procedures (chest tube placement, circumcision, or central venous access)

NEONATAL PAIN ASSESSMENT TOOLS

- Assessing pain in the neonate is mandatory across all hospitals. Common pain assessment tools include the Neonatal Infant Pain Scale (NIPS) and the Premature Infant Pain Profile (PIPPS).
- The NIPS is used in term infants. The infant is scored based on facial expressions, crying and breathing patterns, arm and leg movements, and arousal.
- The PIPPS is used in preterm infants. The infant is scored based on heart rate, oxygen saturation, and facial actions.
- The Neonatal Pain, Agitation, and Sedation Scale (N-PASS) is used in mechanically ventilated patients as well as during a procedure or postoperatively. The infant is scored based on crying, irritability, facial expression, extremity tone, and vital signs (VS).

PAIN MANAGEMENT OF THE NEONATE

- Neonatal pain is best managed using a multidirectional approach to painful procedures in the NICU in a tiered manner, which includes nonpharmacologic and pharmacologic modalities.
- Optimizing pain management in the neonatal population is aimed at reducing the total number of painful events and disrupting the infant throughout the day.

Pharmacologic

- Topical anesthetics such as lidocaine or eutectic mixture of local anesthetics (EMLA)
- Acetaminophen
- Local anesthetics such as lidocaine injections
- Deep sedation including opiates such as morphine and fentanyl ►

Pharmacologic (*continued*)

- Ketamine for procedural sedation
- Midazolam

Nonpharmacologic

- Oral sucrose: A pacifier dipped in oral sucrose is recommended for pain reduction in procedures such as venipuncture and heel sticks.
- Breast milk: Alternatively, a pacifier can be dipped in breast milk, or a mother may breastfeed through the procedure if possible.
- Skin-to-skin can be used during or after painful procedures to reduce pain and soothe the infant.
- Nonnutritive sucking can also be used to soothe the neonate.
- Swaddling or facilitated tucking can be used during painful procedures to comfort the infant.

[⚙]   **ALERT!**

Nonsteroidal anti-inflammatory drugs (NSAIDs) should not be used in infants younger than 6 months old.

[📝]   **POP QUIZ 17.2**

A nurse is preparing to perform a heel stick for a newborn screen on a premature infant. Which intervention would be best practice?

PALLIATIVE CARE OF THE NEONATE

- Palliative care serves as an alternative to intensive care.
- This care continues to provide quality care and grief support while honoring both the baby and the family through prevention and relief of suffering.
- Early assessment and treatment of pain is used along with other physical, psychosocial, and spiritual issues.
- The goal of palliative and bereavement care is to make families and neonates as comfortable as possible. It is important to engage the family in the plan of care and to recognize that each family is unique in their beliefs and wishes.
- Palliative and bereavement care must be considered as standard care.
- The setting for care may be an acute care hospital, an ambulatory care facility, or at home.

Education

- All healthcare professionals who work with pregnant women, neonates, and their families should receive education and demonstrate competence in palliative care.
- Education should include training in how to communicate effectively and empathetically with families.
- Palliative care and bereavement-specific policies should be in place and easily accessible to all staff to ensure a standard of care for all families.
- It is important that staff have a chance to debrief and receive support when working with neonatal loss.

PATIENT SAFETY

Medical Errors

- Misidentification: Using patient armbands is necessary to prevent the wrong treatment being administered, such as blood draws, blood administration, or medication.
- Failure of diagnosis: An example is a failure to diagnose hypoglycemia.
- Medication error: An example is administering the wrong dose or medication.
- Breast milk errors: An example is giving the wrong patient's breast milk to another patient.

Adverse Events

- Adverse events (AEs) are patient injuries resulting from the healthcare provider's intervention rather than as a consequence of the patient's underlying condition.
- Some AEs are the result of errors and others are unavoidable (such as a reaction to an appropriately prescribed medication).
- AEs may be minor events or severe, resulting in death.
- AEs may include IV infiltration from not monitoring an IV properly or nosocomial infections such as a patient contracting methicillin-resistant *Staphylococcus aureus* (MRSA) from a healthcare worker.
- Unplanned extubation may occur when weighing and turning an infant.

Prevention

- Prevention is key to reducing medical errors and AEs in the NICU. The staff should be provided education and competencies in adverse risk areas. The staff should feel safe reporting errors without immediate punitive action.

Tools

- Bundles to prevent hospital-acquired infections (HAIs)
- Hourly IV inspection to prevent infiltration/extravasion
- Barcode scanning for breast milk and medication administration
- Two-nurse identification for potentially harmful medications, breast milk, and blood administration
- Three-way communication for medication, critical situations, and procedural orders
- Using two providers for weighing, turning, and providing kangaroo care to infants at risk of accidental extubation

DISCHARGE PLANNING

Overview

- Discharge planning should begin on the first day of admission. Parents should be continually educated throughout the infant's NICU stay on how to care for their infant in the unit and at home. Barriers to discharge should be recognized early and plans should be put into place by the healthcare team and social worker.

DISCHARGE CONSIDERATIONS

- The AAP recommends discharge of infants from the NICU when they are able to ingest sufficient oral feeding to support appropriate growth; coordinate oral feeding, suck, swallow, and breathing; maintain normal body temperature in a home environment; and have stable cardiorespiratory function.
- Infants requiring increased care at home, such as discharge on home oxygen, tracheostomy, or feeding tube, will be considered for discharge at the discretion of the healthcare team and the comfort and ability to be able to care for the infant at home by the parents.

Parent Education

- Parent education in the NICU should be ongoing and not just at discharge. Healthcare staff should educate parents on how to care for their infant throughout the course of their stay, which will help them feel confident in caring for the infant at home.
- Use a discharge education checklist and allow parents opportunities to practice their skills with direct supervision. Allow rooming-in prior to discharge when possible. Parents should also be provided with a list of helpful supplies they will need at home to care for the baby. ►

Parent Education (*continued*)

- Parents with infants requiring special care will need to be educated on proper procedure and administration of either oxygen, tube feedings, suctioning, and so forth.
- Parents should receive CPR training and any monitor training that may be needed.
- Parents need to be educated on when to call the pediatrician or 911 in emergencies.

SCREENING

- Patients need to have state-mandated metabolic screening testing within 24 to 36 hours of birth. If they are extremely premature, testing will generally be repeated. Infants who are born at term and will be discharged in a few days must have it done prior to leaving the hospital.
- A hearing screening should be completed prior to discharge, with follow-up plans for infants who may require a full audiology assessment.
- A car seat test to assess cardiorespiratory stability in a car seat is recommended for infants born at <37 weeks' gestation or with other risk factors for respiratory compromise.
- All infants should have a screening for critical congenital heart defects (CCHD) when they are at least 24 hours old and must be done prior to discharge.

ASSESSMENTS

- A general assessment should be done to determine if the infant is stable for discharge.
- Assessment includes physical assessment, car seat testing, and hearing screen.
- An assessment should be completed to ensure that the family has the supplies that they need to properly care for the infant at home.

Care Needs of Neonatal Intensive Care Unit Graduates

- Follow-up care is necessary for most NICU graduates. The NICU team needs to collaborate with the family and specialists for follow up and continuity of care.
- The infant will need a primary care pediatrician experienced with infants who have been in the NICU.
- Infants who are at risk of retinopathy of prematurity will need ophthalmology appointments.
- Infants who have intraventricular hemorrhages or neuro issues will need to follow up with neurology.
- Infants with hearing issues will need to follow up with an audiologist.
- Infants with cardiac issues will need to follow up with cardiology, and infants with respiratory issues will need to follow up with pulmonology.
- Infants who are born premature or have neuro conditions should follow up with a developmental pediatrician or clinic.

END-OF-LIFE/HOSPICE CARE

Considerations

- Life-sustaining care and treatment may be ethically withdrawn or withheld in critically ill or dying newborns if doing so is genuinely in the best interests of the infant.
- Clinical considerations for making the decision for end-of-life care involve the healthcare team; specialists such as cardiologists, pulmonologists, or neurologists; social workers; and the parents.
- End-of-life care may be considered when life-sustaining treatment is futile due to a hopeless prognosis or if the burdens of intensive treatment clearly outweigh its benefits. The healthcare team and the parents must come to an agreement and come up with a plan for end-of-life care. ►

Considerations (*continued*)

- Clinical considerations may include significant intraventricular hemorrhage, birth asphyxia resulting in neurologic compromise, multiorgan system failure, CCHD where treatment is futile, and genetic conditions with hopeless prognosis.

Components

- Comfort care involves providing as much comfort as possible until an infant passes, while discontinuation of care usually involves compassionate extubation or withdrawing of care or medications that assist with end of life.
- End-of-life care includes addressing pain and other distressing symptoms in the infant. Pain should be assessed every 15 minutes until it is stabilized, and subsequently at least every 3 hours.
- Nonpharmacologic neonatal comfort measures include swaddling, facilitated tucking, kangaroo care, and nonnutritive sucking with or without oral sucrose.
- Pharmacologic treatment should be given as needed.
- End-of-life respiratory distress may manifest as grunting, retractions, tachypnea, nasal flaring, or gasping. Interventions include positioning such as elevating the head of the bed or positioning the neonate side-lying or prone to attempt to decrease respiratory distress.

In end-of-life care, oxygen is usually not beneficial for patients in respiratory distress.

- Pairing an opioid with a benzodiazepine has been shown to significantly reduce respiratory end-of-life symptoms. Inability to swallow may lead to pooling of saliva in the posterior pharynx and noisy breathing. The family should be educated about what that might sound like and treating only if symptoms become distressing to the neonate. Decreasing or discontinuing hydrating fluids may help decrease secretion production; gentle shallow oral suctioning with a catheter may be done as needed.
- Compassionate extubation or discontinuation of respiratory support in neonates may be offered in patients requiring ventilatory support who are eligible for end-of-life withdraw. It is recommended to initiate opioids with or without benzodiazepine before slowly weaning ventilator settings while monitoring for development of respiratory distress. Parents should be involved and offered all opportunities to comfort if able, including holding, swaddling, and rocking.
- IV fluids and nutrition may not be in the best interest at end of life. They may worsen symptoms and cause fluid overload, respiratory distress, increased abdominal distention, or nausea and vomiting.

RESOURCES

Centers for Disease Control and Prevention. (2022a). *CDC's work on developmental disabilities*. Centers for Disease Control and Prevention. Retrieved December 9, 2022, from https://www.cdc.gov/ncbddd/developmentaldis abilities/about.html

Centers for Disease Control and Prevention. (2022). *Contraindications to breastfeeding or feeding expressed breast milk to infants*. Centers for Disease Control and Prevention. Retrieved December 7, 2022, from https://www.cdc .gov/breastfeeding/breastfeeding-special-circumstances/contraindications-to-breastfeeding.html

Fitri, S. Y. R., Lusmilasari, L., Juffrie, M., & Rakhmawati, W. (2019). Pain in neonates: A concept analysis. *Anesthesiology and Pain Medicine*, 9(4), e92455. https://doi.org/10.5812/aapm.92455. PMID: 31750094; PMCID: PMC6820293.

Goodstein, M. H., Stewart, D. L., Keels, E. L., Moon, R. Y., Committee on fetus and newborn, task force on sudden infant death syndrome. (2021). Transition to a safe home sleep environment for the NICU patient. *Pediatrics.148*(1) e2021052045. https://doi.org/10.1542/peds.2021-052046

Haug, S., Dye, A., & Durrani, S. (2020). End-of-life care for neonates: Assessing and addressing pain and distressing symptoms. *Frontiers in Pediatrics*. 8,574180. https://doi.org/10.3389/fped.2020.574180. PMID: 33072678; PMCID: PMC7542096.

Ilahi, Z., Capolongo, T., DiMeglio, A., Demissie, S., & Rahman, A. (2022). Impact of an infant-driven feeding initiative on feeding outcomes in the preterm neonate. *Advances in Neonatal Care*. https://doi.org/10.1097/ANC .0000000000001033. Epub ahead of print. PMID: 36084170.

Jiménez, B. C., Ferrández, S. F., Sebastián, J. D., & de Pipaon, M. S.(2022). Influence of full oral feeding acquisition on growth of premature infants. *Frontiers in Pediatrics*, *10*. https://doi.org/10.3389/fped.2022.928051

Kenner, C., Press, J., & Ryan, D. (2015). Recommendations for palliative and bereavement care in the NICU: A family-centered integrative approach. *Journal of Perinatology*. *35*(Suppl 1), S19–23. https://doi.org/10.1038/jp .2015.145. PMID: 26597801; PMCID: PMC4660047.

Khan, Z., Sitter, C., Dunitz-Scheer, M., Posch, K., Avian, A., Bresesti, I., & Urlesberger, B. (2019). Full oral feeding is possible before discharge even in extremely preterm infants. *Acta Paediatrica*, *108*(2), 239–244. Retrieved December 7, 2022, from https://www.ncbi.nlm.nih.gov/pmc/articles/PMC6585780/

Kim, S. Y., Yi, D. Y. (2020). Components of human breast milk: From macronutrient to microbiome and microRNA. *Clinical and Experimental Pediatrics*. *63*(8), 301–309. https://doi.org/10.3345/cep.2020.00059. Epub 2020 Mar 23. PMID: 32252145; PMCID: PMC7402982.

Lanzillotti, L. D. S., Seta, M. H. D., Andrade, C. L. T. D., & Mendes Junior, W. V. (2015). Adverse events and other incidents in neonatal intensive care units. *Ciencia & Saude Coletiva*, *20*(3), 937–46. https://doi.org /10.1590/1413-81232015203.16912013. PMID: 25760133.

Maffei, D., Brewer, M., Codipilly, C., Weinberger, B., & Schanler, R. J. (2020). Early oral colostrum administration in preterm infants. *Journal of Perinatology*, *40*(2), 284–287 (2020). https://doi.org/10.1038/s41372-019-0556-x

Mustapha, M., Wilson, K. A., & Barr, S. (2021). Optimising nutrition of preterm and term infants in the neonatal intensive care unit. *Paediatrics and Child Health*, *31*(1), 38–45. https://doi.org/10.1016/j.paed.2020.10.008

Pados, B. F., & McGlothen-Bell, K. (n.d.). Benefits of infant massage for infants and parents in the NICU. *Nursing for women's health*. Retrieved December 7, 2022, from https://pubmed.ncbi.nlm.nih.gov/31059673

Pineda, R., Guth, R., Herring, A., Reynolds, L., Oberle, S., & Smith, J. (2017). Enhancing sensory experiences for very preterm infants in the NICU: An integrative review. *Journal of Perinatology*. *37*(4), 323–332. doi: 10.1038 /jp.2016.179. Epub 2016 Oct 20. PMID: 27763631; PMCID: PMC5389912.

Smith, V. C., Love, K., & Goyer, E. (2022). NICU discharge preparation and transition planning: Guidelines and recommendations. *Journal of Perinatology*. *42*(Suppl 1), 7–21. https://doi.org/10.1038/s41372-022-01313-9. PMID: 35165374; PMCID: PMC9010297.

Soleimani, F., Azari, N., Ghiasvand, H., & Fatollahierad, S. (n.d.). Effects of developmental care on neurodevelopment of preterm infants. *Iranian Journal of Child Neurology*. Retrieved December 7, 2022, from https://pubmed.ncbi .nlm.nih.gov/32256620

Tran, H. T., Nguyen, T. T., & Mathisen, R. (2020). The use of human donor milk. *BMJ*. *371*. m4243 https://doi.org/10 .1136/bmj.m4243

Wellington, A., & Perlman, J. M. (2015). Infant-driven feeding in premature infants: A quality improvement project. *Archives of Disease in Childhood - Fetal and Neonatal Edition*, *100*(6). https://doi.org/10.1136/archdischild-2015 -308296

Witt, N., Coynor, S., Edwards, C., & Bradshaw, H. (2016). A guide to pain assessment and management in the neonate. *Current Emergency and Hospital Medicine Reports*, *4*(1), 1–10. https://doi.org/10.1007/s40138-016 -0089-y. PMID: 27073748; PMCID: PMC4819510.

18 PROFESSIONAL PRACTICE

ETHICAL PRINCIPLES AND PRACTICES

Overview

- *Ethics* refers to the branch of knowledge that pertains to moral principles.
- *Bioethics* is a type of ethics that deals with medicine and healthcare.

FOUR PRINCIPLES OF ETHICS

- *Beneficence* is doing good and providing care that benefits the patient.
- *Justice* is the principle of rendering to others what is due to them.
- *Nonmaleficence* is an obligation to not cause harm or injury.
- *Respect for patient autonomy* acknowledges an individual's right to hold views, make choices, and act based on their own personal values and beliefs.

NEONATAL INTENSIVE CARE UNIT DILEMMAS

- Ethical distress is prevalent in the NICU and can arise from any complex situation; however, the most common causes are end-of-life care, medical futility, periviability, and disagreements on care plans.
- End-of-life care: It typically involves limiting, withdrawing, or withholding lifesaving measures. Transitioning to end-of-life care may be distressing to both the care team members and the parents/ family members. The decision-making process must consider the possibility of prolonged suffering.
- Medical futility: *Futility* refers to a treatment that fails to provide discernible benefit. Concern for quality of life and minimizing suffering is difficult to determine as it may differ across families and the care team. Survival does not equal quality of life.
- Periviability: See Viability under Legal Issues.
- Disagreements on care plans: Disagreements on care plans between members of the care team or between the care team and the parents/family members can occur. The care team must recognize the importance of understanding and respecting the views and values of the patient's family while also keeping in mind the patient's best interest.

PROFESSIONAL–PATIENT RELATIONSHIP

- A professional–patient relationship fosters trust between the patient and the medical professional who is providing treatment.

Informed Consent

- Informed consent can only occur after information about a procedure, surgery, or treatment, including the potential risks and benefits, is given to the patient/family so that they can make their own intelligent, voluntary decision regarding healthcare.
- A newborn's parents or legal guardians must give consent prior to any procedure, surgery, or medical treatment. The family has the right to withdraw their consent at any time.
- A patient's legal guardians are not required to be their parents. They may include grandparents, other family members, or foster parents.
- The healthcare team must ensure a signed consent form is completed prior to starting a procedure or treatment. If a provider obtains verbal consent over the phone, the nurse may serve as a witness. The nurse will verify the person who is giving consent and document the consent as a witness.

Assessment

- Identify cultural and spiritual influences that impact healthcare decisions and practices. Religion impacts many medical decisions, including diet, medications, blood product use, modesty, and preference of gender of their caretakers.
- Assess understanding of language or need for an interpreter. Language barriers can be detrimental to giving and receiving nursing and medical care. Consent should be discussed in the patient's or legal guardian's preferred language.
- Assess the family's ability to understand relevant medical information and their ability to make independent, voluntary decisions. Ask questions of the family prior to giving or signing consent for procedures and treatments to assess understanding.
- When necessary, request translated information and materials in the preferred language or request an interpreter.
- Assess the family's reactions to acute stressors (e.g., hospitalization, new diagnosis, upcoming surgical procedure).
- Assess if the family can identify positive coping strategies.
- Assess whether the family needs time to grieve a new diagnosis, consider new plan of care, evaluate priorities, and participate in discharge planning.
- Understand and address refusal of treatment. Parents can deny treatment for their newborn in certain circumstances. The state may take over medical decisions in some cases.

[⚡] **ALERT!**

The nurse has no legal authority to obtain informed consent. Rather, this is the responsibility of the provider.

[📝] 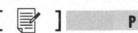 **POP QUIZ 18.1**

The nurse is taking care of a newborn who requires a blood transfusion. The nurse notes that informed consent has not been obtained from the parents. What is the most appropriate action of the nurse?

RESEARCH ETHICS

- Research ethics provides guidelines for the responsible conduct of research.
- Ethical research protects the rights of participants, improves research validity, and maintains scientific integrity.
- Parents or legal guardians are responsible for making informed decisions for their newborns.

ETHICAL DECISION-MAKING

- A shared decision-making model involving both the parents and the clinician is the preferred approach to ethical decision-making. ▶

ETHICAL DECISION-MAKING (*continued*)

- Shared decision-making involves open communication between the parents and the clinicians, including clear, accurate, and unbiased medical evidence about reasonable alternatives and the risks and benefits of each. The provider must have adequate expertise in communicating that evidence and should consider the values, goals, and concerns of the parents.
- This approach promotes informed consent while also allowing physicians to provide treatment recommendations.
- Quality of life is a metric that both parents and clinicians may refer to during the decision-making process for critically ill newborns. Quality of life generally refers to the standard of health, comfort, and happiness experienced by an individual. Parents and clinicians may disagree on what constitutes a "bad" or "good" quality of life for the newborn.

Essential Steps

- Determine whether there is an ethical issue and/or dilemma.
- Identify the key values and principles involved.
- Rank the values or ethical principles which are most relevant to the issue/dilemma.
- Develop an action plan that is consistent with the ethical priorities that have been determined as central to the dilemma.
- Implement the plan, utilizing the most appropriate practice skills and competencies.
- Reflect on the outcomes of this ethical decision-making process.

[📝] **POP QUIZ 18.2**

A term infant has been treated for suspected hypoxic ischemic encephalopathy (HIE) after a traumatic birth. The MRI after rewarming is consistent with severe HIE. The newborn is unresponsive and the EEG is flat. The medical team has a discussion with the family about redirection of care to comfort care. Who is responsible for making the decision to redirect care?

Proxy Decision-Makers

- A *proxy decision-maker* is an adult who has assumed the decision-making capacity for a patient who is incapable of doing so.
- In the NICU, parents or legal guardians are the proxy decision-makers for their newborns.
- If the healthcare team believes that parental decisions are inconsistent with the newborn's best interest, they may consult with the ethical committee.

ETHICS COMMITTEES

- An ethics committee is a group of people appointed by the hospital whose role is to provide guidance and lead discussions on ethical dilemmas, not to make medical decisions.
- The care team may consult with the ethics committee to facilitate communication and support complex decision-making. They can help differentiate between an ethical dilemma and moral distress.

[📝] **POP QUIZ 18.3**

The nurse does not agree with the plan of care because they believe the treatment is futile and is causing the patient to suffer. With whom should the nurse speak to regarding this conflict?

EVIDENCE-BASED PRACTICE

- Evidence-based practice (EBP) allows providers to make informed, evidence-based decisions and provide high-quality care that reflects the values and needs of the patient.
- Using EBP improves survival, decreases morbidity, and promotes long-lasting health for newborns.

Bundles

- Care bundles are a group of evidence-based interventions specific to a disease or care process that, when performed together, result in better outcomes than when applied individually.
- The steps to creating a bundle include identifying a practice theme, identifying up to six interventions within the theme, performing a literature search on each intervention, extraction of evidence, removal of interventions without sufficient evidence, and development of care bundle elements.
- Success of care bundles requires collaboration from all care team members.
- Examples of neonatal care bundles include ventilator-assisted pneumonia (VAP) prevention, intraventricular hemorrhage (IVH) prevention, central line–associated bloodstream infections (CLABSI) prevention, and antenatal corticosteroids for preterm newborns.

FAMILIES IN CRISIS

Overview

- Pregnancy and transition into parenthood are periods of stress and change.
- The birth of a premature or sick newborn presents a unique stress to parents and often leads to familial crisis.
- When in a crisis, parents may be unable to use their typical problem-solving strategies to cope.
- Parents of NICU patients experience a range of emotions, from excitement and joy of meeting their newborn to grief and hopelessness at the thought of losing them.
- During crisis periods, parents may display signs of anxiety, depression, fear, powerlessness, and posttraumatic stress disorder (PTSD).
- The NICU care team plays a key role in anticipating family crises and promoting positive coping strategies.

STEPS OF ATTACHMENT

Attachment theory refers to how the parent–child relationship emerges and influences the child's social, emotional, and cognitive development. There are four stages of attachment:

- Asocial: This occurs at 0 to 6 weeks. Newborns are asocial and produce a positive reaction to many kinds of stimuli (both social and nonsocial).
- Indiscriminate: This occurs at 6 weeks to 7 months. The baby enjoys company and responds equally to any caregiver, and produces negative reaction when interaction stops.
- Specific: This occurs at 7 to 9 months. The baby has a preference for a single attachment individual and seeks out specific people for security and comfort. They display stranger danger and separation anxiety.
- Multiple: This occurs at 10 months onward. The baby has multiple attachments, including parents, grandparents, siblings, and so forth. Stronger attachments are with individuals who respond accurately to the infant's signals.

PARENTAL STRESS IN THE NEONATAL INTENSIVE CARE UNIT

- Newborn's critical status and physical appearance: color, size, cries, movement, stressful/invasive procedures, tubes and wires on or near the newborn
- Physical environment: alarms from monitors and equipment, presence of other critically ill newborns, unfamiliar place
- Staff and parent interactions: conflicting or not enough information from staff, large number of staff, inconsistent care team
- Altered parental roles: parent–child separation, unable to feed/care for the newborn, fear of touching/holding the newborn, feeling helpless/lack of control

FAMILY-CENTERED CARE

- Family-centered care recognizes the family as an important and vital member of the NICU care team.
- Family-centered care promotes parents' ability to understand their newborn's needs to prepare for caregiving at home.
- Parental involvement supports neonatal brain maturation and overall better outcomes.
- Recommendations for supporting parents' role as caregivers in the NICU include providing hands-on care to their newborn, including early and frequent skin-to-skin contact, participating in medical rounds, and having full access to electronic medical records.

Communication With Families

- Miscommunication with families is often reported as one of the biggest stressors in the NICU.
- Care team members should ensure effective communication by updating parents often; being direct about the newborn's status, treatment, and prognosis; avoiding complex terminology and medical jargon; defining terms and diagnoses; being open and sympathetic; and assessing understanding by asking parents for a summarization of the conversation.

Culturally Competent Care

- Cultural competence is the willingness to understand and appropriately interact with people of different cultures, races, and ethnicities.
- Practicing culturally competent care allows the care team to successfully treat patients when patient beliefs or values conflict with those of the medical team.
- There are four components of culturally competent care: awareness, attitude, knowledge, and skills.

Parental Guilt

- Guilt is a common feeling among parents of NICU patients.
- Mothers often feel especially guilty and wonder if they could have changed the outcome by making different decisions during pregnancy.

Coping Strategies for Parents

- Recognize that emotions and feelings are all valid.
- Set realistic expectations.
- Establish a routine.
- Connect with other NICU parents and support groups.
- Reflect on spiritual beliefs and speak with hospital spiritual care staff.
- Keep a journal.
- Exercise if able. ▶

Coping Strategies for Parents (continued)
- Accept that partners may cope differently.
- Be involved with newborn care.
- Practice mindfulness or meditation.
- Speak with a social worker or counselor.

POSTPARTUM MOOD DISORDERS

- *Postpartum mood disorders* are a group of disorders that involve distressing feelings throughout the first year after pregnancy. These may include anxiety, depression, PTSD, psychosis, and obsessive-compulsive disorder (OCD).
- They differ from "baby blues," which is a period of normal adjustment following the birth of a newborn when mothers may feel physically and emotionally overwhelmed. Baby blues are chiefly due to fluctuating hormones. Symptoms last 2 to 3 weeks postpartum.
- Postpartum mood disorders occur when baby blues symptoms last beyond 2 to 3 weeks and become worse or interfere with everyday living.

Risk Factors

Postpartum mood disorders can affect anyone, but the following risk factors may increase the chance of developing one:
- Difficult pregnancy
- Traumatic birth
- Newborn requiring hospitalization after birth through the first year of life
- Personal or family history of depression or anxiety
- History of alcohol or drug use
- Lack of social support
- Stressful life events
- Difficulty breastfeeding

Signs and Symptoms

- Frequent crying
- Poor sleep/insomnia
- Appetite changes
- Inability to think clearly
- Feeling nervous around the newborn
- Mood swings

Nursing Interventions

- All postpartum patients should be screened for postpartum mood disorders at least once during their postpartum period using a standardized, validated tool.
- The Edinburgh Postnatal Depression Scale is the most frequently used screening tool for postpartum depression.

Treatment

- Depends on the type and severity of the mood disorder
- May include therapy, medications, or both

PARENTAL ADAPTION TO THE NEONATAL INTENSIVE CARE UNIT

- Parents of NICU patients must adjust their expectations of a normal postpartum period with their newborn at home.
- Adaptations to having a newborn in the NICU include altered parenting role, being in an unfamiliar and high-stress environment, learning new medical terminology, caring for a premature or sick infant, and balancing time between the hospital, home, work, and family/friends.
- Strategies to promote a positive adaptation include personalizing the NICU space, visiting the NICU often, practicing relaxation both in and out of the NICU, and practicing self-care.

Visiting Guidelines

To promote family-centered care, the NICU should allow 24/7 unlimited visitation access to parents or legal guardians/caregivers. Other visitation guidelines may include:

- A limit to the number of visitors at the bedside at one given time
- A limit to the number of visitors for the duration of the newborn's NICU stay
- An age limit for visitors
- Visitation hours and time limits for visitors other than parents or siblings
- Visitors who may not be given medical information or updates from staff
- Visitors who must follow hand hygiene practices per unit policy

Sibling Involvement

- Siblings may have a difficult time adapting to a NICU hospitalization.
- Siblings require age-appropriate information to understand what is happening.
- The care team should involve a child life specialist before and during the sibling visit.
- Additional ways to include the siblings are to show them pictures of the newborn, read age-appropriate books about the NICU, and encourage the siblings to write cards/letters or draw pictures for the newborn.

Social Work Involvement

- Social workers act as a support resource for both the medical team and the NICU family.
- The role of social work in the NICU is to promote positive developmental outcomes for newborns; assess the family's physical, emotional, social, and financial needs; provide resources for specific needs; and ensure that a family can safely and appropriately care for their newborn upon discharge.

Neonatal Intensive Care Unit Transfers

Common reasons for hospital transfers for newborns may include:

- Requiring a higher level of care from a lower level I/II nursery to a level III/IV NICU
- Requiring specialist care or surgery that is provided at a different hospital
- Graduating from the NICU and transferring to a lower level nursery
- Transferring to a hospital closer to home

Family Considerations

NICU transfers are a source of stress for families. Care team members can help alleviate this stress by:

- Explaining that the newborn will be transferred in an ambulance with trained NICU transport staff
- Offering parents the chance to travel with their newborn, if possible
- Ensuring that the family has accommodations at or around the next hospital

PERINATAL LOSS AND GRIEF

Overview

- Perinatal loss includes miscarriage (<20 weeks' gestation), stillbirth (>20 weeks' gestation), and neonatal death (birth through 28 days of life).
- Perinatal loss often involves the feeling of biological failure and loss of identity.
- Grief after perinatal death resembles other forms of bereavement and may lead to profound depression or PTSD.
- Among family members, feelings of grief may be similar; however, the way these feelings are expressed will vary.
- Factors affecting grief expression include age, gender, culture, coping strategies, life experiences, communication style, personality, and support systems.

Stages of Grief

- Denial
- Anger
- Bargaining
- Depression
- Acceptance

Physical Symptoms of Grief

- Crying
- Fatigue
- Headache
- Palpitations
- Panic attacks
- Loss of appetite
- Difficulty sleeping
- Chronic pain

Emotional Symptoms of Grief

- Sadness/depression
- Guilt
- Fear
- Irritability
- Anger/rage
- Resentment
- Jealousy

Gender Differences in Grieving

While people of any gender can express grief in any given way, there are observed trends and differences in how men and women typically grieve. These generalizations will not apply to each man or woman, and no matter the gender of the person expressing the grief behavior, they must be supported and treated as individuals.

Common Grief Behaviors in Women

- Expressing their emotions outwardly
- Telling their story repeatedly
- Reaching out to friends and family for support
- Questioning or blaming others

Common Grief Behaviors in Men

- Turning inward rather than expressing their emotions
- Avoiding conversation about their loss
- Spending more time working and participating in strenuous or repetitive tasks as a distraction
- Isolating themselves
- Taking control of family needs

Grief Resolution

- *Grief resolution* refers to the conscious choice to accept a loss and learn to live with a new reality.
- It allows sorrow and joy simultaneously.
- There is no timeline for grief resolution; it may take several years for someone to reach this stage.

Characteristics of Grief Resolution

- Feeling relieved
- Renewed energy
- Improved decision-making ability
- Able to laugh and smile again
- Improved eating and sleeping habits
- Improved self-esteem
- Planning for the future

Grief Behaviors to Avoid

While there is no incorrect way to grieve, some common responses to grief that may make it more difficult to process the loss and move forward include:

- Isolating oneself
- Consuming alcohol or drugs
- Making big life decisions or drastic changes
- Neglecting basic self-care
- Ignoring signs of depression
- Not asking for help from family, friends, or providers

Helpful Interventions and Education

- Talk with a trained provider, social worker, grief counselor, or a religious leader.
- Join a support or bereavement group.
- Eat adequate amounts of healthy foods.
- Hydrate.
- Create a routine sleep schedule.
- Limit alcohol consumption.
- Avoid tobacco products.
- Create boundaries with family and friends.

RIGHTS UPON DEATH

The rights of parents after infant death are meant to serve as guidelines for caregivers to ensure that parents are allowed to care for and make memories with their infant in ways that are best for their family.

Parental Rights

- To be given the opportunity to see, touch, hold, and bathe the infant
- To have photographs of the infant taken
- To be given as many memories as possible
- To name and bond with the infant
- To observe cultural and religious practices
- To be with one's support system
- To have alone time with the infant
- To be informed of the grieving process
- To be given the option of tissue/organ donation
- To request an autopsy
- To have information presented in understandable terminology
- To receive information on support resources

Infant Rights

- To be recognized
- To be named
- To be seen, touched, and held
- To have their life ending acknowledged
- To be put to rest with dignity

LEGAL ISSUES

Viability

- Fetal viability is the point at which a fetus can survive outside of the uterus.
- There is no universal definition for fetal viability; it generally considered to be between 22 and 24 weeks' gestation.
- A *periviable birth* refers to a newborn delivery near the limit of viability whose outcomes range from certain or near-certain death to survival with a high chance of serious morbidity.
- The threshold for resuscitation is dependent on each institution.

Neonatal Intensive Care Unit Malpractice

Common areas of malpractice in neonatology include:

- Resuscitation errors
- Breathing assistance errors
- Mismanagement of IVH
- Untreated or improperly treated infections
- Undiagnosed hypoxic ischemic encephalopathy (HIE) and failure to provide therapeutic hypothermic
- Failure to treat seizures
- Failure to diagnose and treat hypoglycemia
- Jaundice mismanagement
- Medication errors
- Central line mismanagement

RESOURCES

Adams, S., Tucker, R., Clark, M., & Lechner, B. (2020). "Quality of life": Parent and neonatologist perspectives. *Journal of Perinatology, 40,* 1809–1820.

American College of Obstetricians and Gynecologists. (2017). *Periviable Birth*. https://www.acog.org/clinical/clinical-guidance/obstetric-care-consensus/articles/2017/10/periviable-birth

American College of Obstetricians and Gynecologists. (2018). *Screening for perinatal depression*. https://www.acog.org/clinical/clinical-guidance/committee-opinion/articles/2018/11/screening-for-perinatal-depression

Carter, J., Mulder, R., & Darlow, B. (2007). Parents stress in the NICU: The influence of personality, psychological, pregnancy and family factors. *Personality and Mental Health. 1*(1), 40–50. https://doi.org/10.1002/pmg.4

Casabianca, S. (2021). Mourning and the 5 Stages of Grief. *PsychCentral*. https://psychcentral.com/lib/the-5-stages-of-loss-and-grief

Craig, J. W., Glick, C., Phillips, R., Hall, S. L., Smith, J., & Browne, J. (2015). Recommendations for involving the family in developmental care of the NICU baby. *Journal of Perinatology. 35*, S5–S8. https://doi.org/10.1038/jp.2015.142

Deering, M. (2022). Cultural competence in nursing. *NurseJournal*. https://nursejournal.org/resources/cultural-competence-in-nursing

Lammert, C. (2008). The rights of parents when a baby dies: Choices or mandates. *National Share Office*. https://nationalshare.org/wp-content/uploads/2021/04/Rights-of-Parents-When-a-Baby-Dies-Choices-or-Mandates.pdf

March of Dimes. (2017). *Dealing with Grief after the Death of Your Baby*. https://www.marchofdimes.org/complications/dealing-with-grief-after-the-death-of-your-baby.aspx

McLeod, S. (2017). Attachment theory. *SimplyPsychology*. https://www.simplypsychology.org/attachment.html

Mills, M., & Cortezza, D. (2020). Moral distress in the neonatal intensive care unit: What is it, why it happens, and how we can address it. *Frontiers in Pediatrics*. https://doi.org/10.3389/fped.2020.00581

National Association of Social Workers. (n.d.) *Essential Steps for Ethical Problem-Solving*. https://www.naswma.org/page/100/Essential-Steps-for-Ethical-Problem-Solving.htm

Professional-Patient Relationship. *Gale Encyclopedia of Nursing and Allied Health*. Retrieved June 6, 2022 from Encyclopedia.com: https://www.encyclopedia.com/medicine/encyclopedias-almanacs-transcripts-and-maps/professional-patient-relationship

Sullivan, A., Cummings, C. (2020). Historical perspectives: Shared decision making in the NICU. *NeoReviews, 21*(4), e217–e225. https://doi.org/10.1542/neo.21-4-e217

Harrison, C., Canadian Paediatric Society (CPS), & Bioethics Committee. (2004). Treatment decisions regarding infants, children and adolescents. *Paediatrics & child health, 9*(2), 99–114. https://doi.org/10.1093/pch/9.2.99

Wilson, B., & Austria, M. (2021). What is Evidence-Based Practice? *University of Utah Health*. https://accelerate.uofuhealth.utah.edu/improvement/what-is-evidence-based-practice

1. When preparing the radiant warmer for a preterm neonate, which action would the nurse implement to ensure that a neutral thermal environment is maintained at the time of delivery?
   A. Avoiding placement of the radiant warmer near the delivery room door
   B. Increasing the ambient temperature in the delivery room
   C. Preheating the radiant warmer in the delivery room

2. Which is the most significant risk factor for respiratory distress syndrome (RDS)?
   A. Female sex assigned at birth
   B. Late preterm birth
   C. Low birth weight

3. An infant born prematurely at 30 weeks' gestation who required supplemental oxygen and prolonged ventilation continues to experience respiratory distress and impaired gas exchange at 38 weeks' post-menstrual age. The infant is now on 40% oxygen via nasal cannula with an oxygen saturation target between 88% and 92%. The infant has been unable to wean off oxygen without increased respiratory effort. What is the likely diagnosis?
   A. Moderate bronchopulmonary dysplasia (BPD)
   B. Persistent pulmonary hypertension of the newborn (PPHN)
   C. Respiratory distress syndrome (RDS)

4. A term neonate is delivered via spontaneous vaginal delivery and is placed on their mother's abdomen for skin-to-skin contact. After breastfeeding for 15 minutes, the nurse examines the neonate and notices a blue tinge to the skin on the hands and feet, as well as to the lips and tongue. A pulse oximetry reading on the right wrist indicates 84% oxygenation. Which diagnostic tool will differentiate the neonate's assessment findings as respiratory or cardiac in origin?
   A. Chest x-ray
   B. EKG
   C. Hyperoxia test

5. After resuscitating a newborn, the nurse will find which observation most concerning?
   A. Apgar score of 8 at 8 minutes of life
   B. Central cyanosis
   C. Oxygen saturation (SpO_2) of 79% at 6 minutes of life

6. The nurse is assessing a term newborn who is the infant of a patient with a history of diabetes. Which clinical finding in the newborn would be attributable to hypoglycemia?
   A. Bradycardia
   B. Depressed Moro reflex
   C. Jitteriness

7. The nurse educates the parents of a term newborn on best practices for bathing. The parents ask why they cannot use the organic soap they prefer to bathe the neonate. Which explanation does the nurse provide?
   A. "The newborn's skin is more acidic and needs protection to guard against damage and breakdown."
   B. "The skin pH of newborns increases in the first 2 to 3 weeks of life; after that you can use organic soap."
   C. "The skin surface of a newborn is typically alkaline, which makes it break down more easily."

8. Inadequate surfactant production, atelectasis, and audible expiratory grunting can be seen in which diagnosis?
   A. Meconium aspiration syndrome
   B. Pneumonia
   C. Respiratory distress syndrome

9. Which disinfectant is preferred for cleansing a newborn's skin before an invasive procedure?
   A. 0.5% chlorhexidine
   B. 10% povidone-iodine
   C. 70% isopropyl alcohol

10. After auscultating a grade 2 harsh systolic murmur at the lower left sternal border, which congenital heart defect (CHD) will the nurse monitor for?
    A. Atrial septal defect (ASD)
    B. Patent ductus arteriosus (PDA)
    C. Ventricular septal defect (VSD)

11. While monitoring the infant with neonatal withdrawal syndrome, the nurse will monitor for excoriation of the skin due to dysfunction of:
    A. The central nervous system
    B. The feeding and gastrointestinal system
    C. Metabolic function and balance

12. Which condition mimics neonatal seizures?
    A. Apnea
    B. Jitteriness
    C. Limb withdrawal

13. After Cesarean delivery under general anesthesia of a postterm neonate with meconium-stained amniotic fluid, the neonate is placed on a radiant warmer, dried, and stimulated. The nurse notes that the newborn has poor tone, peripheral cyanosis, and a heart rate of 90 beats per minute. The newborn is gasping, with periods of apnea. Which intervention will the nurse perform next?
    A. Administering naloxone immediately to counteract the effects of the general anesthesia used during delivery
    B. Continuing to assess the respiratory status to verify that secondary apnea is present before beginning assisted ventilation
    C. Performing oropharynx suctioning to clear secretions before initiating positive pressure ventilation (PPV)

14. Which *initial* intervention will be implemented when a 12-hour-old neonate is confirmed to have hypoxic ischemic encephalopathy?
    A. Initiating head cooling
    B. Maintaining blood glucose levels
    C. Monitoring for electrolyte imbalance

15. Which medication is *least* likely to affect fetal circulation?
    A. Heparin
    B. Protamine sulfate
    C. Warfarin

16. The nurse is about to place an intravenous (IV) catheter into an infant for phenobarbital treatment of seizure activity. Which intervention will the nurse implement to avoid compartment syndrome?
    A. Checking all indwelling lines hourly
    B. Infusing heparinized fluid at a low rate
    C. Using rolled cloths as a footboard

17. Which cardiac condition is considered a normal variant?
    A. Patent foramen ovale
    B. Tetralogy of Fallot
    C. Ventricular septal defect

18. Which statement explains the importance of individualizing fluid and electrolyte therapy for each neonate in the first week of life?
    A. Duration and timing of the glomerular filtration rate (GFR) vary for each individual.
    B. Individualized therapy ensures that the infant receives enough micromolecules when feeding is a concern.
    C. Infants lose weight after birth and need weight-based fluids to maintain weight.

19. A newborn is observed to have central cyanosis that is exacerbated by crying and feeding. Arterial blood gas results show that partial pressure of oxygen (PaO_2), measured at rest on room air, is less than 35 mmHg with metabolic acidosis. The nurse immediately prepares to administer which medication?
    A. Digoxin
    B. Epinephrine
    C. Prostaglandin E1

20. Which congenital heart condition in the neonate is associated with maternal systemic lupus erythematosus (SLE)?
    A. Coarctation of the aorta
    B. Congenital heart block
    C. Patent ductus arteriosus

21. The infant with congestive heart failure (CHF) benefits most from which nutritional intervention?
    A. Burping the infant at the end of the feeding
    B. Limiting feeding time to minimize overexertion
    C. Waiting for the infant to exhibit signs of hunger before offering a feed

22. The NICU nurse, who is present in delivery to assist in a high-risk birth, is viewing the fetal heart rate (FHR) tracing. A tracing that shows accelerations at the time of measurement can exclude which finding?
    A. Heart rate variability
    B. Hypoxic injury
    C. Patent ductus arteriosus

23. For which complication will the nurse assess frequently when caring for a neonate being administered phenytoin for neonatal seizure activity?
    A. Extravasation
    B. Purple glove syndrome
    C. Tachycardia

24. A parent self-identifies as an auditory learner. What teaching format best aligns with this learning style?
    A. Detailed verbal explanations
    B. Handouts that provide instructions in illustrated format
    C. Handouts with step-by-step instructions

25. A 3-day-old infant was born at 39 weeks' gestation via Cesarean section after failed induction of labor and prolonged rupture of the membranes. The infant is exhibiting tachycardia, tachypnea, lethargy, difficulty feeding, and pallor. The neonatologist suspects either sepsis or a critical congenital heart defect. Which physician order will the nurse complete first?
    A. Administering ampicillin intravenously 200 mg/kg/d every 12 hours
    B. Initiating a continuous infusion of prostaglandin E1 (PGE1) at 5 ng/kg/min
    C. Obtaining an echocardiogram

26. Which is the primary behavior denoting an authentically caring presence?
    A. Actively listening
    B. Assisting with basic needs
    C. Providing information

27. During NICU care, a neonate requiring assisted ventilation is prescribed a course of ampicillin and gentamicin. Other medications prescribed include digoxin and furosemide. Discharge planning should include which screening and subsequent follow up related to potential medication adverse effects?
    A. Hearing
    B. Pulse oximetry
    C. Vision

28. What is the ante cibum target glucose level for the first 24 to 48 hours of life when monitoring a newborn receiving intravenous therapy due to symptomatic hypoglycemia?
    A. ≥30 mg/dL
    B. ≥45 mg/dL
    C. ≥60 mg/dL

29. During assessment of a postsurgical wound in a neonate at 37 weeks' gestation, the nurse notes exudate with minimal necrotic tissue. Which action will the nurse take to reduce the risk of bacterial contamination?
    A. Applying silver-containing ointments
    B. Cleansing the wound with antiseptic solution
    C. Irrigating the wound with normal saline

30. While admitting a term newborn to the NICU for respiratory distress, the nurse notes that the infant has visible constriction rings on the fingers. Which finding should the nurse assess for next?
    A. Cleft palate
    B. Elevated blood glucose
    C. Lanugo

31. When providing education to the parent of a neonate diagnosed with cerebral palsy, which method would the nurse use when the parent states that they are a social learner?
    A. Engaging in role-playing activities to encourage advocacy for the neonate
    B. Including critical thinking exercises that simulate various clinical scenarios
    C. Providing hands-on experiences through simulation models and teach-back activities

32. A premature infant whose birth weight was 1,400 grams has developed gastric retention, vomiting, and grossly bloody stool. Bowel sounds are absent, and palpation reveals definite tenderness and a right lower quadrant mass. What radiologic finding might the nurse expect specific to the current disease state?
    A. Ascites
    B. Intestinal dilation
    C. Mild ileus

33. The neonatal team is called to labor and delivery for a newborn with tachypnea, central cyanosis, and poor respiratory effort. When positive pressure ventilation is applied, the nurse notes that there is no chest movement. What should the nurse do *first* to assess the effectiveness of ventilation?
    A. Adjust the mask.
    B. Increase the pressure.
    C. Suction the mouth and nose.

34. When planning care for a term infant in the NICU found to have a watershed injury on MRI, which neuroprotective intervention will be implemented?
    A. Administration of gabapentin
    B. Pain management
    C. Therapeutic hypothermia

35. The nurse is completing the discharge teaching for the parents of a term newborn who spent a few days in the NICU for transient tachypnea of the newborn. The infant is stable, on room air, and breast-feeding every 2 to 3 hours. The infant has a cephalohematoma from birth, and the nurse is including instructions regarding follow up for this condition. What blood test will this infant need a few days after discharge related to the cephalohematoma?
    A. Bilirubin
    B. Complete blood count
    C. Newborn screening

36. Which assessment findings are critical and suggestive of congestive heart failure in the newborn?
    A. Cyanosis with crying, harsh systolic murmur, hypotension, grunting, and retractions
    B. Tachycardia, galloping rhythm, and diaphoresis with feedings
    C. Tachypnea, continuous systolic murmur, bounding peripheral pulses, and tachycardia

37. A newborn is delivered via primary Cesarean section due to being in a breech position and being large for gestational age (LGA). The infant is admitted to the NICU for unstable blood glucose levels. While the nurse is performing a routine assessment, the parent of the infant asks what they are doing. The nurse will best respond by saying:
    A. "I'm performing Barlow's maneuver, which is used to determine infant tone in the limbs."
    B. "I'm performing an ultrasound to assess for growth restrictions of the hip, pelvis, and lower limbs."
    C. "I'm screening for hip dislocation using the Ortolani maneuver."

38. Assessment of an infant reveals features such as epicanthic folds, micrognathia, poor muscle tone, and a transverse palmar crease. Based on these observations, the cardiovascular finding that the nurse will auscultate is grade 3 harsh systolic murmur heard at the:
    A. Lower left sternal border
    B. Mid-left sternal border
    C. Upper left sternal border

39. Which finding immediately follows the transient increase in glomerular filtration rate (GFR) during a newborn's prediuretic phase in the first week of postnatal life?
    A. Return to low baseline GFR, rapid diuresis, and natriuresis regardless of water and sodium intake
    B. Return to low baseline GFR and minimal urine output regardless of water and sodium intake
    C. Slow increase in GFR, with diuresis dependent on salt and water excretion, varying according to intake

40. Cyanosis is first observed in the infant when which condition occurs?
    A. Heart rate over 150 beats per minute
    B. Hemoglobin level of 10 g/dL
    C. Oxygenation of 75% to 85%

41. The nurse performs an assessment on a 2-day-old infant born at term gestation. The infant is currently crying, and assessment findings include abdominal distention, vomiting, and absent bowel sounds. What action should the nurse take first?
    A. Contact the provider.
    B. Draw the morning lab work early.
    C. Feed the crying infant.

42. A primipara patient who is Rh-negative delivers a full-term newborn. The newborn has a positive direct Coombs test. What assessment findings will the nurse expect to see in the first 24 hours after delivery?
    A. Lethargy and jitteriness
    B. Tachypnea and nasal flaring
    C. Yellowing of the eyes and skin

43. An infant is assessed to have notable deformed bilateral upper extremities, with thumbs present and scattered petechiae over the trunk and face. The provider diagnoses the infant with thrombocytopenia-absent radius syndrome (TARS). Which intervention is *most* important when caring for this patient?
    A. Drawing labs via heel stick
    B. Educating parents on feeding options
    C. Handling slowly and gently

44. Which approach is recommended for surfactant replacement therapy?
    A. Administering a preventive dose immediately after delivery of the infant
    B. Combining early nasal continuous positive airway pressure and less invasive administration technique
    C. Using an in–out intubation procedure to instill a single bolus dose

45. Which common extracardiac anomaly is associated with tetralogy of Fallot (TET)?
    A. Diaphragmatic hernia
    B. Intestinal atresia
    C. Renal agenesis

46. Which injury *most commonly* occurs from lateral traction on the shoulders during vaginal delivery?
    A. Median nerve injury
    B. Plexus injury
    C. Spinal cord injury

47. Which is the *best* method for monitoring the oxygenation of a newborn when initiating positive pressure ventilation (PPV) as part of resuscitation efforts at delivery?
    A. EKG
    B. Inspection for signs of central cyanosis
    C. Monitoring of oxygen saturation (SpO_2)

48. Which intervention will the nurse execute to decrease transepidermal water loss (TEWL) in premature infants?
    A. Initiating humidity of at least 50% in the infant's isolette
    B. Limiting the use of adhesive tape on the infant's skin
    C. Using a gelled mattress pad under the infant

49. For which disorder will the nurse monitor in a premature neonate weighing 3 lb. (1.4 kg) who has been exposed to group B *Streptococcus* (GBS)?
    A. Congenital heart defect
    B. Neonatal sepsis
    C. Respiratory distress syndrome

50. Which nursing behavior is the most advanced demonstration of caring practices as defined by the American Association of Critical-Care Nurses (AACN)'s Synergy Model for Patient Care?
    A. Anticipates family needs and acts to meet them
    B. Delivers care based on established standards
    C. Maintains a safe physical environment

51. The parents of a NICU infant inform the nurse that they would like to burn incense in the infant's room in conformance with their spiritual beliefs. The nurse's best initial approach is to:
    A. Contact the spiritual care department to have someone speak to the parents about their needs
    B. Engage in further dialogue with the parents about their request to burn incense
    C. Respect the parents' preferences by allowing them to burn incense in the infant's room

52. A neonate at 28 weeks' gestation has marked denudation of the stratum corneum with weeping. Which priority intervention will the nurse implement?
    A. Administering intravenous fluid replacement
    B. Applying barrier ointment and swaddling
    C. Increasing humidity in the incubator

66. The nurse is caring for a 28-day-old infant who has a history of prematurity and respiratory distress syndrome. The nurse notices that the infant is tachypneic and coughing while the infant's parent is bottle feeding. What can the nurse do to help with bottle feeding?
    A. Encourage the infant's parent to pace the feed.
    B. Place the infant upright for the feed.
    C. Take over the feed and let the infant's parent try again at the next feed.

67. The nurse is assessing a newborn and notes a heart rate of 150 beats per minute, a respiratory rate of 72 breaths per minute, and decreased peripheral pulses. The nurse auscultates the heart and notes a galloping rhythm. Which condition does the nurse suspect?
    A. Congenital heart disease
    B. Patent ductus arteriosus
    C. Respiratory distress syndrome

68. When preparing to care for a neonate born to a patient who has been administered long-term antenatal corticosteroids, the nurse will prepare for:
    A. Hypotension due to placental ischemia
    B. Hypoxia and cardiorespiratory shock due to decreased uterine blood flow
    C. Respiratory complications due to increased lung surfactant production

69. A hyperoxia test has been ordered for an infant suspected to have a cyanotic heart defect. The response to exposure to 100% oxygen for 10 minutes that confirms a cardiac disorder is partial pressure of oxygen (PaO_2) of:
    A. 90 mmHg
    B. 110 mmHg
    C. 150 mmHg

70. A preterm infant in the NICU has been working on bottle feeding with a slow-flow nipple and breastfeeding with pacing. At the next feed, the infant's mother asks for assistance placing the infant in a cross-cradle position to breastfeed. The correct position for the infant is in a side-lying position with the infant's:
    A. Body resting on the bed
    B. Buttocks cradled in the parent's elbow
    C. Head cradled in the parent's elbow

71. Which approach by the nurse will promote a collaborative relationship with the parents of an infant in the NICU?
    A. Listening for intent and feelings as well as content
    B. Offering prompt reassurance about outcomes
    C. Sharing personal opinions and experiences

72. The nurse is caring for a term newborn whose mother has a history of diabetes. The nurse observes jittery movements and slight tremors. Capillary point-of-care (POC) glucose screening reveals a glucose level of 40 mg/dL. Which intervention represents appropriate immediate care for this newborn?
    A. Initiating intravenous glucose infusion
    B. Providing oral feeding
    C. Repeating the POC glucose screen

73. While caring for a neonate diagnosed with congestive heart failure (CHF), the nurse will monitor for signs of heart enlargement and increased pressure of the heart and:
    A. Brain
    B. Liver
    C. Spleen

74. Which action fosters effective collaboration within the interdisciplinary team?
    A. Direct patient care
    B. Multidisciplinary rounds
    C. Professional presentations

75. In determining whether central cyanosis has a cardiac origin or a pulmonary origin, which assessment finding best confirms a cardiac origin?
    A. Central cyanosis that does not improve with administration of 100% oxygen
    B. Circumoral cyanosis that improves with crying
    C. Pulse oximetry of 80% in a neonate with normal hemoglobin

76. Which statement best explains how the addition of xanthine therapy aids in the treatment of neonatal apnea?
    A. Respiratory activity is stimulated by the mechanism of these drugs for short durations.
    B. Xanthines are metabolized to caffeine, which acts to increase respiratory drive.
    C. Xanthines prevent the development of tachycardia and tachypnea, common complications of apnea treatment.

77. The NICU nurse is called to labor and delivery to assist with the delivery of an infant. Upon the nurse's arrival, the infant is under the radiant warmer with the labor and delivery nurse. What is the first question the nurse should ask when arriving at the room?
    A. "How long has the infant been in distress?"
    B. "Is the infant term?"
    C. "What is the Apgar score?"

78. The nurse is caring for a newborn after prolonged labor and a difficult, vacuum-assisted, vaginal delivery. Upon admission, the infant had a caput succedaneum, but now has generalized edema of the scalp, which has spread to the eyelids and is discolored. The infant is tachycardic and tachypneic. The nurse calls the attending provider to the bedside for an exam. After reviewing the current assessment, the provider orders a head CT. Which complication from delivery does the nurse suspect?
    A. Depressed skull fracture
    B. Subdural hemorrhage
    C. Subgaleal hemorrhage

79. The nurse assesses the neonate for which clinical sign when congestive heart failure (CHF) is suspected?
    A. Bradycardia
    B. Failure to thrive
    C. Polyuria

80. Which action describes the function of expiratory grunting?
    A. Decreases intrapulmonary pressure
    B. Keeps alveoli open
    C. Reduces residual lung gas volume

81. The nurse auscultates a harsh grade 5 murmur at the left mid- and upper sternal border. The infant exhibits severe cyanosis and dyspnea with feedings and has episodes of rapid, deep respiration, irritability and crying, and increased cyanosis. Blood gas results show partial pressure of carbon dioxide ($PaCO_2$) and pH in normal ranges, while partial pressure of oxygen (PaO_2) is low according to the degree of right-to-left shunting. An EKG indicates right ventricular hypertrophy. To assist the provider in determining a diagnosis, which study will the nurse prepare the infant for?
    A. Cardiac catheterization
    B. Chest x-ray
    C. Echocardiogram

82. Which learning theory asserts that the parents of a neonate receiving inpatient care education are motivated by the perceived usefulness of the content?
    A. Cognitive field
    B. Humanistic
    C. Stimulus response

83. Respiratory syncytial virus (RSV) presents the greatest threat to which patient?
    A. A neonate born at 33 weeks' gestation with a standard NICU course
    B. A full-term neonate born to a patient with asthma and gestational diabetes
    C. An 11-month-old infant with a history of bronchopulmonary dysplasia

84. Delivery room assessment of an infant at 36 weeks' gestation known to have umbilical cord prolapse reveals a temperature of 96.9°F (36.1°C) after the infant has been dried with and wrapped in warmed towels. Which intervention will the nurse implement?
    A. Initiation of skin-to-skin care
    B. Maintenance of infant on radiant warmer
    C. Placement of infant in preheated incubator

85. A premature infant presents with respiratory grunting and a respiratory rate of 70 breaths per minute. The nurse determines that the infant is suffering from a respiratory disorder after noting which additional primary finding?
    A. Central cyanosis
    B. Edema of extremities
    C. Intercostal retractions

86. Clinical signs of respiratory distress in the newborn include grunting, nasal flaring, tachypnea, and which other clinical sign?
    A. Hypertension
    B. Shrill cry
    C. Substernal retractions

87. A 6-month-old infant in the NICU follow-up clinic exhibits increased muscle tone, stiffened legs, and an overextended back when picked up. The nurse determines that the clinical presentation is indicative of which neurodevelopmental impairment?
    A. Quadriplegia
    B. Spastic diplegia
    C. Spastic hemiplegia

88. The nurse assesses an infant with neonatal herpes simplex virus (HSV) who is experiencing an outbreak of symptoms. How will the nurse document their findings?
    A. Coppery, maculopapular rash on the palms and soles
    B. Fluid-filled vesicles across the trunk
    C. Petechiae and purpura present on the extremities

89. In preparation for delivery, the nurse increases the temperature in the delivery room. This nursing action will prevent heat loss in the newborn through:
    A. Convection
    B. Evaporation
    C. Radiation

90. When an infant is born with atrioventricular (AV) block associated with structural heart disease, the nurse will most likely prepare for:
    A. Neonatal demise
    B. Sinus node dysfunction
    C. Sustained tachycardia

91. The nurse is caring for an infant with an amniotic band constriction ring to the right arm. What assessment finding would require notifying the provider?
   A. Absence of a right radial pulse
   B. Brachial plexus palsy of the right shoulder
   C. Capillary refill of 3 seconds

92. The nurse is caring for a newborn admitted to the NICU following early delivery due to preeclampsia. The parent is confined to their bed in labor and delivery (L&D) and cannot visit the newborn for several days. What action can the NICU nurse take to best involve the parent in the newborn's care?
   A. Asking the parent's L&D nurse to update the parent on the infant
   B. Bringing a photo of the infant to L&D and providing updates to the parent
   C. Encouraging the parent to pump breast milk as soon as possible

93. What is the *main objective* of treating primary hypertension of the newborn?
   A. Providing adequate oxygenation
   B. Reducing pulmonary vascular resistance
   C. Treating associated pathology

94. An important nursing intervention specific to medication therapy in the treatment of patent ductus arteriosus (PDA) is to:
   A. Closely monitor urine output
   B. Maintain daily weights
   C. Promote fluid intake

95. The parents of a neonate diagnosed with seizure disorder have four other children at home, two of whom also have seizure disorder. The parents have been dividing their time spent in the NICU to maintain normalcy for the family at home. When providing discharge education, which approach would best fit the parents' situation?
   A. Allowing the parents to self-direct learning needs
   B. Keeping teaching brief and to the point
   C. Offering to follow up with a phone call at home

96. Pulse oximetry results show a difference in partial pressure of oxygen (PaO$_2$) between the upper and lower extremities. Pulses in the upper extremities are easily palpated, but they are difficult to discern in the lower extremities, and the systolic blood pressure is higher in the right upper extremity than in the lower extremities. Which study results will the nurse evaluate to support suspected coarctation of the aorta?
   A. Arterial blood gases
   B. Echocardiography
   C. EKG

97. The nursing team assigned to determine satisfaction of the NICU staff and the care provided has determined an initial process to gather data. How can the team ensure the process will be implemented effectively and successfully?
    A. By defining goals and implementing process based on boundaries related to professional roles
    B. By ensuring commonly shared understanding of information and goals among all team members
    C. By maintaining traditionally accepted professional hierarchies to divide workload and responsibilities

98. Maternal administration of neuraxial analgesia is most likely to affect the neonate in which way?
    A. Difficulty breastfeeding
    B. Neonatal hypertension
    C. Tachycardia

99. At the time of delivery of a neonate at 41 weeks' gestation, the pregnant patient is determined to have maternal chorioamnionitis. When the neonate is delivered with thick meconium amniotic fluid, the nurse will prepare to perform which nursing action for the neonate *first*?
    A. Drying with warm towels and placing on the warmer
    B. Performing oral and nasal suctioning using a bulb suction
    C. Moving the neonate to the NICU immediately

100. Which characteristic identifies periodic breathing versus apnea of prematurity?
    A. Absent respiratory effort
    B. Apnea duration of 5 to 10 seconds
    C. Bradycardia

101. When integrating family-centered care (FCC) into the nursing plan of a preterm infant admitted to the NICU, which primary principle should be included?
    A. Promoting acceptance of the neonatal prognosis
    B. Enabling and empowering parents as members of the interdisciplinary team
    C. Providing sympathy and compassion to the family while promoting coping skills

102. When assessing a neonate with low hemoglobin levels for indications of congenital heart lesions, the nurse will assess the tongue for:
    A. Cyanosis
    B. Gag reflex
    C. Muscle tone

103. Which assessment finding suggests that patent ductus arteriosus is present in the newborn?
    A. Bounding peripheral pulses
    B. Central cyanosis
    C. Low oxygen saturation

104. Following the preterm birth of a neonate at 36 weeks' gestation, the nurse notes physical evidence of abuse in the neonate's mother, who also becomes upset when the other parent visits the NICU. To promote optimal safety of both the neonate's mother and the neonate, the nurse will first:
    A. Discuss safety options with the neonate's mother and the interdisciplinary team
    B. Make a referral to social services after reporting the abuse to local authorities
    C. Provide a nesting location for the neonate's mother and the neonate

105. An infant diagnosed with coarctation of the aorta (COA) has become symptomatic, exhibiting signs such as dyspnea, tachycardia, and diminished femoral pulses. Which pharmacotherapy will the nurse prepare to administer?
    A. Digoxin
    B. Dopamine/dobutamine
    C. Furosemide

106. The nurse is caring for an infant who received a ventriculoperitoneal shunt 1 day earlier. The nurse assesses that the infant has developed a shrill cry, a shiny scalp, and increased head circumference. What action will the nurse take?
    A. Raising the head of the infant's bed
    B. Turning the infant as ordered and reassessing at the next care time
    C. Notifying the provider

107. The nurse caring for a patient in active labor at 38 weeks' gestation interprets the fetal heart rate baseline as 150 beats per minute (bpm), with minimal variability. The fetal heart baseline rises to 165 bpm for 20 seconds during digital scalp stimulation, and moderate variability is noted. The nurse can expect the cord blood gas to show that the newborn is:
    A. Acidotic
    B. Hypoxic
    C. Well-oxygenated

108. While assessing a neonate born at 29 weeks' gestation on day 2, the nurse notes jaundice of the skin and eyes. The neonate is not latching on and has not taken to a bottle. For which pathophysiologic event would the nurse investigate?
    A. Infiltration of melanin-forming cells into the dermal skin
    B. Reduced ability of the liver to filter bilirubin
    C. Vasomotor instability

109. When assessing a neonate born to a patient with substance use disorder, which multisystem impact would the nurse monitor as a priority?
    A. Gastrointestinal
    B. Integumentary
    C. Urinary

110. The nurse is caring for a 5-week-old preterm infant with a history of late metabolic acidosis who was recently weaned from oxygen to room air and is now taking feeds by mouth. The nurse performs a weight check and notices that the infant's weight has decreased over the last few days. Which long-term complication is the nurse concerned for?
    A. Developmental delays
    B. Poor skeletal growth
    C. Vision impairment

111. Assessment of a newborn reveals irritability, hyperactive reflexes, a high-pitched cry, fever, diarrhea, and mottling skin color. Maternal history includes drug rehabilitation with methadone. The recommended toxicology test for this newborn is analysis of:
    A. Hair
    B. Meconium
    C. Urine

112. In premature infants, the principal factor in the development of respiratory distress is:
    A. Gestational age
    B. Sex assigned at birth
    C. Surfactant deficiency

113. A patient with persistent pulmonary hypertension of the newborn (PPHN) is on high-frequency oscillatory ventilation and nitric oxide. What should the nurse do to facilitate treatment of this patient?
    A. Promote minimal stimulation of the infant.
    B. Provide fixed fraction of inspired oxygen (FiO_2) per provider order.
    C. Take frequent blood draws.

114. Which is a criterion indicating the need for supplemental oxygen?
    A. Capillary refill time greater than 3 seconds
    B. Partial pressure of oxygen (PaO_2) of 80 mm Hg
    C. Peripheral cyanosis

115. The nurse is providing teaching to the parents of an infant who is having a ventriculoperitoneal (VP) shunt placed. Which statement made by the parents *best* indicates that the teaching was successful?
    A. "We must be careful that the tubing doesn't get snagged on anything when we are dressing our baby."
    B. "We should follow up with our family care provider to make sure the shunt is working correctly."
    C. "We will need to call the doctor immediately if there is any redness or if our baby has a fever."

116. When caring for a very-low-birthweight newborn on mechanical ventilation, the nurse works to prevent which clinical manifestation?
    A. Bronchopulmonary dysplasia (BPD)
    B. Diaphragmatic hernia
    C. Persistent pulmonary hypertension in the newborn (PPHN)

117. Which neonatal disorder could potentiate long-term respiratory difficulty with possible cystic lung changes?
   A. Bronchopulmonary dysplasia
   B. Congestive heart failure
   C. Pneumonia

118. Which action by the NICU nurse best represents the concept of an authentically caring presence when working with the family of a neonate being discharged home with a poor prognosis?
   A. Creatively solving problems related to at-home care
   B. Ensuring the family understands all discharge instructions
   C. Preserving the family's faith and hope while honoring inner life

119. The nurse is admitting a newborn with a history of nuchal cord during birth and an Apgar score of 4 at 1 minute of age. The nurse will monitor the patient for an increased risk for which complication needing immediate intervention?
   A. Hyperbilirubinemia
   B. Hypocalcemia
   C. Hypoglycemia

120. When assessing a neonate with suspected congestive heart failure (CHF), for which clinical finding will the nurse evaluate as a contributing factor for cardiomegaly?
   A. Anemia
   B. Tachycardia
   C. Volume overload

121. The nurse is caring for a patient with a diagnosis of meconium aspiration syndrome. On assessment, the nurse notices decreased breath sounds on the right side and increased respiratory effort despite respiratory support. Which diagnosis will the nurse suspect?
   A. Persistent pulmonary hypertension
   B. Pneumothorax
   C. Pulmonary hemorrhage

122. Visible signs of respiratory distress in an infant include:
   A. Acrocyanosis
   B. Retractions
   C. Tachycardia

123. The nurse is caring for a neonate who is undergoing therapeutic hypothermia treatment for perinatal asphyxia. The nurse implements which interventions to prevent kidney injury?
    A. Avoiding nephrotoxic medications, minimizing fluid intake, and ensuring strict intake and output recordings
    B. Careful fluid management, limiting use of nephrotoxic drugs, and promptly treating any hemodynamic or respiratory issues
    C. Increasing vital sign frequency, decreasing stimulation of the infant, weighing diapers for output, and weaning of oxygen as oxygen saturation reaches normal limits

124. During assessment of a 2-day-old preterm neonate, the nurse notices a sudden onset of atypical swimming motions of the legs along with tongue thrusting and fluttering eyelids. What does the nurse suspect the neonate is experiencing?
    A. Hypoxic ischemic encephalopathy
    B. Neonatal jitteriness
    C. Subtle seizure activity

125. The provider is at bedside with the nurse performing transillumination of the patient's chest wall, which shows a translucent glow. What does the nurse expect to see on the chest x-ray?
    A. Accumulation of air in the pleural space
    B. Coarse, patchy infiltration
    C. "Sail sign"

126. The nursing team has been working with the parents of a neonate diagnosed with neonatal compartment syndrome (NCS) to prepare them for the extensive healthcare needs of the near future. When formulating a parent education plan, what action will the nurse take to create a comprehensive approach to teaching the parents how to address their infant's unique healthcare needs?
    A. Assessing the parents' current knowledge of the disorder and providing teaching on the missing information
    B. Coordinating learning activities and resources that include all team members and are geared to both neonatal and parental needs
    C. Providing content centered on professional resources and allowing time for inquiry with each team member who has cared for the neonate

127. The nurse finds extravasation at the intravenous (IV) site on the infant's right hand. Which action will the nurse take *first*?
    A. Administering hyaluronidase
    B. Flushing with saline wash
    C. Removing the IV needle

128. While the nurse is preparing a postpartum patient and a neonate at 38 weeks' gestation for discharge, the neonate is found to be mildly jaundiced and to have difficulty feeding due to upper lip tie. Which primary intervention will the nurse provide during discharge education to prevent hyperbilirubinemia?
    A. Breastfeeding and lactation education and support
    B. Directions for implementing phototherapy at home
    C. Discussion of phenobarbital administration and follow-up lab work

129. What is the most definitive symptom of central nervous system (CNS) dysfunction in newborns?
    A. Hypotonia
    B. Poor feeding
    C. Seizures

130. A term newborn with a history of difficult vaginal delivery is admitted to the NICU at 3 hours of life. The infant has swelling of the scalp that is firm and crosses the suture lines. The admission vital signs are heart rate of 170 beats per minute, respirations of 68 breaths per minute, blood pressure of 42/23 mmHg, temperature of 98.2°F (36.8°C) axillary, and pulse oximetry of 96% on room air. The infant is pale and lethargic, and capillary refill is sluggish. Which neurologic, birth-related complication does the nurse suspect is occurring?
    A. Caput succedaneum
    B. Cephalohematoma
    C. Subgaleal hemorrhage

131. An infant receiving care in the NICU exhibits gaze aversion and a minimal quiet alert state. The infant becomes hypotonic with caregiving. Which neuroprotective intervention is likely to be the *most* beneficial?
    A. Protected sleep
    B. Stress management
    C. Supportive activities of daily living

132. Which assessment findings would first alert the nurse to the development of respiratory distress syndrome (RDS) in the newborn?
    A. Acrocyanosis due to impaired lung perfusion
    B. Hypotension and bradycardia
    C. Tachypnea and intercostal retractions with expiratory grunting

133. The NICU nurse is assisting with the delivery of a low-birthweight preterm neonate. Which step that is specific to this newborn should be performed after delivery to limit heat loss?
    A. Neonatal abstinence scoring
    B. Thorough drying of the head
    C. Wrapping in occlusive wrap

134. The concentration of bicarbonate (HCO_3) is elevated in a preterm neonate who is demonstrating wheezing and decreased lung compliance. During assessment, the nurse would evaluate for which organ dysfunction?
    A. Heart
    B. Kidney
    C. Liver

135. The nurse is aware that in the event of a Cesarean delivery, fetal lung fluid will be excreted from the lungs via which mechanism?
    A. Increased diuresis
    B. Pulmonary lymph system
    C. Thoracic squeezing

136. Which outcome reflects the rationale for the use of prostaglandin E1 (PGE1) in the treatment of newborns with dextro-transposition of the great arteries (d-TGA)?
    A. Corrected metabolic acidosis
    B. Maintenance of patency of the ductus arteriosus
    C. Reduction of systemic blood pressure and improved perfusion

137. Which prenatal maternal diagnosis increases an infant's risk of developing respiratory distress syndrome?
    A. Asthma
    B. Gestational diabetes
    C. Hypertension

138. While monitoring the administration of intravenous nafcillin in a neonate at 36 weeks' gestation, the nurse will prioritize assessment for:
    A. Infection
    B. Infiltration
    C. Pain and discomfort

139. The nurse is caring for a term newborn with a severe spinal cord injury following a traumatic breech delivery. The nurse is preparing the parents for discharge home. The neonate will be discharged with a ventilator, feeding tube, and catheter. Which statement made by the parents indicates the need for additional teaching?
    A. "Our baby will be able to walk and do all the things other babies do as they get older."
    B. "Our baby will need lifetime complex care, and we will need home healthcare to help us."
    C. "Our baby will need the ventilator and specialized medical care around the clock."

140. A nurse is caring for an infant born at 27 weeks' gestation and is starting enteral feeds via a nasogastric tube. The infant's mother is producing small amounts of breast milk, and the nurse has an order to supplement with donor milk. The nurse knows that donor milk varies from breast milk because it has:
    A. Decreased lactose
    B. Increased insulin-like growth factors
    C. Lower nutrient value

141. A neonate is born at 38 weeks' gestation as a result of uncontrollable preeclampsia in the neonate's mother. The neonate is determined to be small for gestational age (SGA). When determining outcomes for the nursing care plan, the nurse will determine:
    A. Degree of asymmetrical SGA
    B. Fetal growth trajectory
    C. Relative risk for respiratory infection

142. A nurse is assisting with the delivery of an infant who requires oxygen at birth. At how many minutes of life should the nurse expect the preductal target oxygen saturation (SpO$_2$) to be above 85%?
    A. 3
    B. 5
    C. 10

143. The nurse is caring for a neonate whose parents are from a different cultural background from the nurse and who speak a different language from the nurse. The parents appear to be emotionally distressed. What is the nurse's most appropriate action?
    A. Providing prewritten communication in the parents' language that explains the care the neonate may receive
    B. Requesting an interpreter to communicate the neonate's diagnosis and prognosis and the parents' concerns
    C. Requesting that the hospital's spiritual care department send someone to help comfort the parents

144. Delayed sponge-bathing in the preterm newborn is beneficial because it:
    A. Allows additional time for newborn assessment
    B. Prevents evaporative heat loss and temperature variability
    C. Reduces the risk of cold stress

145. The nurse palpates a neonate's abdomen and notes absence of abdominal muscles and cryptorchidism. Voiding cystourethrogram (VCUG) confirms Eagle-Barrett syndrome with unilateral obstruction, for which the provider has ordered prophylactic antibiotics in preparation for orchiopexy. While preparing the patient for surgery to take place the following day, the nurse's primary action is to:
    A. Assess for abdominal distention
    B. Monitor intake and output for kidney function
    C. Obtain blood for lab testing

146. Pulse oximetry test results reveal a right upper extremity (RUE) oxygen saturation of 95% and a right lower extremity (RLE) oxygen saturation of 90%. Which is the nurse's next step?
    A. Documenting the result as normal
    B. Initiating the process to transfer to NICU
    C. Repeating the test in 1 hour

147. When introducing the parents of a neonate being admitted to the NICU to the team, which activity demonstrates the nurse's respect and care for the family as individuals?
    A. Addressing the parents and the patient by name when discussing care
    B. Being alert to the parents' nonverbal responses and cues
    C. Ensuring that the parents understand processes in the unit

148. The nurse is preparing to provide feeding through a nasogastric tube to an appropriate for gestational age (AGA) infant at 30 weeks' gestation who is being treated for respiratory distress syndrome. The parent asks why the nurse placed the infant in a prone position for feeding. What response from the nurse will provide education to the parents?
    A. "Laying an infant on the stomach during tube feeding helps with digestion."
    B. "Lying on the stomach reduces the risk for tube displacement."
    C. "Placing the infant on the stomach alleviates pressure on the lungs while feeding."

149. What may indicate an acute hypoxic intrapartum event?
    A. Cord pH of 6.7
    B. Oxygen saturation of 89% at 6 minutes of life
    C. Respiratory acidemia

150. When providing discharge instructions to the parents of a neonate with a surgical dressing that must be changed and monitored for infection, which approach will the nurse use to ensure that the parents are knowledgeable and comfortable providing care?
    A. Printed instructions for home use
    B. Simulation-based learning
    C. Teach-back method

151. When assessing a neonate born prematurely to a patient who has had no prenatal care, the nurse observes notable vernix, lanugo present on the shoulders and arms but not the face, embryonic vessels present in the ocular lens, and observable but not fully developed testes. The nurse determines the neonate to be approximately how many weeks' gestation?
    A. 28 to 30
    B. 32 to 34
    C. 36 to 38

152. What factor places premature neonates at higher risk of developing acute kidney injury (AKI)?
    A. Antibiotic use
    B. Decreased serum calcium after birth
    C. Increased renal perfusion

153. An infusion of prostaglandin E1 to an infant with transposition of the great vessels has been initiated. Which *immediate* management intervention would the nurse implement?
    A. Administering fluids
    B. Assessing vital signs
    C. Monitoring for infection

154. The nurse is caring for a 49-day-old infant with a history of preterm birth at 32 weeks' gestation and subsequent bronchopulmonary dysplasia. The infant recently began to have difficulty with feeding, abdominal distention, poor weight gain, and episodes of cyanosis. The most recent vital signs reflect a fever. The nurse performs a bedside urine dip and notes nitrates and protein in the sample. The provider is notified and additional labs are ordered. Based on the information given, what is the likely diagnosis for this infant?
    A. Group B *Streptococcus* (GBS) pneumonia
    B. Necrotizing enterocolitis (NEC)
    C. Urinary tract infection (UTI)

155. While assessing a preterm neonate who is fussy, febrile, and grunting, the nurse will first assess which system as a primary area of infection?
    A. Gastrointestinal tract
    B. Heart
    C. Lungs

156. When working with a team member who is opposed to nesting in the NICU, how will the group ensure that collaborative care is implemented?
    A. Implement professional development training for maintenance of professional roles.
    B. Provide an organizational chart for clear delineation of authority and decision-making in the unit.
    C. Remove barriers by reviewing shared goals and decision-making.

157. A neonate is most likely prescribed antibiotics as a result of:
    A. Contraction-induced hypoxia
    B. Preterm premature rupture of membranes (PPROM)
    C. Twin reversed arterial perfusion (TRAP) sequence

158. While providing assistance with a delivery, the nurse notes a category 2 tracing based on decreased fetal heart rate and decreased variability on electronic fetal monitoring of a fetus found to have large nuchal translucency on the 10-week ultrasound. The nurse implements which *immediate* action?
    A. Administration of high-concentration oxygen to the patient
    B. Repositioning of the patient to hands and knees
    C. Preparation of a bolus of crystalloid fluid for intravenous administration

159. A nurse is preparing to discharge an infant with a diagnosis of phenylketonuria (PKU). What can the nurse expect to educate the parents on?
    A. Dietary restrictions
    B. Nutritional supplementation with herbal remedies
    C. Side effects of pegvaliase

160. A NICU nurse is caring for a critically ill, premature, 32-week-old infant on extracorporeal membrane oxygenation. The multidisciplinary team has consulted palliative care. The parent is at the bedside and is distressed, asking "Are they coming because my baby is dying?" Which response will the nurse provide?
   A. "The team has been notified to help develop a plan of care in case your baby's status deteriorates."
   B. "The team helps make sure the needs of your baby and family are met while helping coordinate your baby's medical care."
   C. "Your baby's prognosis is poor, and the palliative care team will help make an appropriate plan of care to prevent any further distress or pain."

161. When assessing a neonate after a traumatic birth, on which joint will the nurse concentrate?
   A. Acromion process
   B. Cranial sutures
   C. Symphysis pubis

162. The nurse is caring for a term infant suspected of having hypoxic ischemic encephalopathy (HIE) a few hours after delivery at a different facility. Passive cooling was started while waiting for transport and continued for 72 hours after arrival. MRI now indicates a white matter injury. After the provider updated the parents on the infant's prognosis, they became distraught and began to argue with the medical team, stating that the child did not have brain damage before arriving at the NICU. Which nursing action would be most appropriate?
   A. Asking the parents if they would like to have a member of the spiritual care department come to meet with them
   B. Listening to the parents for a few minutes, telling them to come to the bedside to see their infant when they are ready, and then leaving to offer privacy
   C. Offering reassurance that the NICU is the best place for the infant and stating that the injury could have been much worse if not for the cooling therapy

163. At 4 days of age, an infant born at term has developed pallor, cyanosis, and diaphoresis. Heart sounds reveal a gallop rhythm with an audible murmur heard at the mid-left sternal border. Rectal temperature is 98°F (36.6°C), heart rate is 170 beats per minute, and respiratory rate is 68 breaths per minute with audible grunting. The nurse's *first* action will be to:
   A. Monitor intake and output (I&O)
   B. Obtain an oxygen saturation (SpO$_2$) level
   C. Obtain blood for a complete blood count (CBC)

164. Which clinical sign is considered a strong indicator of neonatal sepsis?
   A. Hyperactive reflexes
   B. Rectal temperature ≤95°F (35°C)
   C. Respiratory rate <30 breaths per minute

165. Which situation presents the most significant risk of an infant being born with a congenital heart defect (CHD)?
    A. Family history of a sibling with CHD
    B. Fetal diagnosis of Turner syndrome
    C. Maternal history of gestational diabetes with poor glycemic control

166. The *best* plan of care for a breastfeeding neonate whose mother is prescribed a potentially transmissible medication would be to:
    A. Administer the medication to the mother after the infant's feeding time
    B. Encourage the mother to continue pumping and discarding to maintain milk supply
    C. Establish feeding times based on the medication's half-life

167. A neonate born at 30 weeks' gestation weighing 3.1 lb. (1.4 kg) is being evaluated in the NICU due to perinatal asphyxia. Upon assessment, the patient is exhibiting significant intercostal retractions with expiratory grunting and nasal flaring. For which increased risk will the nurse monitor this patient?
    A. Meconium aspiration syndrome (MAS)
    B. Respiratory distress syndrome (RDS)
    C. Transient tachypnea of the newborn (TTN)

168. Assessment reveals that the systolic blood pressure in the newborn's right upper extremity is 10 mmHg greater than the systolic blood pressure in the lower extremity. Which condition does this finding suggest?
    A. Coarctation of the aorta
    B. Persistent pulmonary hypertension
    C. Transposition of the great vessels

169. Parents have just experienced the death of their newborn and are grieving the loss. Which intervention by the nurse values the parents' grieving process?
    A. Avoiding discussion of the loss until the parents mention it
    B. Offering grief education to the parents
    C. Providing distraction from the loss to the parents

170. Arterial blood gas testing after exposure to 100% oxygen for 10 minutes reveals a partial pressure of oxygen (PaO$_2$) level of 85 mmHg. Which diagnostic study should be ordered next?
    A. Chest x-ray
    B. Echocardiography
    C. EKG

171. Which action demonstrates how cooling the newborn reduces the severity of hypoxic ischemic encephalopathy (HIE)?
    A. Controlling cerebral edema and offering neuroprotection
    B. Lowering the oxygen demand
    C. Reducing the incidence of intraventricular hemorrhage

172. A newborn's inability to effectively dilute urine is a result of:
   A. Heightened aldosterone sensitivity
   B. Minimized extracellular volume
   C. Reduced glomerular filtration rate

173. Educating parents on strategies to prevent sudden infant death syndrome (SIDS) is critical. Which position for the infant would the nurse caution against because it is unsafe?
   A. On the stomach while awake and supervised
   B. Prone in the crib with a loose blanket when it is time for sleep
   C. Supine in the crib and wrapped in a snug swaddle when it is time for sleep

174. Which of the following is associated with an increased risk of respiratory distress syndrome (RDS) in the neonate?
   A. Absence of phosphatidylglycerol
   B. Increase in lecithin before delivery
   C. Presence of fetal lung fluid during delivery

175. An infant is admitted to the NICU for tachypnea and stridor and also has Pierre Robin syndrome. Oxygen saturation levels range from 91% to 93%. What intervention will the nurse perform first?
   A. Applying oxygen via nasal cannula
   B. Placing the infant prone
   C. Preparing for oral intubation

1. **A) Avoiding placement of the radiant warmer near the delivery room door**

   A neutral thermal environment maintains the infant's temperature through a stable metabolic state and minimal oxygen and energy expenditure. The nurse would avoid placing the radiant warmer near the delivery room door because cool drafts in the ambient air from opening and closing the door can lead to loss of heat from convection. Increasing the ambient temperature in the delivery room and preheating the radiant warmer are actions to reduce heat loss in the newborn from convection and conduction, respectively.

2. **C) Low birth weight**

   Low birth weight (<1,200 grams) is one of the two most significant risk factors associated with RDS, along with gestational age younger than 30 weeks. The incidence of RDS related to late preterm birth is 5% at 34 weeks of gestation and less than 1% at 37 weeks of gestation. Male, not female, sex assigned at birth is considered a risk factor.

3. **A) Moderate bronchopulmonary dysplasia (BPD)**

   Target oxygenation of infants with BPD is lower than the standard 95% (or higher) that would be expected in a newborn without BPD. The infant would have a history of prolonged ventilation and continue to require ongoing oxygen therapy. RDS is a short-term diagnosis that progressively improves as the disease process is managed. PPHN occurs in term or near-term infants and is also a short-term diagnosis.

4. **C) Hyperoxia test**

   A hyperoxia test is used to differentiate respiratory disease from cyanotic heart disease. To perform a hyperoxia test, arterial blood gases are obtained at room air and after administration of 100% supplemental oxygen for 5 to 10 minutes. If the partial pressure of oxygen (PaO_2) is greater than 150 mmHg, the most likely cause of central cyanosis in the neonate is respiratory disease. A chest x-ray can identify cardiomegaly and pulmonary edema; however, it cannot determine whether the pulmonary edema is caused by primary lung disease or a congenital heart defect. A neonatal EKG is useful in the diagnosis of cardiac dysrhythmias, not structural heart defects. Neonatal EKG results are commonly within normal limits despite significant structural cardiac defects. The echocardiogram is the ideal tool used to define cardiac anatomy and assess cardiac physiology in diagnosing congenital heart defects.

5. B) Central cyanosis

Central cyanosis may be indicative of hypoxia and would be a concerning observation requiring further investigation. Apgar scores of 7 and below are likely to require some type of intervention. At 8 minutes of life, an Apgar score of 8 is considered acceptable. Likewise, at 6 minutes of life, an SpO_2 reading of 79% is not concerning. A newborn may take up to 10 minutes or more to achieve SpO_2 readings over 90%.

6. C) Jitteriness

Symptoms of hypoglycemia include jitteriness, tremors, tachycardia, pallor, cyanosis, and an exaggerated Moro reflex.

7. C) "The skin surface of a newborn is typically alkaline, which makes it break down more easily."

The mean pH measurement of a term infant's skin is 6.34, making it relatively alkaline compared with mature skin's pH of closer to 5.5. An alkaline skin surface reduces stratum corneum integrity and increases susceptibility to skin breakdown. In the first weeks of life, skin pH decreases, making it more acidic and bringing it closer to 5.5. Until this happens, a sponge bath with warm water and a mild, pH-neutral soap should be used.

8. C) Respiratory distress syndrome

Respiratory distress occurs in premature infants with a lack of surfactant in their lungs. This leads to collapse of the alveoli in the lung, causing grunting, tachypnea, nasal flaring, and cyanosis. Pneumonia and meconium aspiration syndrome have similar outward signs, but neither is associated with surfactant production.

9. B) 10% povidone-iodine

Use of povidone-iodine is the preferred method of skin disinfectant due to its efficacy in preventing infection and its low incidence of side effects such as blisters and burns. While chlorhexidine and isopropyl alcohol are both recognized as effective skin disinfectants, neither is preferred for neonates due to the risk of skin irritation, burns, and blistering associated with their use.

10. C) Ventricular septal defect (VSD)

VSD is the most common CHD, with clinical presentation of a grade 2 to 3/4 harsh systolic murmur heard at the lower left sternal border. ASD is less common; heart sounds may not be detectable in infancy, but they occur at the upper left sternal border. PDA primarily affects premature infants and presents with a grade 1 to grade 3/4 murmur over the upper left sternal border.

11. B) The feeding and gastrointestinal system

Excoriation of the skin results from loose, watery stools that are often present in the gastrointestinal dysfunction associated with neonatal withdrawal syndrome. Metabolic and central nervous system disturbances are associated with different sets of symptoms in neonatal withdrawal syndrome, such as fever and mottling, as well as hypo- or hypertonia, seizures, and jitteriness.

12. **B) Jitteriness**

Seizures are more subtle in neonates than in older infants and children. Neonatal jitteriness can mimic seizure activity and make it difficult to determine the proper diagnosis. The quickest way to assess for seizure is to see if the activity calms with touch; if it does, it is jitteriness and is not seizure related. Apnea may be seen in neonates experiencing seizure activity, as well as in many other underlying medical issues in the newborn. However, apnea does not resemble a seizure itself. Limb withdrawal is a form of pain response in a neonate and it is not similar in appearance to seizure.

13. **C) Performing oropharynx suctioning to clear secretions before initiating positive pressure ventilation (PPV)**

After assessment of the newborn, the next nursing action would be to clear the newborn's nose and mouth of any secretions that could prevent proper ventilation. The nurse would then begin PPV. Historically, endotracheal intubation and suctioning have been used in newborns with meconium-stained amniotic fluid to minimize the risk of meconium aspiration syndrome (MAS). However, these procedures are no longer recommended because they have not been shown to reduce the risk of MAS but have been shown to cause negative impacts from delaying ventilation. Any signs of observed apnea should be treated with immediate resuscitation efforts because the onset of acidosis is generally unknown and could be either primary or secondary in origin. Naloxone is not recommended for newborns with respiratory depression in the delivery room during initial resuscitation. For a newborn with respiratory depression after maternal drug exposure, the focus needs to remain on effective ventilation and airway support for the persistently apneic newborn.

14. **A) Initiating head cooling**

Hypoxemia and ischemia are significant causes of brain injury in the neonate because delivery of both oxygen and glucose to cerebral tissue is impaired. The initial treatment to be implemented would be to induce mild hypothermia by head cooling or whole-body cooling to provide neuroprotein protection of injured central nervous system cells and prevent cerebral edema, thus lowering the risk of neurodevelopmental disability. Once cooling protocol has been carefully implemented, additional treatment and interventions include ventilation support, maintaining blood glucose levels, and monitoring for electrolyte imbalance.

15. **A) Heparin**

Due to its comparatively large molecular size, heparin is unable to cross the placenta into the fetal circulation and is least likely to affect fetal circulation. Warfarin is a common anticoagulant, and protamine sulfate is administered to neutralize heparin. Both of these medications cross the placenta into the fetal circulation.

16. **C) Using rolled cloths as a footboard**

Footdrop, or compartment syndrome, is caused by positioning of a footboard along the lateral aspect of the fibula, preventing movement and constraining intravenous (IV) fluids to a restricted space. To avoid this, the nurse will used rolled cloths as a footboard or will pad an IV board extensively to avoid restricting the area. Indwelling lines should be checked for signs of extravasation, but this measure will not prevent compartment syndrome. Infusing heparinized fluid at a low rate is done when medications will be administered intermittently, not to avoid compartment syndrome.

17. **A) Patent foramen ovale**

A patent foramen ovale allows the foramen ovale, a flap-like opening in the atrial septum, to remain open, permitting blood flow between the left atrium and the right atrium. The foramen ovale usually closes after birth due to increased pulmonary blood flow; however, 20% of adults have a patent foramen ovale with no consequences. Thus, a patent foramen ovale is considered a normal variant and requires no medical treatment. Tetralogy of Fallot is a combination of four heart defects that prevent oxygen-rich blood from flowing through the body and is managed symptomatically during the neonatal period. Surgical correction is performed during the first year of life. A newborn with a ventricular septal defect, a hole in the heart wall of the lower chambers, can be medically treated with diuretics, digoxin, caloric supplementation, and afterload reducers. Surgical correction of a ventricular septal defect is needed for those who continue to experience failure to thrive with medical management.

18. **A) Duration and timing of the glomerular filtration rate (GFR) vary for each individual.**

It is imperative that intravenous fluid and electrolyte therapy be individualized for each neonate in the first week of life because the duration and timing of each GFR phase vary. GFR in the fetal kidney is significantly lower than in the adult kidney and increases with gestational age. If insensible fluid losses are overestimated during the prediuretic phase, excess fluid intake could result in dilutional hyponatremia, whereas inadequate fluid intake during the diuretic phase leads to dehydration and hypernatremia. This is especially significant in preterm and low-birthweight infants. Fluids are not given due to water loss after birth; infants can typically manage this loss through feeding. Care providers must ensure that the infant is getting the proper nutrients, including both macro- and micromolecules, but this is not the specific reason that fluid and electrolyte therapy needs to be individualized.

19. **C) Prostaglandin E1**

A PaO_2 of <35 mmHg on room air indicates severely inadequate intracardiac mixing, as seen with transposition of the great vessels, in which there is little to no communication between the left and right side of the heart unless other anomalies are present. Immediate administration of prostaglandin E1 is indicated to maintain the patency of the ductus arteriosus. Neither digoxin nor epinephrine is indicated at this time.

20. **B) Congenital heart block**

Newborns of patients with SLE are at risk of congenital heart block, which can be significant and may require placement of a cardiac pacing device. Coarctation of the aorta is a common congenital heart defect associated with newborns who have Turner syndrome. A patent ductus arteriosus is a congenital heart defect associated with Down syndrome.

21. **B) Limiting feeding time to minimize overexertion**

In CHF incidence, it is important to limit the infant's feeding time. This ensures that the infant does not expend too much energy on oral feeds. Feeding time should be limited to 15 to 20 minutes if the infant is symptomatic, and the remainder of the meal should be given via gavage. While burping the infant is vital to minimizing emesis and nutritional loss, it is best to burp the infant more frequently during feeding, preferably after every half-ounce. Waiting until the infant shows signs of hunger is not advisable because it is often too late, and the infant may expend unnecessary energy in crying. It is generally advised to offer food to infants before they show outward signs of hunger, especially in the case of CHF, when reserving energy is crucial.

22. B) Hypoxic injury

Accelerations in heart rate indicate adequate oxygenation and exclude fetal hypoxia at the time of measurement. Variability refers to accelerations and decelerations in fetal heart rate. FHR tracings do not suggest the presence or absence of a patent ductus arteriosus.

23. A) Extravasation

Phenytoin is administered to neonates with seizure activity via intravenous (IV) mixture with normal saline. However, due to the high-acid pH of the medication, extravasation may be a complication; therefore, the nurse will monitor for this frequently to avoid damage to the skin. Purple glove syndrome is seen in adults who receive phenytoin via IV in the back of the hand. Bradycardia, not tachycardia, is a possible adverse effect of the medication.

24. A) Detailed verbal explanations

According to the VARK model of learning, the four primary learning styles are visual, auditory, reading/writing, and kinesthetic. Auditory learners prefer receiving information vocally. Text instructions are of greatest benefit to reading/writing learners, and graphical representations are preferred by visual learners. Most people learn through a combination of modes, so the most effective teaching includes a variety of formats.

25. B) Initiating a continuous infusion of prostaglandin E1 (PGE1) at 5 ng/kg/min

In a newborn whose condition worsens clinically in the first days of life, the differential diagnosis of a critical heart defect must always be considered along with a suspected diagnosis of sepsis. This means that in cases of uncertainty, therapy with PGE1 in a low dosage should be initiated. Continuous infusion of PGE1 in a low dosage of 5 to 10 ng/kg/min is recommended. Treatment should be started immediately in any newborn whose condition worsens clinically in the first days of life. Infusion would be initiated while awaiting echocardiogram to confirm heart dysfunction. This recommendation is also true when sepsis is suspected or even confirmed by laboratory data. The basic therapeutic goal is the stabilization of the infant with restoration of the fetal parallel circulatory physiology and optimization of pulmonary and systemic resistance. Secondary to maintaining adequate circulation would be confirming a sepsis diagnosis and beginning antibiotic treatment.

26. A) Actively listening

The primary behaviors denoting a caring presence are the practice of active listening, providing positive regard, and a nonjudgmental approach toward the patient. Assisting with basic needs speaks to establishing a helping and trusting relationship. Providing information clearly and honestly facilitates the patient's right to make informed decisions about their own healthcare concerns.

27. A) Hearing

The infant should be screened for hearing loss prior to discharge, with follow-up screening at 1 to 3 months of age. Factors associated with risk of hearing loss include NICU care for 5 or more days, assisted ventilation, and ototoxic medications such as gentamicin and furosemide. Pulse oximetry screening has been recommended related to the high incidence of postdischarge diagnosis of critical congenital heart disease (30%–50%), but it would not be indicated for potential adverse effects. Vision screening is recommended for infants born at less than 30 weeks' gestation or with a birth weight of less than 1,500 grams, but it is not needed in correlation with potential adverse effects from medication.

28. **B) ≥45 mg/dL**

Current guidelines recommend a target glucose level of 45 mg/dL or greater in the first 24 to 48 hours of life, and then a level of greater than 70 mg/dL after 48 hours of age.

29. **C) Irrigating the wound with normal saline**

The first step to reduce the risk of bacterial contamination and thus infection is to irrigate the wound with normal saline using a 20- to 60-mL syringe and a blunt intravenous catheter. Once the area has been irrigated, debridement of necrotic tissue may be needed. Cleansing the wound with antiseptic solutions and applying silver-containing ointments are not recommended in the treatment of neonates.

30. **A) Cleft palate**

Infants with amniotic band syndrome and constriction rings often present with craniofacial defects, such as cleft lip and/or palate. Elevated blood glucose is not associated with amniotic bands. Lanugo is not important to assess for in an infant with amniotic bands.

31. **A) Engaging in role-playing activities to encourage advocacy for the neonate**

Social learners best process information by relating with others, so they would benefit from an interactive approach such as role-playing activities that encourage advocating for the patient. Logical learners will benefit from critical thinking activities, and kinesthetic learners will do well with the inclusion of hands-on experiences.

32. **A) Ascites**

The symptoms that the infant is experiencing indicate moderate necrotizing enterocolitis (NEC), which would be confirmed by the presence of ascites on x-ray. Mild ileus and intestinal dilation are seen at the earlier stages of NEC.

33. **A) Adjust the mask.**

When assessing the effectiveness of ventilation, the nurse should use the acronym MR SOPA. This starts with *m*ask readjustment on the face, *r*epositioning the airway to sniffing position, *s*uctioning the mouth and nose for secretions, *o*pening the mouth slightly with the jaw lifted forward, *p*ressure increase, and *a*irway alternative such as intubation. The steps should be done in this order because the adjustments go from the least to the most invasive.

34. **C) Therapeutic hypothermia**

A watershed injury found in full-term neonates is often due to hypoxic ischemic encephalopathy, which is treated with therapeutic hypothermia to reduce the risk of cerebral edema and protect the neuroproteins in the brain from further injury. Pain management would not be indicated in this patient, and gabapentin would not be a typical course of treatment unless seizures were present.

35. **A) Bilirubin**

A common complication in infants with a cephalohematoma is hyperbilirubinemia. Breastfeeding infants typically receive less volume with their feeds and are at higher risk of hyperbilirubinemia. This infant would need a bilirubin level drawn within a few days of discharge. A complete blood count is not necessary after hospital discharge unless the infant is presenting with signs of infection or anemia. The newborn screening test is a more comprehensive assessment performed after 24 hours of life and before discharge of the infant, although some states also mandate a repeat screening for all infants after discharge.

36. **B) Tachycardia, galloping rhythm, and diaphoresis with feedings**

Tachycardia, galloping rhythm, diaphoresis with feedings, and cardiac enlargement are critical assessment findings associated with congestive heart failure. Cyanosis with crying, harsh systolic murmur, hypotension, grunting, and retractions are assessment findings associated with persistent pulmonary hypertension in the newborn. Tachypnea, continuous systolic murmur, bounding peripheral pulses, and tachycardia are assessment findings associated with a patent ductus arteriosus.

37. **C) "I'm screening for hip dislocation using the Ortolani maneuver."**

The Ortolani and Barlow maneuvers are useful in diagnosing developmental dysplasia of the hip (DDH), which can be an outcome in infants born in the breech position and in LGA infants. The Ortolani maneuver is used to determine hip dislocation in the infant—a type of DDH. The Barlow maneuver is not used to determine tone. Ultrasound can help confirm the diagnosis of DDH in infants born breech, but it is not used to assess for growth restriction. Additionally, it is not typically done as a routine assessment.

38. **A) Lower left sternal border**

Assessment findings are consistent with trisomy 21 syndrome, or Down syndrome, which is associated with a risk of congenital heart disease (CHD). The most common CHD is a ventral septal defect (VSD). VSD presents with a grade 2 to grade 6 murmur heard at the lower left sternal border. Heart sounds associated with pulmonary stenosis include a grade 2 to grade 6 murmur heard at the upper left sternal border; this is a CHD associated with trisomy 18. Turner syndrome is associated with tetralogy of Fallot and presents with a grade 2 to grade 6 murmur heard at the mid-left sternal border.

39. **B) Return to low baseline GFR and minimal urine output regardless of water and sodium intake**

During the first week of postnatal life, the infant's GFR goes through three distinct phases to maintain fluid and electrolyte homeostasis. The prediuretic phase, in the first 24 hours of life, is characterized by a transient increase in the GFR followed by a return to low baseline GFR and minimal urine output regardless of water and sodium intake. This phase can be prolonged for up to 36 hours with a preterm infant. The diuretic phase follows, in which the infant experiences a rapid increase in GFR, rapid diuresis, and natriuresis regardless of water and sodium intake. The postdiuretic phase typically starts around day 4 of life, at which time the GFR slowly begins to increase with maturation, and salt and water excretions vary according to intake.

40. **C) Oxygenation of 75% to 85%**

Cyanosis, a blue discoloration of the skin indicating hypoxia, is first observable when oxygenation levels are maintained between 75% and 85%. A heart rate over 150 beats per minute is considered normal in a newborn and does not indicate hypoxia or precede cyanosis. Hemoglobin levels coincide with oxygen delivery. Although a hemoglobin level of 10 g/dL is considered low in a newborn, one of the first clinical manifestations of this condition would most likely be pallor due to lack of oxygen delivery, not cyanosis.

41. A) Contact the provider.

Abdominal distention, vomiting, and absent bowel sounds can be indications of a serious gastrointestinal problem for which the provider should be notified immediately. The infant should not be fed until evaluated by the provider. Drawing lab work outside of the order time is beyond a nurse's scope of practice.

42. C) Yellowing of the eyes and skin

Yellowing of the eyes and skin is a cardinal sign of jaundice associated with hyperbilirubinemia. A positive Coombs test indicates that the neonate's blood has the mother's antibodies attached, thus increasing the risk of jaundice due to hemolytic disease, including erythroblastosis fetalis. Lethargy and jitteriness are associated with hypoglycemia, which can be caused by multiple factors, including growth restriction, hypothermia, poor feeding, respiratory distress syndrome, and sepsis. Tachypnea and nasal flaring are signs of respiratory distress, which can be caused by respiratory distress syndrome, transient tachypnea of the newborn, sepsis, aspiration, or pneumothorax.

43. C) Handling slowly and gently

Slow, gentle handling of an infant with TARS is important to avoid bruising due to decreased platelets. Educating parents on feeding options should be included in the nursing care plan but is not the most important intervention. Drawing labs by heel stick should be avoided, if possible, in an infant with TARS. Blood should be collected via a placed intravenous line or with special pediatric butterfly equipment.

44. B) Combining early nasal continuous positive airway pressure and less invasive administration technique

The recommended approach to surfactant replacement therapy consists of early initiation of nasal continuous positive airway pressure combined with the less invasive surfactant administration technique, via a thin catheter, allowing dispersion by the infant's spontaneous breaths with continuous positive airway pressure support. Studies comparing preventive administration of surfactant in the delivery room with early nasal continuous positive airway pressure and selective surfactant administration indicate no apparent advantages of prophylactic administration. Similarly, there is no benefit to the in–out intubation technique when early nasal continuous positive airway pressure plus less invasive surfactant administration is implemented.

45. A) Diaphragmatic hernia

Common extracardiac anomalies associated with TET include diaphragmatic hernia, cleft lip/palate, and omphalocele. Extracardiac anomalies not associated with TET include tracheoesophageal fistula, renal agenesis (unilateral or bilateral), and intestinal atresia.

46. B) Plexus injury

Plexus injuries are more common than spinal cord injuries and result from lateral traction on the shoulders during vertex, vaginal deliveries, or on the head during breech vaginal births. Median nerve injuries are mostly postnatal and are the result of brachial or radial arterial punctures. Spinal cord injuries are an uncommon occurrence and may result from traction on the head or neck during delivery.

47. **C) Monitoring of oxygen saturation (SpO$_2$)**

Upon initiation of PPV, it is recommended that SpO$_2$ monitoring be established for optimal monitoring of the newborn's oxygenation during resuscitation. Visual inspection for cyanotic changes in the newborn is unreliable in assessing oxygenation levels. EKG is recommended in extended resuscitation efforts for more accurate heart rate readings. It is used in conjunction with SpO$_2$ monitoring to provide both audio and visual monitoring.

48. **A) Initiating humidity of at least 50% in the infant's isolette**

Premature infants are at increased risk of TEWL because they have fewer stratum corneum layers. The stratum corneum is responsible for protecting the infant from environmental toxins and helps maintain body temperature. The use of increased humidity in a premature infant's isolette helps decrease the incidence of TEWL by reducing evaporative heat loss. While limiting adhesive tape on the skin and using gelled mattress pads for premature infants are recommended interventions, they are not implemented with the intent of reducing TEWL.

49. **B) Neonatal sepsis**

Sepsis is the most common cause of death in infants under 1,500 grams (3.3 lb.) of birth weight. This is typically due to not only gestational age and birth weight, but also exposure to bacterial microorganisms such as GBS, metabolic acidosis, and hypothermia. Exposure to GBS is not a causative factor in congenital heart defects, which are primarily due to gene expression along with maternal factors during pregnancy (e.g., smoking, medication use). While GBS exposure can cause some respiratory disorders, such as pneumonia, respiratory distress syndrome is related to a surfactant deficiency.

50. **A) Anticipates family needs and acts to meet them**

Under the AACN's Synergy Model for Patient Care, caring practices cover all nursing activities that support a therapeutic, supportive, and compassionate environment. Anticipating a family's needs before they communicate them is an example of advanced caring practice. Delivering care based on established standards and maintaining safety, while important, are examples of basic caring practice.

51. **B) Engage in further dialogue with the parents about their request to burn incense**

Hospital policy will likely state that no candles or other burning substances, such as lit incense, are allowed for the safety of everyone in the building. However, by engaging in further dialogue with the parents about their request, the nurse can gain insight into their beliefs and practice preferences, allowing the nurse and the parents to work together to find an acceptable alternative. Although the spiritual care department may eventually play a role in finding or implementing that alternative, the nurse should first attempt to gain an understanding to provide appropriate family-centered care.

52. **C) Increasing humidity in the incubator**

Marked denudation of the stratum corneum with weeping in an extremely preterm neonate increases the risk of fluid and electrolyte loss due to lack of fatty tissue. The first step to address the loss is to increase the humidity in the incubator. Intravenous fluids would not be a priority intervention until the skin thickens over the first week. Applying barrier ointments and swaddling are not appropriate until later, when adipose tissue has formed.

53. C) Transient tachypnea of the newborn (TTN)

The observation of this neonate is most consistent with factors associated with TTN: male sex assigned at birth, term or late preterm gestation, Cesarean section delivery, and onset of symptoms between 2 and 6 hours of age. Differentiating factors associated with RDS include preterm gestation with immediate signs of respiratory compromise. Differentiating factors for MAS would include postterm delivery, antenatal hypoxia, and meconium-stained amniotic fluid.

54. A) Metabolic acidemia

The umbilical artery provides the most accurate information for determining neonatal acid–base status at birth. Metabolic acidemia may occur with prolonged disruption of fetal oxygenation, resulting in anaerobic metabolism and buildup of lactic acid greater than the fetal capacity to buffer acids. Decreased pH and bicarbonate, increased base deficit, and decreased base excess are reflective of this process. Respiratory alkalosis involves an increase in pH, a decrease in $PaCO_2$, and normal bicarbonate and base excess.

55. B) Encouraging kangaroo care whenever possible with individualized support for the father

Kangaroo care fosters the relationship between parents and infants. It is always helpful to encourage parents to participate in kangaroo care to promote bonding with the infant, but because the mother's health is declining, encouraging the father to participate is particularly important. Educating the family support system on care of the neonate and the father is important, but this is not an action that would be taken to ensure bonding of the father and the neonate. While it is important for the father to spend time bonding with the infant, it would be unreasonable and insensitive to recommend that they spend all their time with the infant when they likely also wish to spend time with their partner.

56. A) After at least 24 hours of life

Waiting to perform the test until at least 24 hours after the infant's birth can avoid many false-positive CCHD results. It is not generally recommended to perform the study before that time, and waiting 1 to 2 weeks is not advisable. The test should be performed prior to the infant's discharge from the hospital to alert medical staff to cardiac abnormalities or any other abnormalities that may affect cardiac function and show up on CCHD testing.

57. C) Respiratory rate 62 breaths per minute

Tachypnea (respiratory rate of 60 breaths per minute or more) after the first hour of life is the earliest sign of respiratory disease. It is an indication that the neonate is attempting to maintain alveolar ventilation and gas exchange. Further assessment for signs of respiratory compromise is indicated. Periodic breathing is common among preterm infants due to their immature central nervous systems. This breathing pattern involves cycling between apnea (5–10 seconds) and ventilation (10–15 seconds). A heart rate in the range of 120 to 160 beats per minute is a normal finding in a preterm infant.

58. C) Shunt failure

In cases of VP shunt failure, patients will display signs of increased intracranial pressure. These symptoms include increasing head circumference, full or tense fontanelle, sutures that are more separated by palpation, high-pitched or shrill cry, irritability or sleeplessness, vomiting or poor feeding, nystagmus, sunset sign of the eyes, shiny scalp with distended vessels, and hypo- or hypertonia. The infant is exhibiting many of these signs. Although postfeed emesis may be present in an infant with an ileus, the child would have additional signs of a gastrointestinal issue, such as abdominal distention as noted by increasing abdominal measurements and absence of bowel sounds. Signs of infection in the VP shunt would include redness or drainage at the site, temperature instability, lethargy or irritability, pallor, poor feeding, and poor weight gain. Based on the nurse's assessment, the infant likely is experiencing a VP shunt failure.

59. C) Polycythemia
Living at a high altitude increases maternal and fetal hemoglobin production due to decreased oxygen pressure in the atmosphere. Prematurity and intrauterine growth restriction are also common in infants born at high altitudes. Anemia is seen in multiparity greater than three, and hypoglycemia can be seen in infants of diabetic patients.

60. B) Ensuring that home caregivers for the infant have been trained in CPR
The home caregivers for the infant must be trained in CPR prior to discharge due to the complex medical histories of NICU patients. It is crucial to the infant's health and safety to identify a healthcare professional trained in the care of former NICU patients as early in the admission as possible to facilitate regular communication regarding the infant's medical course and ensure continuation of care after discharge. However, a 1-week evaluation is not the optimal time frame for ensuring postdischarge success and safety. For preterm infants, the attainment of minimum weight is no longer the criterion for discharge; the infant must be able to maintain physiologic stability, and the family must demonstrate the ability to care for the infant's physiologic and developmental needs.

61. B) EKG PR interval of >0.16 seconds
One of the earliest signs of digoxin toxicity is the prolongation of the PR interval. Bradycardia (heart rate of less than 90 beats per minute) is another early sign. Digoxin level should be less than 2.0 ng/mL.

62. C) "My baby will feel less stress if one parent is the primary kangaroo care provider."
Kangaroo care aids the development of a healthy parent–infant relationship. For parents, it promotes bonding, helps establish the routine of parental involvement in the infant's care, and increases maternal oxytocin levels. Benefits to the infant include stress reduction, improved sleep, and greater success in feeding. If the infant has two parents, benefits are maximized when both parents are involved in providing kangaroo care. Limiting regular care to one parent does not reduce the infant's stress; involving both parents increases the amount of time during which the child receives benefits.

63. A) 22
The currently accepted lower limit for viability is set at 23 weeks' gestation. A "gray zone" for periviability is a range of 22 to 25 weeks' gestation, during which time treatment decisions may be based on provider and/or parental preferences and are typically limited to comfort care. At 25+ weeks' gestation, the provider will recommend more intensive therapy, although parental authorization is required.

64. B) Establishing family-to-professional partner relationships and mutual respect
The goal of FCC is to support optimal family functioning during the NICU experience and then promote the discharge of the intact family unit as the newborn's issues resolve. Some of the key elements of FCC are facilitating the family-to-professional partner relationship and collaboration at all levels of care; encourag-

ing family-to-family support and networking; and recognizing that family is a constant, whereas providers are constantly changing. NICU visitation policies should be revised to allow parents, but not the extended family, to be with the infant. Likewise, revising visitation policies to address nonfamily support members is important, but these support members are not included as participants in care.

65. C) Clinically benign

Respiratory acidemia is common in newborns and is considered clinically benign. It is not associated with neurologic injury in newborns. Lactic acid buildup in the tissues causes metabolic acidosis, not respiratory acidosis.

66. A) Encourage the infant's parent to pace the feed.

The nurse should encourage pacing with the bottle to give the infant frequent breaks during the feed. The infant should not be placed upright for the feed, but should be placed in a side-lying position for the best control of milk flow into the mouth. The nurse would educate the infant's parent on how to bottle-feed the infant and should avoid taking over to complete the feed.

67. A) Congenital heart disease

In the United States, an estimated 40,000 infants are expected to be affected by congenital heart disease annually. Heart defects are among the most common congenital disabilities, and symptoms include tachypnea, respiratory distress, galloping heart rhythm, decreased peripheral pulses, mottled extremities, tachycardia, hepatomegaly, and poor feeding. Respiratory distress syndrome would not include a galloping rhythm, and a patent ductus arteriosus would have bounding pulses and a heart rate greater than 170 beats per minute.

68. C) Respiratory complications due to increased lung surfactant production

Long-term corticosteroid use increases surfactant in neonates, which can lead to respiratory complications for which the nurse should be prepared. Hypoxia, cardiorespiratory shock, and hypotension are not associated with long-term use of corticosteroids but are associated with decreased blood flow in either the uterus or the placenta from other complications.

69. A) 90 mmHg

A hyperoxia test—exposure to 100% oxygen for 10 minutes—can help differentiate between cardiac disease and pulmonary disease. With cyanotic heart disease, the PaO_2 typically changes very little and does not exceed 100 mmHg. Conversely, with pulmonary disease, the PaO_2 will increase to 100 mmHg or more.

70. B) Buttocks cradled in the parent's elbow

For an infant who requires pacing and a slow-flow nipple, orienting the infant on the side is preferred to allow indirect flow of breast milk into the mouth instead of directly toward the throat. In the cross-cradle hold, the parent holds the newborn in the side-lying position with the newborn facing the parent's chest. The parent cradles the newborn's buttocks in the elbow, and the parent's cupped palm supports the back of the infant's head. The infant's head being cradled in the elbow is the cradle-hold position. Resting the newborn's body on the bed in a side-lying position would not be recommended for an infant who needs pacing because the parent is unable to frequently unlatch the infant.

71. **A) Listening for intent and feelings as well as content**

    Active listening—listening for intent as well as content, and understanding feelings—is an essential component of establishing a collaborative relationship. It is important that parents feel heard and understood. Offering reassurance about outcomes may be counterproductive rather than helpful. Rather than discussing personal opinions and experiences, it is important for the nurse to keep the focus on the parents' concerns, feelings, and questions.

72. **A) Initiating intravenous glucose infusion**

    Newborns with symptoms of hypoglycemia and a low POC glucose level (35–45 mg/dL) should immediately be treated with an intravenous glucose infusion, especially with neurologic signs such as jitteriness and tremors. Oral feeding will not be an appropriate intervention because it is not the most effective method of quick glucose administration. Rather than repeat the POC glucose screening, the nurse should send a venous blood sample to the lab for glucose level evaluation.

73. **B) Liver**

    Due to the excess fluid present in CHF, blood often backs up and increases pressure not only in the heart but also in the hepatic system, causing hepatomegaly. The nurse will monitor for hepatomegaly by palpating the abdomen to determine the size of the liver. CHF does not result in increased size or pressure of the brain or the spleen.

74. **B) Multidisciplinary rounds**

    During multidisciplinary rounds, all team members are able to share information in a timely manner and are able to address all facets of patient care, expressing their concerns and questions. Each discipline may not be involved in a specific or direct patient care event, and professional presentations typically address a specific topic that limits collaboration due to the manner of presentation.

75. **A) Central cyanosis that does not improve with administration of 100% oxygen**

    Central cyanosis that does not improve with administration of oxygen therapy is indicative of a cardiac origin. Cyanosis that improves with crying or oxygen therapy administration indicates a pulmonary origin. Pulse oximetry of less than 80% to 85% in a neonate with normal hemoglobin will result in centralized cyanosis, but this does not differentiate the origin of the cyanosis.

76. **B) Xanthines are metabolized to caffeine, which acts to increase respiratory drive.**

    Xanthine therapy is a form of therapy that includes drugs like theophylline and theobromine, which metabolize into a less stimulating form of caffeine. While the exact mechanism is unclear, this mild form of stimulation acts as an anti-inflammatory and also improves central respiratory drive. While the duration of action varies in each neonate, it is necessary to monitor closely for tachycardia and tachypnea. The long-term effects of this form of therapy have yet to be substantiated, but data do suggest that there is no long-term damage to learning and behavioral activities.

77. B) "Is the infant term?"

According to the Newborn Resuscitation Program (NRP), the first questions the nurse should ask upon arrival are "Is the infant term?" "Is the infant breathing or crying?" and "Is there good muscle tone?" While the Apgar score and time of distress are important, the nurse should follow the recommended questions outlined in the NRP.

78. C) Subgaleal hemorrhage

Subgaleal hemorrhage is a serious complication which can lead to death if left untreated. It is caused by trauma at birth, a shearing force to the scalp that causes tearing of the large emissary veins. This injury is most common after an instrumental vaginal birth, especially with a vacuum-assisted delivery. The large space of the galea aponeurotica, or subaponeurotic space, can contain the entire blood volume of the newborn if left untreated. Although a depressed skull fracture can occur from birth trauma, it does not cross suture lines and would present as an indentation of the skull, not edema. Subdural hemorrhage can also occur in difficult vaginal deliveries and is similar to subgaleal hemorrhage in that there is a slow increase in the size of the hematoma. However, decreased level of consciousness, seizure activity, and asymmetry of motor function are more commonly seen with this type of hemorrhage.

79. B) Failure to thrive

Difficulty feeding and failure to thrive are common clinical presentations of CHF. In the incidence of CHF, the infant's heart rate is likely to increase, resulting in tachycardia, not bradycardia. Due to fluid retention, the infant is likely to have a decrease in urinary output, not an increase (i.e., polyuria).

80. B) Keeps alveoli open

The function of expiratory grunting is to keep the alveoli open, allowing greater time for gas exchange to occur. In addition, grunting serves to increase intrapulmonary pressure and create residual lung gas volume.

81. C) Echocardiogram

An echocardiogram is considered diagnostic for tetralogy of Fallot, helping to define the degree and level of related anomalies and mapping blood flow through the cardiovascular system. Chest x-ray is not helpful in the newborn because the results will appear essentially normal. Cardiac catheterization is not typically indicated for a patient in this situation.

82. B) Humanistic

The humanistic learning theory asserts that the learner is motivated by the perceived usefulness of the content and that learning is acquired through the act of doing. The learner's values are paramount, and learning will not occur if the learner does not value the content or the skill involved. The cognitive field learning theory assumes that individuals learn and develop insights by analyzing their own interactions with their environment. The stimulus response learning theory is based on negative versus positive reinforcement and thus on providing immediate feedback on learner performance.

83. **C) An 11-month-old infant with a history of bronchopulmonary dysplasia**

    For the first 2 years of life, infants with a history of chronic lung disease of prematurity, including bronchopulmonary dysplasia, are at increased risk of severe complications from respiratory infections such as RSV. Likewise, infants born before 29 weeks' gestation are at an increased risk of complications from RSV. An infant born at 33 weeks' gestation with a standard NICU course would not be considered to have an exceptionally elevated risk of severe RSV infection. While maternal asthma and gestational diabetes present other risks during pregnancy and in newborns, these conditions do not increase the risk of severe RSV infection.

84. **A) Initiation of skin-to-skin care**

    Hypothermia in the neonate is determined when there is a core body temperature of less than 97.7°F (36.5°C). For mild hypothermia, also known as cold stress (96°F–97.6°F [36°C–36.4°C]), the infant can be rewarmed by skin-to-skin care (i.e., placing the infant directly on the mother's bare chest and covering both with a blanket). Early skin-to-skin care for the first 24 hours of life, or 48 hours for late preterm and term infants, can reduce hypothermia. With moderate hypothermia (89.6°F–96.7°F [32°C–35.9°C]), the infant can be rewarmed in a preheated incubator or radiant warmer. With severe hypothermia (<89.6°F [32°C]), the infant should be maintained on a radiant warmer with servo control over several hours.

85. **B) Edema of extremities**

    Respiratory disorders manifest as tachypnea, which is a respiratory rate of 60 breaths per minute or more and is the earliest sign of respiratory disease in the neonate. Respiratory grunting and intercostal retractions along with nasal flaring are additional primary indications of respiratory disorder. Cyanosis is a late-occurring sign, which makes its presence or absence an unreliable sign of respiratory compromise in neonates. Edema of the extremities is also a manifestation that occurs during later stages of respiratory distress.

86. **C) Substernal retractions**

    Clinical signs of respiratory distress may be present at birth or may occur at any time in the early neonatal period. These signs include grunting, nasal flaring, retractions, tachypnea, and cyanosis. Hypertension is not associated with respiratory distress. A shrill cry can be associated with neonatal abstinence syndrome. A newborn in respiratory distress would be saving their respiratory reserve and would not cry.

87. **B) Spastic diplegia**

    The clinical signs are consistent with spastic diplegia, characterized by spasticity in both lower extremities and mild or minimal involvement of upper extremities. Spastic diplegia is the most common form of cerebral palsy (CP) in preterm infants. Quadriplegia is the most severe form of CP, affecting both upper and lower extremities, with the lower extremities being the most affected. Spastic hemiplegia involves one side of the body, with greater involvement of the upper extremities than the lower extremities.

88. **B) Fluid-filled vesicles across the trunk**

    HSV is characterized by the presence of fluid-filled vesicles or groups of vesicles on the skin. The presence of a copper-tinted rash on the palms and soles indicates the presence of congenital syphilis. Petechiae and purpura are visible in more than half of symptomatic cytomegalovirus infections in infants.

89. A) Convection

Convective heat loss results from exposure to cooler ambient air. Evaporative heat loss occurs when liquid on the skin converts to vapor. Radiant heat loss occurs when heat is drawn away by a cooler surface that is near, but not in contact with, the body.

90. A) Neonatal demise

More than 75% of infants with AV block associated with structural heart disease will not survive. Sinus node dysfunction can be the result of various intrinsic or extrinsic processes but is not known to be a result of AV heart block. In the case of AV heart block, the infant will present with sustained bradycardia, not tachycardia.

91. A) Absence of a right radial pulse

The absence of a right radial pulse indicates obstructed blood flow to the limb with an amniotic band restriction ring and needs to be assessed by the provider immediately. Brachial plexus palsy in the neonate, referred to as neonatal brachial plexus palsy, is due to a compression of the cervical or thoracic nerves, not a constriction of the arm. Capillary refill of up to 3 seconds indicates adequate blood flow.

92. B) Bringing a photo of the infant to L&D and providing updates to the parent

Regular updates and photographs from the infant's nurse are given to the parent to improve parental involvement and morale. Encouraging breast milk expression as soon as possible may not be a viable option due to the medications the parent may be taking and the additional stress it places on the parent. Updating parents through other staff is not the best way to help them feel involved with the care team.

93. C) Treating associated pathology

The primary objective of treatment of primary hypertension of the newborn is treating the associated cause, for example, by administering antibiotics for sepsis or pneumonia. The secondary and tertiary goals are providing oxygenation and reducing pulmonary vascular resistance. Additional goals include increasing systemic vascular resistance and preventing a right-to-left shunt.

94. A) Closely monitor urine output

Indomethacin and acetaminophen are first- and second-line treatments for PDA. These treatments require consistent urine output measurement to ensure adequate kidney function. While maintaining daily weights would be advisable in any ill infant, this intervention is not specifically geared toward the treatment of PDA. Rather than promoting fluid intake, fluids would be restricted until kidney function is established.

95. A) Allowing the parents to self-direct learning needs

While many approaches are viable, it is important to understand that the adult learner is primarily self-directed, especially when there is experience in the subject matter. By allowing the parents to self-direct learning needs, the nurse can provide information in context and fill in the missing information as assessment of learning unfolds. Conversely, when the learner is dependent, it is important to keep teaching to primary points that are subject-centered. A follow-up phone call helps determine whether there are additional teaching needs, but it does not replace discharge teaching.

96. **B) Echocardiography**

The echocardiogram is considered diagnostic for coarctation of the aorta, showing the area of constriction with color flow mapping. Arterial blood gases may be essentially normal as long as the ductus arteriosus is open. An EKG may reveal right ventricular hypertrophy or may be normal.

97. **B) By ensuring commonly shared understanding of information and goals among all team members**

Attributes of an effective collaborative team include communication skills that will ensure shared understanding of information across differing disciplines. An effective collaborative team promotes role interdependence and symbiosis, rather than defending strict boundaries, while respecting individual autonomy. Rather than assigning authority based on traditional roles, the team shares authority and responsibility based on mutual respect and trust.

98. **A) Difficulty breastfeeding**

Analgesic and anesthetic drugs are most likely to affect the fetus by transplacental passage. Effects on the neonate may result in difficulty initiating breastfeeding due to lingering anesthetic effects of the drugs. Neuraxial analgesia is known to cause maternal hypotension, but not neonatal hypertension or tachycardia.

99. **B) Performing oral and nasal suctioning using a bulb suction**

The neonate is already at a higher risk of infection, including sepsis, and will need immediate attention. While meconium amniotic fluid is common in postterm deliveries due to advanced maturity of the fetus, a decrease in amniotic fluid volume can add to the thick consistency of the meconium, which increases the risk of infection. During labor, an amnioinfusion can be used to thin the fluid and reduce the risk of meconium aspiration syndrome. However, when meconium is thick at the time of delivery, the priority nursing action is to suction the newborn's nasal and oral cavities immediately using a bulb syringe to eliminate as much meconium as possible before initiating breathing to avoid meconium aspiration syndrome. Drying the newborn can stimulate respiration and should be avoided until suctioning has been completed. Once the airway has been cleared of all visible meconium, the nurse should dry and warm the infant and stimulate respirations. The neonate would then be taken to the NICU to be further assessed and monitored.

100. **B) Apnea duration of 5 to 10 seconds**

Periodic breathing is characterized by a cyclic breathing pattern of apnea for 5 to 10 seconds and ventilation for 10 to 15 seconds. With apnea of prematurity, the duration of the cessation of breathing is 20 seconds or more, possibly resulting in bradycardia. Respiratory effort is absent during apnea episodes for both periodic breathing and apnea of prematurity.

101. **B) Enabling and empowering parents as members of the interdisciplinary team**

The FCC model focuses on addressing and encouraging parent involvement. One of the primary principles involves enabling and empowering the parents as members of the interdisciplinary team. Enabling refers to building on a family's strengths to create opportunities and ways they can use their abilities to learn how to meet the needs of the neonate and the family. Empowering means acknowledging and respecting the family's strengths and capabilities and building on those to support the family in meaningful decision-making that develops or maintains the family's sense of control over their own lives. This produces positive change. While parents may need to accept the neonatal prognosis, this is not a principle of FCC. There may be times when sympathy and compassion are appropriate, but these are not the focus of the FCC model.

102. A) Cyanosis

In the incidence of congenital heart lesions, pulmonary blood flow obstruction often results in cyanosis. To distinguish central cyanosis from acrocyanosis, the nurse will assess the tongue. While the nurse may assess the tongue's muscle tone to determine if the neonate is capable of breastfeeding, this assessment is unrelated to congenital heart disease. Similarly, gag reflex is unrelated to congenital heart disease.

103. A) Bounding peripheral pulses

Due to their rapid upstroke and wide pulse pressure, peripheral pulses are easily palpated and bounding. In patent ductus arteriosus, the predominant shift is from left to right, resulting in the absence of central cyanosis and normal oxygen saturation.

104. A) Discuss safety options with the neonate's mother and the interdisciplinary team

When physical abuse is identified, all steps should be taken to ensure patient and neonate safety by first discussing a plan with the neonate's mother and the interdisciplinary healthcare team. Providing a room for nesting may aid in keeping the patient and the neonate safe, but this should be done only after consultation with the patient and the rest of the team. Referral to social services may be needed, and reporting to local authorities may be a legal requirement, but the nurse's initial efforts should be focused on providing safety until these groups can become involved.

105. A) Digoxin

Medical management for COA primarily centers on infusion of digoxin—or, alternatively, prostaglandin E1—to keep the ductus arteriosus open or to stimulate reopening. Inotropes such as dopamine and/or dobutamine, and diuretics such as furosemide, may be prescribed with symptoms of congestive heart failure.

106. C) Notifying the provider

A shrill cry, a shiny scalp, and increased head circumference are signs of increased intracranial pressure or shunt failure. The provider should be notified immediately. Raising the head of the infant's bed could increase the intracranial pressure further due to ventricular collapse, which could lead to hemorrhage of the brain. Turning the infant and reassessing at the next care time would result in a delay in care and potentially adverse outcomes.

107. C) Well-oxygenated

Because fetal heart tracings do not show how well the infant is oxygenating, interventions such as digital scalp stimulation and vibroacoustic stimulation can help prevent unnecessary testing or interventions for an infant who is not in distress. Accelerations of the fetal heart rate that are at least 15 bpm above the baseline and with a duration of at least 15 seconds correlate highly with a normal fetal acid–base status. The lack of acceleration during stimulation can be a sign of hypoxemia or acidemia and should be managed accordingly.

108. B) Reduced ability of the liver to filter bilirubin

The presence of jaundice is associated with reduced ability of the newborn's liver to filter bilirubin, resulting in an increase in indirect bilirubin in the blood (hyperbilirubinemia) and a yellowish appearance in the skin and sclera of the eyes. Elevation of bilirubin is common even in a healthy infant; however, when it is found in a neonate who is at risk of dehydration or malnutrition, it can be deadly. Vasomotor instability in the neonate is associated with acrocyanosis, a condition that results in a bluish hue in the skin of the extremities due to poor circulation to these areas. Infiltration of melanin-forming cells into the dermal skin results in the appearance of slate-gray nevi. An increase in the production of bilirubin in the neonate is considered pathologic jaundice if it occurs within the first 24 hours after birth.

109. A) Gastrointestinal

Exposure to dependency-producing substances can have a multisystem impact on the neonate, with the gastrointestinal and central nervous systems being the primary systems affected. While monitoring urinary and integumentary systems is important, they would not be considered a priority.

110. B) Poor skeletal growth

Late metabolic acidosis develops after the first week of life because the net excess of acid intake exceeds the capacity for acid excretion. Late metabolic acidosis is usually more pronounced in the preterm infant or in those on parenteral nutrition, but it usually resolves after the first month of life due to renal maturation. If metabolic acidosis is persistent past that point, it can result in poor weight gain and poor skeletal growth. There is no evidence that persistent late metabolic acidosis leads to developmental delays or vision impairment.

111. B) Meconium

Meconium toxicology analysis is considered the highest standard because it is conducted postpartum and will detect in-utero exposure for the last two trimesters of the pregnancy. A urine sample may be the easiest to obtain but may not provide the most accurate results. While hair analysis is more accurate, the newborn may not have a sufficient quantity of hair on which to perform the test.

112. C) Surfactant deficiency

Respiratory distress is most often due to immature development of lung tissue, especially surfactant deficiency. Sex assigned at birth and gestational age are not principal factors in the development of respiratory distress.

113. A) Promote minimal stimulation of the infant.

Since the infant has PPHN and is on high-frequency oscillatory ventilation and nitric oxide, the infant is of higher acuity. The nurse would want to promote minimal stimulation of the infant because in PPHN the pulmonary arteries are highly reactive and can fluctuate significantly when the infant is handled. This can increase vasoconstriction and impact the infant negatively. For the same reason, the nurse would cluster blood draws for this patient. Fixed FiO_2 is not required for patients with PPHN.

114. **A) Capillary refill time greater than 3 seconds**
The criteria indicating the need for supplemental oxygen include a capillary refill time greater than 3 seconds. Other criteria for supplemental oxygen include PaO_2 of less than 60 mmHg and central cyanosis. Central cyanosis is located in the periorbital, perioral, regional, and mucous membranes, including the gums and lips.

115. **C) "We will need to call the doctor immediately if there is any redness or if our baby has a fever."**
It is important for the parents to be able to recognize signs of infection, as well as the symptoms of shunt failure. Both complications need urgent treatment to prevent further severe complications. The shunt will be placed under the skin of the scalp, so while it will be palpable it will not be visible or potentially catch on objects. This infant will need to be closely followed by the neurology team and other specialists throughout childhood and likely for life. Although regular well-baby visits are still appropriate, a family practitioner is not qualified to provide sole management of this issue.

116. **A) Bronchopulmonary dysplasia (BPD)**
BPD is seen in very-low-birthweight newborns who require long-term mechanical ventilation. The pathogenesis is multifactorial, including damage from hyperinflation, oxygen toxicity, inflammatory response, and edema. This acute lung injury results in the characteristic signs of BPD, including airway obstruction, emphysema-atelectasis, pulmonary edema, pulmonary hypertension, fibrotic tissue damage, and decreased number of alveoli. Careful management of inspiratory pressures and oxygen concentrations used with mechanical ventilation in the very-low-birthweight newborn can help prevent BPD development. A diaphragmatic hernia is a hole in the diaphragm of the newborn that can result in displacement of the abdominal organs and can be the result of asymmetrical chest wall movement and associated unilateral lesions of the diaphragm. PPHN results from hypoxemia secondary to right-to-left shunting of blood at the foramen ovale and ductus arteriosus.

117. **A) Bronchopulmonary dysplasia**
Bronchopulmonary dysplasia is a chronic lung disease affecting premature infants who experienced mechanical ventilation for respiratory distress syndrome. The disease increases the risk of cystic lung changes during infancy. Congestive heart failure and pneumonia also occur later in infancy but are not characterized by cystic lung changes.

118. **C) Preserving the family's faith and hope while honoring inner life**
Caring presence refers to mutual trust and connectedness between the nurse and the patient or family. An authentically caring presence requires preserving faith and hope and acknowledging and honoring the inner life of oneself and others. Ensuring that the family fully understands discharge instructions is an important component of competent care but is not related to caring presence. Creative problem-solving is an essential nursing attribute, but it is not a factor in caring presence.

119. **C) Hypoglycemia**
A history of nuchal cord and an Apgar score of 5 or less indicates an increased risk of development of hypoglycemia due to the increased utilization of glucose related to stress. While hypocalcemia and hyperbilirubinemia may develop as a result of perinatal asphyxia, these are not the most immediate potential problems.

120. C) Volume overload

Volume overload in CHF can cause hypertrophy and cardiomegaly. While anemia and tachycardia are also present in CHF, neither process directly contributes to cardiomegaly.

121. B) Pneumothorax

A pneumothorax is a potential complication of meconium aspiration syndrome. It is due to the overinflation and air trapping that occurs in the lungs. The nurse will suspect pneumothorax with infants on respiratory support who exhibit decreased breath sounds and increased respiratory effort. The nurse will further assess for hypotension and skin mottling. Pulmonary hemorrhage has an acute presentation with pink frothy secretions from the mouth and is not seen with meconium aspiration. Persistent pulmonary hypertension of the newborn can be seen in meconium aspiration patients, but the patient will not have decreased breath sounds and will have cyanosis and tachypnea instead.

122. B) Retractions

Retractions observed on and around the infant's chest are an indicator that the infant is working harder to ventilate the lungs. This is typically a sign of respiratory distress. Cyanosis in the hands and feet shortly after birth, known as acrocyanosis, is considered normal and does not indicate the presence of respiratory distress. Additionally, the presence or absence of cyanosis in a newborn is generally not a reliable indicator of the infant's respiratory status. Tachycardia, while often a symptom of respiratory distress in infants, is not directly observable by the clinician. Diagnosing tachycardia would require auscultation by the clinician or the use of monitoring equipment.

123. B) Careful fluid management, limiting use of nephrotoxic drugs, and promptly treating any hemodynamic or respiratory issues

Prevention of acute kidney injury (AKI) in a high-risk infant, such as one receiving hypothermia therapy or having a history of perinatal asphyxia, should include careful fluid management, limited use of nephrotoxic medications unless the risks outweigh the benefits, prompt recognition and treatment of respiratory or hemodynamic instabilities, and maintenance of an adequate circulatory volume to prevent further insult to the infant and their kidneys. Completely avoiding nephrotoxic drugs may be difficult because some treatments may be needed, and the benefits will outweigh the damages. There is no need to restrict fluid intake as this could lead to further complications. There is no need to increase the frequency of vital signs more than with any other infant. A neonate undergoing therapeutic hypothermia protocol would already be on continuous oxygen saturation readings with weaning to room air as possible and frequent vital signs measurement, strict input and output recordings, weighing of diapers, and decreased stimulation; these are not specifically reserved for those at greater risk for AKI.

124. C) Subtle seizure activity

Subtle seizures are the most common type of seizure among neonates. These seizures are often overlooked because they are inconspicuous, consisting of signs such as rapid onset of swimming or peddling motion of the legs, horizontal deviation of the eyes, repetitive blinking or fluttering of the eyelids, sucking, or tongue thrusting. It is often difficult to discern between these and neonatal jitteriness, which is often associated with a startle reflex but does not manifest with ocular or oral repetitiveness. Hypoxic ischemic encephalopathy is a combination of hypoxemia and ischemia due to impaired placental or pulmonary function, and symptoms are noticeable and determinable, unlike subtle seizures.

125. A) Accumulation of air in the pleural space

Accumulation of air in the pleural space is indicative of a pneumothorax. Transillumination is a method used to see if a patient has a pneumothorax prior to receiving chest x-ray. For transillumination, the light is pressed to the skin of the chest wall, and a translucent glow will be noted. A "sail sign" is seen with a pneumomediastinum due to air outlining the undersurface of the thymus gland. While a pneumomediastinum can accompany a pneumothorax, it will not be seen through transillumination. Coarse, patchy infiltrates are seen in infants with meconium aspiration syndrome and are visible with radiography, not transillumination.

126. B) Coordinating learning activities and resources that include all team members and are geared to both neonatal and parental needs

A comprehensive approach to unique healthcare needs involves a wide range of methods, including assessing knowledge and providing information. However, to build a plan around comprehensive approaches, the nurse must coordinate learning activities and resources that address both neonatal and parental needs while including all team members in the approach.

127. C) Removing the IV needle

When extravasation is noticed, the first action is to remove the IV needle from the area and elevate the hand. Once this is done, hyaluronidase will be administered with or without saline wash.

128. A) Breastfeeding and lactation education and support

Initiation of breastfeeding in the first 4 hours after delivery helps establish lactation and set a pattern of frequent feedings. This has been shown to reduce peak bilirubin levels due to a decrease in intestinal transit time and a decrease in enterohepatic circulation. However, when an infant has difficulty latching on, the nurse will provide education on how to help the neonate obtain nutrition through continued breastfeeding and on the importance of pumping to continue lactation. The neonate can be fed breast milk through a bottle with special nipples if needed, and this would be discussed in the discharge education. While phototherapy is used to treat newborns with diagnosed hyperbilirubinemia, it is not the primary intervention. Administration of phenobarbital is often an intervention for neonates diagnosed with Crigler–Najjar syndrome and is a treatment used in conjunction with phototherapy, so this would not be a primary intervention in this patient.

129. C) Seizures

Seizure activity is one of the most common signs, and sometimes the only clinical sign, of CNS dysfunction in newborns. Seizures occur more frequently during the neonatal period than in any other period of life. They should be investigated to determine the underlying cause. While hypotonia may be a symptom of CNS dysfunction in a neonate, it can be difficult to determine the cause. Hypotonia is easily confused with muscle weakness, and therefore the cause must be investigated to determine whether it is neurologic or musculoskeletal in nature. Poor feeding is not specifically attributed to CNS dysfunction and is more often due to ankyloglossia or thermoregulation issues.

130. C) Subgaleal hemorrhage

This infant is showing several signs of hypovolemic shock as a result of a subgaleal hemorrhage. A subgaleal hemorrhage initially presents as scalp swelling that is firm and crosses suture lines; the edema may progress down to the neck. This type of injury causes bleeding to collect under the aponeurosis, which may continue for several hours after birth; the space has the capacity to fill with the infant's entire blood volume. This is a life-threatening injury and needs interventions such as blood and volume replacement and treatment of shock. Infants with caput succedaneum have soft, pitting edema of the scalp that crosses suture lines. Caput succedaneum does not require any treatment; it is self-limiting and should resolve within a few days after birth. Infants with cephalohematoma present with a firm, tense collection of blood that does not cross suture lines. This is often from the use of a vacuum in delivery, and sometimes a fracture is also present. Although cephalohematoma is self-limiting, parents of infants with the condition should be warned that the swelling may worsen after birth and may remain for up to a few months before resolving.

131. A) Protected sleep

Protected sleep addresses the importance of the behavioral state and the need for adequate rest to support state regulation and physiologic stability. Sleep deprivation exerts a long-term effect on behavior and brain function. The effectiveness of subsequent measures, such as stress and pain management and supportive activities of daily living, is contingent on establishing physical, behavioral, and emotional readiness for caregiving activities by providing protected sleep.

132. C) Tachypnea and intercostal retractions with expiratory grunting

Tachypnea—a newborn respiratory rate of greater than 60 breaths per minute—and intercostal retractions are signs of acute RDS in the newborn and should be further evaluated and treated. Expiratory grunting is a sign of RDS because it is a manifestation of tachypnea and intercostal retractions. Acrocyanosis is a normal finding in the first 48 hours after birth and is not specific to impaired lung perfusion. Hypotension in the newborn is associated with blood loss or cardiac anomalies. Bradycardia in the newborn can be a late sign of hypoxia, but it can also be associated with hypothermia, hypovolemia, and hemothorax and would be further evaluated to rule out any differential diagnosis.

133. C) Wrapping in occlusive wrap

While drying and stimulating are critical components of thermoregulation in a newborn and should be routinely performed after every delivery, the low-birthweight neonate should be wrapped in a medical-grade plastic bag or an occlusive wrap. Neonatal abstinence scoring is indicated in situations where there is suspected maternal drug use or when the infant is showing clinical symptoms of withdrawal.

134. B) Kidney

The kidneys are responsible for controlling the concentration of HCO_3, which is directly correlated to lung function and oxygenation. The liver does not play a direct role in the acid–base balance of the lungs or in oxygen delivery. The heart plays an important role in moving oxygen through the blood to other organs, but it is not a primary factor in controlling HCO_3 levels.

135. B) Pulmonary lymph system

The pulmonary lymph system will be the main source of excreting fetal lung fluid in the event of a Cesarean delivery because a mechanical squeezing of the infant's chest and lungs will not occur as it does during a vaginal delivery. The infant will not experience higher levels of diuresis following a Cesarean delivery; this is not a mechanism for removal of fetal lung fluid in healthy newborns. Thoracic squeezing is experienced by the infant in a vaginal, not Cesarean, delivery.

136. **B) Maintenance of patency of the ductus arteriosus**

Before surgery for d-TGA, a PGE1 medication such as alprostadil may be given to increase blood flow and improve the mixing of oxygen-poor and oxygen-rich blood through maintenance of the patency of the ductus arteriosus. Metabolic acidosis in newborns with d-TGA is treated with administration of sodium bicarbonate and fluid replacement. Angiotensin-converting enzyme (ACE) inhibitors can be used to reduce systemic blood pressure and improve perfusion in newborns with d-TGA.

137. **B) Gestational diabetes**

A prenatal diagnosis of gestational diabetes increases an infant's risk for respiratory distress syndrome. While comorbidities such as asthma and hypertension can complicate pregnancy and present problems during delivery, neither is directly related to increased risk of respiratory distress syndrome in the newborn.

138. **B) Infiltration**

Medications such as nafcillin can be irritating to the veins and the surrounding skin, so the nurse will monitor for infiltration into the tissue and extravasation as priority assessments. Pain and discomfort, as well as infection, are important to monitor but would not be considered the priority assessment.

139. **A) "Our baby will be able to walk and do all the things other babies do as they get older."**

It is imperative that parents of infants with severe spinal injuries understand the implications of the injuries and that recovery may be minimal to nonexistent. The parents should be given realistic information about the implications of their infant's injuries. They need to know that the child may require lifelong, specialized care. The parents will need extensive teaching and counseling throughout the hospital stay to prepare them for a successful discharge home. They will likely be overwhelmed by the complexity of their newborn's condition and need emotional, financial, and educational support.

140. **C) Lower nutrient value**

Donor milk has differing nutrient content and energy value due to the pasteurization process it goes through. This reduces immunoglobulin A, lactoferrin, lysozyme, insulin-like growth factors, hepatocyte growth factor, water-soluble vitamins, and antioxidant activity. Pasteurization does not decrease oligosaccharides, long-chain polyunsaturated fatty acids, lactose, or fat-soluble vitamins. Although the contents of donor milk vary from a mother's own breast milk, it is still preferred over formula for premature infants.

141. **A) Degree of asymmetrical SGA**

To determine prognosis, it is important to determine the degree of asymmetrical SGA because this is most common in patients with preeclampsia. This form of SGA typically has a poorer outcome than symmetrical SGA, so determining the degree is critical. Fetal growth trajectory is an important factor in perinatal mortality of neonates with intrauterine growth restriction (IUGR) who are classified as very small for gestational age, but it would not be used to determine the goals and outcomes for an SGA neonate. Relative risk correlated to the degree of IUGR is a factor in respiratory illnesses of preterm neonates but is not specific to SGA neonates at 38 weeks' gestation.

142. C) 10

The nurse should expect the preductal target SpO_2 to be above 85% at 10 minutes of life. If the infant is below 85% at 10 minutes of life, they will need their oxygen to be increased. At 5 minutes of life, the nurse should expect the target SpO_2 to be between 80% and 85%, and at 3 minutes of life the saturation should be between 70% and 75%.

143. B) Requesting an interpreter to communicate the neonate's diagnosis and prognosis and the parents' concerns

The most appropriate action to provide the best possible care for the patient is to request an interpreter who can communicate diagnosis and prognosis to the parents and allow the parents to convey preferences, concerns, and culturally appropriate care to the nurse. Providing prewritten communication may be helpful if an interpreter is currently unavailable, but an interpreter will be better able to facilitate discussion between the parents and the NICU staff. Providing spiritual care may be appropriate if the parents express a need for it, but a member of that department would be unable to convey all of the necessary health information that a trained interpreter could.

144. C) Reduces the risk of cold stress

The practice of delayed bathing after birth allows for the neonate to achieve temperature stability, reducing the risk of comorbidities from cold stress. It also permits earlier skin-to-skin contact with the parents, which can reduce stress and immediately promote bonding, and it results in reduced risk of infection through preservation of the vernix. The delay in bathing is not intended to allow additional time for assessment. Evaporative heat loss and thermal variability are addressed by drying the newborn immediately following delivery and again when bathing begins.

145. B) Monitor intake and output for kidney function

Eagle-Barrett syndrome, also known as prune belly syndrome, is managed through the neonatal period by urinary tract drainage, management of renal insufficiency, and antibiotic prophylaxis to prevent urinary tract infection. Surgical repair is not typically indicated with unilateral obstruction; however, the provider is planning surgery to correct cryptorchidism. The nurse will monitor intake and output to monitor for renal insufficiency and urinary tract infection as a primary intervention. While assessment of the abdomen may be needed, as well as obtaining blood for lab testing in preparation for surgery, it is not the primary action the nurse will take for this patient because renal function is the primary concern.

146. C) Repeating the test in 1 hour

Pulse oximetry screening should be repeated in 1 hour if both RUE and RLE are between 90% and 94%, or if the difference between the two is greater than 3%. If the second screening test is not negative, a further diagnostic evaluation is indicated; possible transfer to the NICU would also be indicated.

147. A) Addressing the parents and the patient by name when discussing care

Using the parents' and the patient's names demonstrates the nurse's awareness of each person's worth and dignity. An awareness of the patient's and parents' responses serves to guide the nurse toward therapeutic intervention. Ensuring that the parents fully understand their situation facilitates their right to informed choices regarding their own healthcare needs and those of their infant.

148. A) "Laying an infant on the stomach during tube feeding helps with digestion."

Positioning infants with respiratory distress syndrome in the prone position during enteral feeding helps with gastric emptying. Parents should receive accurate, direct explanations of care that help to educate them for care at home when needed. The positioning is not intended to alleviate lung pressure or prevent tube displacement.

149. A) Cord pH of 6.7

A cord pH below 7.0 is a sign of metabolic acidemia and thus is an indicator of an acute hypoxic event. Respiratory acidemia is considered benign and does not indicate an acute hypoxic event. At 6 minutes of life, oxygen saturation of 89% is not cause for concern. Healthy infants can take up to 10 minutes to maintain oxygen saturation over 90%.

150. C) Teach-back method

One of the most effective approaches to ensuring that patients and their parents fully understand and can implement teaching is to allow them to "teach back" the material to the nurse, thus providing both practice for the patient or the parents and confirmation to the nurse that the teaching was successful. Printed instructions should also be sent home, but this does not allow the nurse to confirm that the teaching is effective and that the parents are capable of providing care. Simulation-based learning is not always available, and parents often feel awkward working with an inanimate object, which may inhibit learning.

151. A) 28 to 30

Using the Ballard system of determining gestational age, the nurse determines that this neonate has signs of physical development of approximately 28 to 30 weeks' gestation. Observable vernix, presence of lanugo on the shoulders but not the face, and observable embryonic vessels and testes are all signs of a preterm neonate in this gestational age range. Vernix will begin to disappear as the neonate develops and is closer to term. Lanugo begins to disappear from the face and anterior trunk at around 28 weeks' gestation but is still present over the shoulders. As the fetus develops, the lanugo will eventually be reduced to only patches across the shoulders. Embryonic vessels are not present before week 27 or after week 34. Male testes begin to descend from the abdomen and are noticeable in the scrotum at 28 weeks' gestation. By week 37, they have fully descended unless cryptorchidism is present.

152. A) Antibiotic use

Infants prescribed antibiotics in the NICU are at higher risk of developing AKI because many drugs in this class of medication are nephrotoxic. Because premature infants have immature renal tubes, medications that are excreted by the kidney have a prolonged half-life, causing them to circulate through the body and kidneys for a longer period of time, elevating the risk of AKI. Infants at risk of AKI have impaired renal perfusion. Serum calcium concentration decreases naturally after birth in a premature infant due to elevated serum phosphate concentration.

153. A) Administering fluids

Once prostaglandin E1 infusion has begun, fluids would need to be initiated to ensure that arterial pressure is maintained. Assessing vital signs and monitoring for infection are steps to take after initiating fluids.

154. C) Urinary tract infection (UTI)

During the first few months of life, the presentation of a UTI is nonspecific and subtle. Symptoms include feeding difficulties, poor weight gain, temperature instability, cyanosis, fever, abdominal distention, hepatomegaly, and jaundice. The presence of protein, blood, nitrates, and leukocytes in the urine dipstick is indicative of a UTI. UTI in infants is common and can complicate a NICU course and lead to long-term sequelae if not treated properly and promptly. Given the symptoms and timing, GBS pneumonia or NEC is not likely the source of this neonate's new health issue. These complications typically occur within the first few weeks of life rather than later in the NICU course.

155. C) Lungs

The neonate is demonstrating signs of group B *Streptococcus* infection, and the nurse will need to assess for sepsis and respiratory infections because the lungs are the most common site of primary infection in newborns. While infections do occur in other areas, such as the heart and the gastrointestinal tract, in newborns those sites are less common primary sites of infection.

156. C) Remove barriers by reviewing shared goals and decision-making.

Elements essential to the effectiveness of interdisciplinary collaboration include shared goals and decision-making processes, as well as removal of barriers. Therefore, reviewing the unit's shared goals and decision-making processes will help remove barriers such as resistance from other team members. Rather than a central authority, shared power or authority among the team is critical, requiring respect for, and trust in, team members' skills and expertise. While providing professional development is important for maintaining professional roles, collaboration involves overlaps in competencies that may cross the traditionally accepted lines of professional roles—again, requiring mutual trust and respect.

157. B) Preterm premature rupture of membranes (PPROM)

Antibiotics are most likely prescribed when PPROM occurs because this condition could introduce microorganisms into fetal circulation. TRAP sequence occurs in twins when arterial perfusion is reversed and one twin's heart provides circulation for both fetuses. TRAP sequence is treated surgically, not directly by antibiotic therapy. Contraction-induced hypoxia occurs during delivery and does not require antibiotic therapy.

158. A) Administration of high-concentration oxygen to the patient

The tracing is nonreassuring, indicating a risk for hypoxia and necessitating administration of high-concentration oxygen to the patient. Thickened or large nuchal translucency on ultrasound is the trademark sign for early detection of aneuploidy in utero, which is associated with various developmental abnormalities, including those affecting the cardiovascular system. Repositioning would be indicated if the fetus was showing signs of umbilical cord prolapse, such as recurrent variable decelerations and bradycardia. Intravenous crystalloid fluids would be needed in a patient with hypotension due to neuraxial anesthesia.

159. A) Dietary restrictions

The primary treatment for PKU is dietary restriction of phenylalanine, and infants with the disorder will be placed on a phenylalanine-free formula. Pegvaliase is approved for treatment of PKU in adults, but it has not been approved for pediatric therapy, so its use would not be discussed. Although medications such as sapropterin have been approved for pediatric patients, including infants, herbal remedies are not supported or recommended.

160. **B) "The team helps make sure the needs of your baby and family are met while helping coordinate your baby's medical care."**
Palliative care may be consulted when the neonate is diagnosed with a life-threatening or life-limiting condition. The team focuses on the needs of the infant and family—both physical and psychosocial—rather than just the prognosis of the infant's condition. The team's involvement is not necessarily an indication that death is imminent. The nurse should not indicate that the team's involvement suggests a poor prognosis or an anticipated decline; rather, the nurse should help the parent understand the team's role and allow the provider and team to discuss the nature of the infant's condition.

161. **B) Cranial sutures**
Cranial sutures are important to assess for proper growth and development of the infant. Following traumatic birth, injury to the skull is possible, and the nurse must assess for it. While shoulder dystocia is possible in traumatic birth, the acromion process—the bony extension of the scapula toward the front of the body—is not a primary concern for evaluation. Symphysis pubis would not be a primary concern in evaluating for trauma because this is the area least likely to experience damage.

162. **C) Offering reassurance the NICU is the best place for the infant and stating that the injury could have been much worse if not for the cooling therapy**
Parents in this situation are likely to be upset, anxious, hopeless, or angry and may be looking to place blame. They need the nurse to support and comfort them at this time. The nurse can do this by restating what happened in a different way and focusing on the positive. Stating that the parents did the right thing by consenting to transfer of the infant to a higher level of care, which subsequently prevented a potentially worse brain injury, will offer some reassurance. The parents do need someone to listen to them, but it is best not to leave them alone after a few minutes unless they request it. While offering to contact a person of faith to sit with the parents may demonstrate caring, it is not the most appropriate response to the parents' concerns.

163. **B) Obtain an oxygen saturation (SpO_2) level**
Onset of cardiovascular symptoms at 2 days of age is most likely due to the presence of ductus-dependent congenital heart disease, precipitated by closure of the ductus arteriosus. Therefore, the nurse's first action will be to obtain an accurate SpO_2 through pulse oximetry, followed by capillary refill testing in the extremities. Blood should be obtained for a CBC to determine electrolytes and glucose levels; arterial blood gas testing will also be needed to determine acidosis. Monitoring of I&O is needed but is not the first action of the nurse.

164. **B) Rectal temperature ≤95°F (35°C)**
Given the neonate's inability to maintain temperature, hypothermia in particular is considered a strong indication of neonatal sepsis, especially in preterm infants. Additional clinical signs associated with sepsis include tachypnea and/or apnea, lethargy, and hypoactive reflexes.

165. **B) Fetal diagnosis of Turner syndrome**

Fetal diagnosis of Turner syndrome is associated with an increased risk of CHD. More than 50% of neonates diagnosed with Turner syndrome will have coarctation of the aorta, bicuspid aortic valve, aortic aneurysm, atrial septal defect, or ventricular septal defect. Maternal history of uncontrolled type 1 or type 2 diabetes mellitus is associated with an increased risk of CHD; however, this risk is not associated with gestational diabetes. A genetic link accounts for a lower risk, 3% to 5%, of recurrence among siblings.

166. **C) Establish feeding times based on the medication's half-life**

The best practice and safest plan of care is to establish feeding times based on the medication's half-life to avoid exposure to the neonate. Feeding times may be planned for when the drug concentrations begin to decline or for just prior to the next dosage. Another safe alternative is to administer the drug, pump immediately afterward, and discard the milk. The breastfeeding patient continues this practice until they are no longer taking the medication to maintain a milk supply while keeping the infant safe. However, this limits the amount of actual breast milk the neonate will be able to ingest. Administering the drug immediately after the infant's feeding time may not always be appropriate because feeding times are not necessarily aligned with the timing of medication dosages.

167. **B) Respiratory distress syndrome (RDS)**

The incidence of RDS is greater at lower gestational ages, with 30% of infants born between 28 and 34 weeks' gestation experiencing reduced lung compliance as characterized by cyanosis, nasal flaring, sternal or intercostal retractions, expiratory grunting or whining, and often edema in the extremities. MAS is seen in approximately 10% of all newborns and is characterized by tachypnea, gasping respirations, and often wheezing or rales. TTN is the presence of unabsorbed lung fluid that is seen in term or close-to-term infants and is characterized by increased respiratory rate but minimal intercostal retractions and grunting.

168. **A) Coarctation of the aorta**

Coarctation of the aorta is a localized constriction of the aorta, usually occurring at the junction of the transverse aortic arch and the descending aorta near the ductus arteriosus. This constriction causes significant differences in blood pressure in the right upper extremity when compared with the lower extremities based on circulatory pathways. Persistent pulmonary hypertension is seen in newborns with abnormally elevated vascular resistance. This syndrome does not cause abnormal blood pressure. Transposition of the greater vessels is a condition in which the aorta, which should arise from the left ventricle, arises from the right ventricle, and the pulmonary artery, which should arise from the right ventricle, arises from the left ventricle. While it affects oxygenation, this condition does not affect blood pressure.

169. **B) Offering grief education to the parents**

Offering grief education, emotional support, and attention to grieving parents can be helpful. Avoiding talking about the loss and distracting the parents from the loss are both powerful ways to deny that the infant ever existed, and they inhibit the healing process.

170. **B) Echocardiography**

The hyperoxia test result of a PaO_2 below 100 mmHg is suggestive of congenital heart disease and should trigger an echocardiographic examination. Two-dimensional echocardiography is the definitive noninvasive test to determine the presence of congenital heart disease because it can identify the presence, degree, and direction of the cardiac shunt. A chest x-ray may be useful for identifying unique findings related to cyanotic cardiac diseases, such as heart shape or size, but it is not the priority next step. An EKG measures the electrical activity of the heart, revealing problems such as cardiac rhythm disturbances, inadequate coronary artery blood flow, and electrolyte disturbances.

171. **A) Controlling cerebral edema and offering neuroprotection**

Inducing moderate hypothermia in neonates with suspected HIE provides neuroprotection of the injured central nervous system cells and decreases cerebral edema. Therapeutic cooling has been shown to improve the outcomes of newborns with HIE and lower the rate of developmental disability. Reduced oxygen demand is not a benefit of cooling therapy; in fact, complications of cooling include respiratory distress (increased oxygen demand and support), as well as cardiac issues (bradycardia and hypotension), coagulation issues, jaundice, electrolyte imbalance, and sepsis. Therapeutic cooling does not decrease the incidence of intraventricular hemorrhage.

172. **C) Reduced glomerular filtration rate**

The glomerular filtration rate of newborns is low, resulting in reduced ability to dilute urine. Neonates have a decreased, not increased, sensitivity to aldosterone. Neonates have large extracellular volume in comparison with adults.

173. **B) Prone in the crib with a loose blanket when it is time for sleep**

To prevent SIDS, the American Academy of Pediatrics (AAP) recommends placing infants supine for every sleep, using firm sleep surfaces, keeping soft objects and loose bedding out of the crib, and using a separate sleep surface that is close to the parents' bed. "Tummy time," or placing the newborn on their stomach while awake and monitored, is safe and is encouraged by the AAP.

174. **A) Absence of phosphatidylglycerol**

Phosphatidylglycerol, a component of lung surfactant, appears around the gestational age of 36 weeks and is associated with a lower risk of RDS. The absence of this fluid is a key indicator of RDS in neonates, especially those born preterm. Lecithin concentrations rise after week 32 of gestation, resulting in an increase in the lecithin to sphingomyelin ratio in the amniotic fluid. Low ratios are associated with increased risk of RDS. All infants continuously produce fetal lung fluid while in utero. Fetal lung fluid is normal and will usually be expelled during a vaginal delivery or will be removed via the pulmonary lymphatic system.

175. **B) Placing the infant prone**

Infants with Pierre Robin syndrome have a small chin with the potential for airway occlusion by the tongue. The nurse should try to alleviate tachypnea and stridor by placing the infant prone and bringing the tongue forward to prevent occlusion of the airway. If this does not alleviate the symptoms, the nurse would then prepare the infant for oral intubation. Oxygen would be indicated if the infant had low oxygen saturation, which would be a level below 90%.

21 POP QUIZ ANSWERS

CHAPTER 2
Pop Quiz 2.1
Infants of diabetic patients are more likely to develop respiratory distress syndrome (RDS) and exhibit signs such as tachypnea, retractions, and nasal flaring. Maternal hyperglycemia appears to delay surfactant synthesis, which inhibits fetal lung maturation.

Pop Quiz 2.2
Magnesium sulfate is not recommended in patients with myasthenia gravis (MG) as it can precipitate a myasthenic crisis. The nurse should attempt to treat with antihypertensives. If the fetus is considered to be at a safe gestational age for delivery, delivery of the fetus may be the best option.

CHAPTER 3
Pop Quiz 3.1
Low for gestational age (LGA) infants are frequently born to diabetic patients with poor glucose control. Maternal hyperglycemia results in fetal hyperglycemia and hyperinsulinemia. High insulin levels act as fetal growth hormone, which causes macrosomia and causes hypoglycemia in the infant after birth.

Pop Quiz 3.2
The nurse should first administer positive pressure ventilation (PPV) before considering further interventions to treat this infant's low heart rate. Hypoxia and inadequate ventilation are the most frequent cause of bradycardia in a newborn.

Pop Quiz 3.3
The nurse should assess the infant. If there is breathing or crying, positive pressure ventilation (PPV) should be stopped. The nurse should stop ventilating if the infant is breathing at greater than 30 times per minute or if the infant is not drawing in their chest. The nurse should continue to monitor the infant every 15 minutes.

CHAPTER 4
Pop Quiz 4.1
Rapid infusion of vancomycin may cause anaphylactoid reactions, including wheezing, hypotension, dyspnea, hypotension, and urticaria. The infant may also experience flushing of the upper body ("red neck/red person syndrome") or muscle spasms and pain in the back and chest. The infant may need to have an antihistamine or corticosteroid administered.

Pop Quiz 4.2

Furosemide can cause depletion of electrolytes, especially potassium. Neonates receiving frequent furosemide may need potassium supplementation. The nurse should be sure to monitor the patient's output and renal function.

Pop Quiz 4.3

The dosage should be 0.8 mL. Use either the ratio proportion method or the formula method to calculate.

CHAPTER 5

Pop Quiz 5.1

Abnormalities in both respiratory (carbon dioxide [CO_2] >45) and metabolic (bicarbonate [HCO_3] <21) components in combination with acidosis (pH <7.35) represent mixed respiratory and metabolic acidosis.

Pop Quiz 5.2

Administer supplemental oxygen, perform a chest x-ray, monitor respiratory effort and the need for respiratory support such as continuous positive airway pressure (CPAP), assess the need for surfactant replacement, and establish intravenous (IV) access for fluid administration while the newborn is NPO (nothing by mouth).

Pop Quiz 5.3

The nurse should notify the provider as tachycardia is an adverse effect of caffeine citrate. Serum drug level should be taken to assess for caffeine toxicity prior to administering the scheduled dose.

CHAPTER 6

Pop Quiz 6.1

The neonate may have poor lower extremity pulses, be pale in color, have a heart murmur, and have a blood pressure discrepancy >15 mmHg between the upper and lower extremities. Diagnostic testing will be done to determine the severity of the coarctation. Parents should be informed of the needed interventions as soon as possible.

Pop Quiz 6.2

The degree of cyanosis depends on the amount of mixing between the pulmonary and systemic circulations. Oxygenated pulmonary blood returns to the lungs, while deoxygenated systemic blood returns to the body. There must be some mixing to allow oxygenated blood to reach the body and deoxygenated blood to reach the lungs.

Pop Quiz 6.3

These are signs and symptoms of tetralogy of Fallot. The first step is to try to calm the infant down and put them on oxygen. Anticipate an order for an opioid, such as morphine, and propranolol.

CHAPTER 7

Pop Quiz 7.1

The nurse should contact the practitioner to decide if the residual should be refed or discarded. Actions would be to hold the feed, obtain an order for an abdominal x-ray, and evaluate for possible necrotizing enterocolitis (NEC).

Pop Quiz 7.2

The nurse should immediately contact the practitioner and place a nasogastric tube to decompress the stomach and prevent further vomiting and aspiration. The practitioner may order a Replogle to intermittent suction.

Pop Quiz 7.3

Duodenal atresia. The double bubble sign represents dilatation of the proximal duodenum and air in the stomach.

CHAPTER 8

Pop Quiz 8.1

A loop diuretic such as furosemide can be used. Loop diuretics prevent the reabsorption of sodium and potassium in the loop of Henle and directly increase urinary potassium excretion.

Pop Quiz 8.2

This might be the case of strangulated hernia. The infant is experiencing a strangulated hernia in which the blood supply of the contents of the hernia is cut off. Symptoms include severe pain, vomiting, no appetite, fever, bloody stool, and redness or bruising around the bulge. Emergent surgery would be necessary.

Pop Quiz 8.3

Peritonitis is suspected and a provider order for antibiotics should be started immediately. Peritoneal dialysis should be temporarily terminated if tolerated.

CHAPTER 9

Pop Quiz 9.1

In the absence of pathologies such as hydrocephalus or craniosynostosis, brain growth is best assessed by weekly measurements of head circumference.

Pop Quiz 9.2

The nurse should ensure a slow withdrawal of blood from the arterial catheter to minimize changes in blood pressure. This is especially important for this neonate, as most intraventricular hemorrhages occur within the first few days of life.

Pop Quiz 9.3

The nurse should position the infant prone, apply warm, sterile saline-soaked gauze to the defect, and cover it with plastic wrap to keep the defect area clean and prevent heat loss.

CHAPTER 10

Pop Quiz 10.1

These results should be interpreted as positive Barlow and Ortolani tests. The infant should be referred to an orthopedist for further evaluation.

Pop Quiz 10.2

Excessive hip adduction, femoral shortening on the affected side, asymmetrical thigh, and gluteal folds, and positive Ortolani and Barlow tests.

Pop Quiz 10.3

The nurse should assess the neurovascular status of the affected foot and compare it with the unaffected foot and report any neurovascular compromise to the provider. The nurse should also assess pain level.

CHAPTER 11

Pop Quiz 11.1

The nurse can ensure that the delivery room temperature is increased to ≥78.8°F (26°C). Upon delivery, the infant will be placed in a polyurethane bag up their necks with their head covered before being dried. The infant should be transported to the NICU in the bag inside of an incubator before being placed on a radiant warmer bed in the NICU.

Pop Quiz 11.2

The nurse should have the physician assess for *Candida* and obtain an order for nystatin to be applied with every diaper change.

Pop Quiz 11.3

Classic signs of acute wound infection include heat, swelling, pain, erythema, edema, and loss of function.

CHAPTER 12

Pop Quiz 12.1

The nurse should use a specialized nipple for infants with cleft palate. The patient should be placed at a 30° to 45° angle when feeding, and their respiratory rate and effort should be monitored continuously.

Pop Quiz 12.2

Eye drops need to be applied every 2 hours in the early postoperative period. Not adhering to this schedule may result in inflammation, which can have permanent adverse effects on the child's vision.

Pop Quiz 12.3

The condition is tracheoesophageal fistula. Infants with tracheoesophageal fistula may have round, full abdomen due to gas being trapped. The fistula makes it impossible to pass a nasogastric tube. The nurse should alert the physician so further testing can be conducted.

CHAPTER 13

Pop Quiz 13.1

Crush the pill and mix it in milk, formula, or water; do not give levothyroxine with soy, fiber, or iron because these can interfere with the absorption process; laboratory samples are expected to be drawn at frequent intervals.

Pop Quiz 13.2

A goiter can compress and obstruct the airway. The nurse should position the infant with slight neck extension and elevate the head of the bed to help maintain a patent airway.

Pop Quiz 13.3

The nurse should anticipate giving a D10W bolus at 2 mL/kg and rechecking the glucose 30 minutes after.

CHAPTER 14
Pop Quiz 14.1
Because the neonate is anemic and symptomatic, the nurse should anticipate placing a peripheral intravenous (IV) and administering packed red blood cells (PRBCs).

Pop Quiz 14.2
The most likely diagnosis is hemophilia. It is an X-linked recessive disorder in which females are carriers and males exhibit the disease. There is a 75% chance of another male family member having the disease. Bleeding after circumcision is the most common site. Hemophilia presents with prolonged PTT, and normal PT and platelet count.

Pop Quiz 14.3
The nurse should explain that newborns with hyperbilirubinemia are already mildly dehydrated, and phototherapy can further increase dehydration via insensible water loss. Intravenous (IV) fluids in addition to regular feedings will promote adequate hydration until the newborn's bilirubin levels are in acceptable range.

CHAPTER 15
Pop Quiz 15.1
The infant would be suspected to have a *Chlamydia trachomatis* infection. A precipitous delivery of an infant without prenatal care would not allow time for sexually transmitted infection (STI) testing in the mother prior to birth. The infant should be tested and treated with azithromycin.

Pop Quiz 15.2
Prophylactic erythromycin ophthalmic ointment administered to all infants post delivery has markedly reduced gonococcal conjunctivitis in neonates.

CHAPTER 16
Pop Quiz 16.1
The nurse should suspect maple syrup urine disease, would alert the physician, and perform a newborn screening if not already obtained.

Pop Quiz 16.2
Pregnant women should avoid hot tubs and saunas and vigorous exercise that increase the core body temperature significantly. Pregnant women should also try to control fevers when they are sick to not rise above 102.2°F (39°C).

CHAPTER 17
Pop Quiz 17.1
The infant would benefit from prone positioning until they outgrow their airway obstruction or surgical intervention.

Pop Quiz 17.2
The infant should be swaddled and offered an oral sucrose-dipped pacifier. EMLA (eutectic mixture of local anesthetics) cream is not recommended in heel lancing or with extremely preterm infants.

CHAPTER 18

Pop Quiz 18.1

The nurse should notify the provider that informed consent has not been obtained and not to administer the blood transfusion until consent is obtained.

Pop Quiz 18.2

The parents or legal guardians are the legal decision-makers and are the only people who may make the decision to redirect care.

Pop Quiz 18.3

The nurse should speak with the ethics committee, who can provide support and objectivity. They can help facilitate communication between the nurse, the medical team, and the family.

INDEX

Page entries that appear in italics refer to content in the practice test and practice test answer chapters.